Nanoplatforms for Cancer Imaging

Online at: https://doi.org/10.1088/978-0-7503-5864-4

IPEM–IOP Series in Physics and Engineering in Medicine and Biology

About the Series

The series in Physics and Engineering in Medicine and Biology will allow the Institute of Physics and Engineering in Medicine (IPEM) to enhance its mission to 'advance physics and engineering applied to medicine and biology for the public good'.

It is focused on key areas including, but not limited to:

- clinical engineering
- diagnostic radiology
- informatics and computing
- magnetic resonance imaging
- nuclear medicine
- physiological measurement
- radiation protection
- radiotherapy
- rehabilitation engineering
- ultrasound and non-ionising radiation.

A number of IPEM–IOP titles are being published as part of the EUTEMPE Network Series for Medical Physics Experts.

A full list of titles published in this series can be found here: https://iopscience.iop.org/bookListInfo/physics-engineering-medicine-biology-series.

Nanoplatforms for Cancer Imaging

Edited by
Nanasaheb D Thorat
Department of Physics and Bernal Institute, Limerick Digital Cancer Research Centre (LDCRC), University of Limerick, Castletroy, Ireland

Sandeep B Somvanshi
Department of Physics and Bernal Institute, Limerick Digital Cancer Research Centre (LDCRC), University of Limerick, Castletroy, Ireland

IOP Publishing, Bristol, UK

ISBN 978-0-7503-5864-4 (ebook)
ISBN 978-0-7503-5862-0 (print)
ISBN 978-0-7503-5865-1 (myPrint)
ISBN 978-0-7503-5863-7 (mobi)

DOI 10.1088/978-0-7503-5864-4

Version: 20250401

IOP ebooks

British Library Cataloguing-in-Publication Data: A catalogue record for this book is available from the British Library.

Published by IOP Publishing, wholly owned by The Institute of Physics, London

IOP Publishing, No.2 The Distillery, Glassfields, Avon Street, Bristol, BS2 0GR, UK

US Office: IOP Publishing, Inc., 190 North Independence Mall West, Suite 601, Philadelphia, PA 19106, USA

Contents

Preface

The rapid advancement of nanotechnology has opened new avenues in the field of biomedicine, particularly in cancer diagnosis and treatment. This book, *Nanoplatforms for Cancer Imaging*, is a timely and essential contribution to this rapidly evolving area. By providing a comprehensive understanding of nanoplatforms and their integration with biomedical imaging, this work explores cutting-edge approaches to improving cancer diagnosis and treatment outcomes. Cancer, one of the most significant global health challenges, demands innovative solutions for early detection and effective treatment. Traditional imaging techniques, while indispensable, face limitations in terms of sensitivity, specificity, and resolution when used independently. Nanotechnology-based platforms address these limitations by offering precise, multifunctional, and adaptable solutions. This book serves as a crucial resource for researchers, clinicians, and students interested in the intersection of nanotechnology and biomedical imaging.

The content of this book is organized into four chapters, each addressing a critical aspect of nanoplatform-based imaging for cancer diagnosis and therapy. The opening chapter provides an introduction to the concept of nanoplatforms in biomedical imaging. It explores the basics of nanotechnology, the principles of imaging modalities, and their integration for cancer diagnosis. By establishing a foundational understanding, this chapter sets the stage for readers to delve deeper into the nuances of the subject.

The second chapter focuses on the core principles that govern nanoplatform-based imaging, discussing the physicochemical properties of nanomaterials, their interaction with biological systems, and the mechanisms that enable their effectiveness in imaging applications. This chapter also outlines the challenges associated with designing and implementing these platforms in cancer diagnosis.

The third chapter provides a detailed analysis of the latest trends and innovations in the field. Advances in nanotechnology and imaging modalities, such as quantum dots, gold nanoparticles, and multifunctional nanocomposites, are examined. This chapter also delves into the integration of artificial intelligence and machine learning to enhance imaging outcomes.

Bridging the gap between laboratory research and clinical application, the fourth chapter examines the translation of nanoplatform-based imaging technologies into clinical settings. It highlights the progress made in regulatory approvals, clinical trials, and real-world applications, while case studies illustrate the impact of these technologies on patient care and treatment outcomes. The concluding chapter focuses on the therapeutic potential of nanoplatforms. It explores the concept of image-guided therapy, where imaging and treatment are seamlessly integrated, discussing topics such as targeted drug delivery, photo-thermal therapy, and the role of nanoplatforms in minimizing off-target effects. This chapter underscores the future prospects of nanotechnology in personalized medicine and precision oncology.

This book is designed to foster scientific knowledge, inspire innovation, and promote multidisciplinary collaboration. Its content is relevant to both academic and industrial communities, bridging the gap between fundamental research and practical applications. By integrating insights from nanotechnology, imaging science, oncology, and clinical medicine, the book provides a holistic understanding of the subject. Furthermore, it emphasizes innovation as a driving force in the fight against cancer and includes clinical advances and case studies to ensure that the content is grounded in real-world applications. By serving as a comprehensive guide for students and early-career researchers, the book provides foundational knowledge alongside advanced insights into nanoplatform-based imaging. By discussing future directions and challenges, the book inspires continued research and innovation in this promising field.

This book is intended for a diverse audience, including researchers in nanotechnology, biomedical imaging, and oncology, who will find it a valuable resource for understanding the latest advancements and identifying areas for further research. Clinicians, including oncologists, radiologists, and other medical professionals, will benefit from the clinical insights and case studies presented in the book. Graduate and postgraduate students, as well as educators in related fields, can use this book as a comprehensive reference for coursework and independent study. Moreover, professionals in the pharmaceutical, biotechnology, and medical imaging industries will gain insights into the potential applications of nanotechnology in cancer diagnosis and treatment.

The development of this book would not have been possible without the collaborative efforts of contributors from various disciplines. We extend our gratitude to the authors of individual chapters, who have shared their expertise and insights. We also acknowledge the support of the institutions and organizations that facilitated this work. Special thanks are due to the editorial team at IOP Publishing for their guidance and commitment to excellence.

Nanoplatforms for Cancer Imaging is not merely a collection of chapters but a concerted effort to advance the understanding of a critical area in oncology. As the field continues to evolve, we hope this book serves as a foundation for future discoveries and innovations. By bridging the gap between technology and medicine, we can work towards a future where cancer diagnosis and treatment are more effective, accessible, and personalized. It is our sincere hope that this book inspires readers to contribute to this dynamic field and ultimately improves the lives of those affected by cancer.

Acknowledgments

The project leading to this work received funding from the Science Foundation Ireland and Irish Research Council (SFI-IRC) pathway program (21/PATH-S/9634). The research conducted in this publication was funded by the Irish Research Council under grant number GOIPD/2024/588.

Editor biographies

Dr Nanasaheb D Thorat

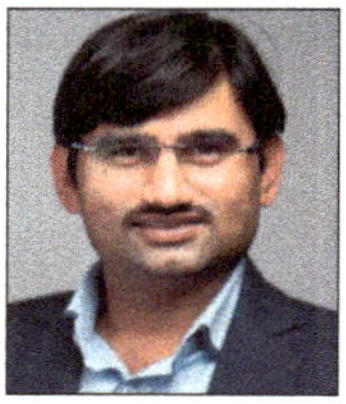

Dr Nanasaheb D Thorat is Associate Professor at Department of Physics, Bernal Institute, jointly associated with Limerick Digital Cancer Research Centre (LDCRC) UL, Ireland. He is a Fellow of the Royal Society of Medicine London. He specializes in cancer nanotheranostics and developed an award-winning cancer theranostics approach within the 'NANOCARGO' MSCA-PF project. This novel technology received the European Commission's innovation Radar 'Grand Prix 2020' for developing groundbreaking technology for breast cancer theranostics. He is a three-time awardee of the MSCA-PF, GF in the year 2016 (Wroclaw University of Science and Technology, Poland), 2019 (University of Oxford, UK), and 2022 MSCA-GF (Harvard Medical School, USA). He subsequently secured a Science Foundation Ireland (SFI — €592 207) and Irish research council (IRC — €117 113) grant to establish his own cancer nanomedicine lab at the Bernal Institute & LDCRC in UL. He has raised more than €1.7 M funding from various agencies during his early research career. Dr Thorat was involved in an innovation partnership research project to develop Raman spectroscopy analysis to probe a drug–material interface that involved four world-leading pharmaceutical companies, Jansen, GSK, Pfizer, and MSD. He has published more than 135 international scientific publications, including 110 research papers, 7 books, 25 book chapters, 1 patent filed, and 2 innovations registered in the European Commission's innovation Radar project. His work has been cited by many authors, with 6000 citations, and his H-index is 43, while his i-10 index is 85. He currently leads the well-established Cancer Nanomedicine Group with four PhDs and two postdocs based in the Biomaterials Research Cluster at the Bernal Institute & LDCRC, UL. He is on the board of the leadership team under the early career scientist scheme of a €40 million flagship institute, the Bernal Institute. Dr Thorat is also an invited member of the consortium that designs the policies for the 'EU Beating Cancer by 2030' mission and contributed to developing the cancer research roadmap for the next 10 years.

Dr Sandeep B Somvanshi

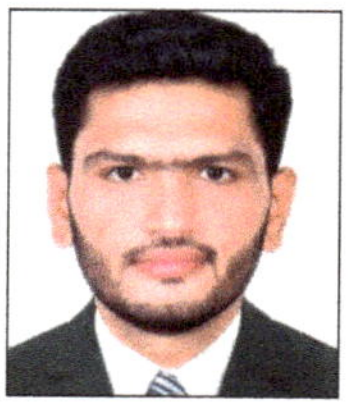

Dr Sandeep B Somvanshi is working as a IRC Fellow at the Department of Physics, University of Limerick, Ireland. He has published more than 60 research papers in peer reviewed journals and seven book chapters. His major research interests include magnetism and magnetic nanomaterials, magnetic fluid hyperthermia for cancer treatment, magnetic resonance imaging, drug delivery systems, silica aerogels, nanocatalysts, and photocatalysts, etc. He has reviewed several research papers from reputable publishers, such as ACS, RSC, Elsevier, IOP, and Springer-Nature. He is the recipient of many prestigious awards, such as TUM Global Postdoctoral Fellowship, Young Scientist Award by Lindau Nobel Laureate Foundation in the 69th Lindau Nobel Laureate Meeting held at Lindau, Germany, DST-DFG Award for Post Lindau Nobel Laureate Meeting Tour, Young Scientist Award by DST, Govt of India for participation in the 5th BRICS Young Scientist Conclave, DST-Inspire Fellowship by Govt of India, Overseas Doctoral Fellowship by Government of India and several merit scholarships.

List of contributors

Srijani Dasgupta
Department of Pharmaceutical Sciences, Jharkhand Rai University, Jharkhand 834010, India

Harshit Dubey
Fergana Medical Institute of Public Health, Fergana 150100, Uzbekistan

Swati Dubey
Department of Applied Chemistry, Samrat Ashok Technological Institute, Vidisha 464001, Madhya Pradesh, India

Ketan P Gattu
Department of Nanotechnology, Dr Babasaheb Ambedkar Marathwada University, Aurangabad 431004, Maharashtra, India

Alluru Gopala Krishna
Department of Mechanical Engineering, Jawaharlal Nehru Technological University Kakinda, Nagamallithota, Kakinada 533003, Andhra Pradesh, India

Umesh Kumar
Department of Biosciences, IMS Ghaziabad, Grand Trunk Rd, Industrial Area, Lal Kuan, Ghaziabad 201009, Uttar Pradesh, India

Shakti Prasad Pattanayak
School of Medicine, Woods Building, W408, Case Western Reserve University, 10900 Euclid Ave, Cleveland, OH 44106, USA
Department of Pharmacy, School of Health Sciences, Central University of South Bihar, Patna 824236, India

Gaurav Ranjan
Department of Pharmacy, School of Health Sciences, Central University of South Bihar, Patna 824236, India

Eravalli Sudhakar Rao
Department of Pathology, Government Medical College and Hospital, Khaleelwadi, Nizamabad 503001, Telangana, India

C Chandrasekhara Sastry
Department of Electronics and Communication Engineering, Indian Institute of Information Technology Design and Manufacturing, Jagannathagattu Hill, Kurnool 518008, Andhra Pradesh, India

Raje Sengar
Department of Applied Chemistry, Samrat Ashok Technological Institute, Vidisha 464001, Madhya Pradesh, India

Dola Sundeep
Department of Electronics and Communication Engineering, Indian Institute of Information Technology Design and Manufacturing, Jagannathagattu Hill, Kurnool 518008, Andhra Pradesh, India

Priyashree Sunita
School of Medicine, Woods Building, W408, Case Western Reserve University, 10900 Euclid Ave, Cleveland, OH 44106, USA
Government Pharmacy Institute, Dept. of Health, Medical Education and Family Welfare, Bariatu, Ranchi 834009, India

Mulukala Swetha
Department of Pathology, Kakatiya Medical College, Warangal 506007, Telangana, India

Kovuri Umadevi
Department of Pathology, Osmania Medical College, Koti, Hyderabad 500095, Telangana, India

Eswaramoorthy K Varadharaj
Department of Electronics and Communication Engineering, Indian Institute of Information Technology Design and Manufacturing, Jagannathagattu Hill, Kurnool 518008, Andhra Pradesh, India

Abhay Kumar Yadav
Department of Chemistry, School of Physical and Chemical Sciences, Central University of South Bihar, Patna 824236, India

Chapter 1

Introduction to nanoplatform-based biomedical imaging

Ketan P Gattu, Sandeep B Somvanshi and Nanasaheb D Thorat

Nanoplatforms are becoming a valuable tool in the realm of biomedical imaging. Advances in nanoplatform-based biomedical imaging have been rapidly evolving, driven by innovations in nanotechnology, materials science, and biomedical engineering. The dimensions of nanoplatforms with a diameter of 1–100 nm are similar to those of biological functional units. Numerous nanoplatforms have the potential to serve as probes for the early detection of cancer-like diseases because of their surface chemistry, distinctive magnetic characteristics, adjustable absorption and emission capabilities, and recent improvements in the synthesis and engineering of different nanoplatforms. Nanoplatforms now have more promise as molecular imaging probes due to their easy surface functionalization. The continuous advancement of nanoplatform-based biomedical imaging holds great promise for improving disease diagnosis, monitoring, and treatment, ultimately leading to better patient outcomes and healthcare outcomes. This chapter provides an in-depth exploration of nanoplatform-based biomedical imaging, offering a comprehensive overview of this rapidly advancing field.

1.1 Introduction

1.1.1 Scope and importance of nanoplatform-based biomedical imaging

Nanoplatforms in biomedical imaging are revolutionizing how we visualize and understand biological systems at the nanoscale [1, 2]. These platforms typically involve the integration of nanoparticles with imaging techniques to provide high-resolution images with enhanced contrast and sensitivity. Nanoplatform-based biomedical imaging stands at the forefront of medical innovation, poised to revolutionize healthcare delivery. By harnessing the power of nanoparticles, this cutting-edge technology offers a multifaceted approach to disease management, emphasizing early detection, precise diagnosis, and tailored therapeutic interventions [3, 4]. A brief introduction to the relevant concepts is given below:

doi:10.1088/978-0-7503-5864-4ch1

- **Nanoparticles**: these are tiny particles, often ranging from 1 to 100 nm in size, with unique physical and chemical properties. They can be engineered to carry specific functionalities, such as targeting ligands, imaging agents, or therapeutic payloads.
- **Biomedical imaging techniques**: various imaging modalities are used in biomedical research and clinical practice, including optical imaging, magnetic resonance imaging (MRI), computed tomography (CT), positron emission tomography (PET), and ultrasound imaging. Each modality has its advantages and limitations in terms of resolution, depth of penetration, and sensitivity.
- **Integration of nanoparticles with imaging techniques**: nanoparticles can be tailored to enhance the performance of imaging techniques. For example, fluorescent nanoparticles can be used in optical imaging to visualize cellular and molecular processes with high sensitivity. Magnetic nanoparticles can serve as contrast agents in MRI, improving the visualization of tissues and organs. Similarly, nanoparticles can be functionalized with radioactive isotopes for PET imaging or with heavy elements for enhanced contrast in CT imaging.
- **Targeting and delivery**: one of the key advantages of nanoplatforms is their ability to target specific cells or tissues. Surface functionalization of nanoparticles with targeting ligands enables them to selectively bind to molecular markers that are overexpressed in diseased tissues, improving the specificity of imaging. Moreover, nanoparticles can be used as carriers for therapeutic agents, allowing for targeted drug delivery in addition to imaging.
- **Multimodal imaging**: nanoplatforms can also enable multimodal imaging, where multiple imaging techniques are combined to provide complementary information about biological systems. For example, a single nanoparticle could incorporate both fluorescent and magnetic properties, allowing for simultaneous optical and MRI imaging.
- **Challenges and future directions**: despite their promise, the development and clinical translation of nanoplatforms face several challenges, including concerns about biocompatibility, toxicity, and regulatory approval. Additionally, there is ongoing research to improve the stability, targeting efficiency, and imaging performance of nanoparticles.

Nanoplatforms based on nanoparticles offer exciting opportunities to advance biomedical imaging by providing enhanced sensitivity, resolution, and specificity [5]. By integrating these platforms with existing imaging techniques, researchers and clinicians can gain deeper insights into complex biological processes and improve the diagnosis and treatment of various diseases [6].

1.1.1.1 Scope

Nanoplatforms represent a paradigm shift in biomedical imaging, offering a multitude of advantages over conventional techniques:

- **Enhanced sensitivity and specificity:** engineered nanoparticles equipped with targeting ligands exhibit a remarkable ability to bind selectively to diseased cells or tissues, enabling the detection of minute anomalies with unprecedented accuracy.

- **Improved resolution:** the diminutive size of nanoparticles facilitates deep tissue penetration, granting researchers access to cellular and sub-cellular structures previously beyond the reach of traditional imaging methodologies.
- **Multimodality:** nanoplatforms are not bound by the constraints of single imaging modalities. Instead, they can be tailored to accommodate multiple imaging techniques, such as fluorescence, MRI, CT, ultrasound, and PET, thereby furnishing clinicians with a comprehensive overview of pathological processes.
- **Theranostics:** a hallmark feature of nanoplatforms is their capacity for dual functionality, seamlessly integrating diagnostic and therapeutic capabilities. These versatile constructs enable both the visualization of disease pathology and the targeted delivery of therapeutic agents, heralding a new era of personalized medicine.

1.1.1.2 Importance

The significance of nanoplatform-based biomedical imaging is underscored by its potential to:

- **Elevate disease diagnosis:** by affording heightened sensitivity and specificity, nanoplatforms facilitate the early identification of pathological changes, thereby minimizing diagnostic ambiguity and expediting treatment initiation.
- **Pioneer early intervention:** timely detection of diseases translates into improved prognoses and enhanced treatment outcomes. Nanoplatforms empower clinicians to intervene preemptively, mitigating disease progression and optimizing patient care.
- **Facilitate precision medicine:** in an era characterized by a growing emphasis on personalized healthcare, nanoplatforms are emerging as indispensable tools for tailoring therapeutic regimens to individual patient profiles. By virtue of their targeted drug delivery capabilities, these platforms minimize systemic side effects while maximizing therapeutic efficacy.
- **Promote healthcare economics:** the judicious application of nanoplatform-based imaging holds the promise of substantial cost savings by circumventing the need for resource-intensive treatments necessitated by late-stage disease presentations.

In summary, the burgeoning field of nanoplatform-based biomedical imaging epitomizes the convergence of cutting-edge science and clinical utility. As research endeavors continue to unravel the full spectrum of its capabilities, the transformative impact of this technology on modern healthcare delivery is poised to become increasingly pronounced. Figure 1.1 shows the different types of nanoparticles used in bio-applications.

1.1.2 Overview of this chapter

This chapter provides an in-depth exploration of nanoplatform-based biomedical imaging, offering a comprehensive overview of this rapidly advancing field. It begins

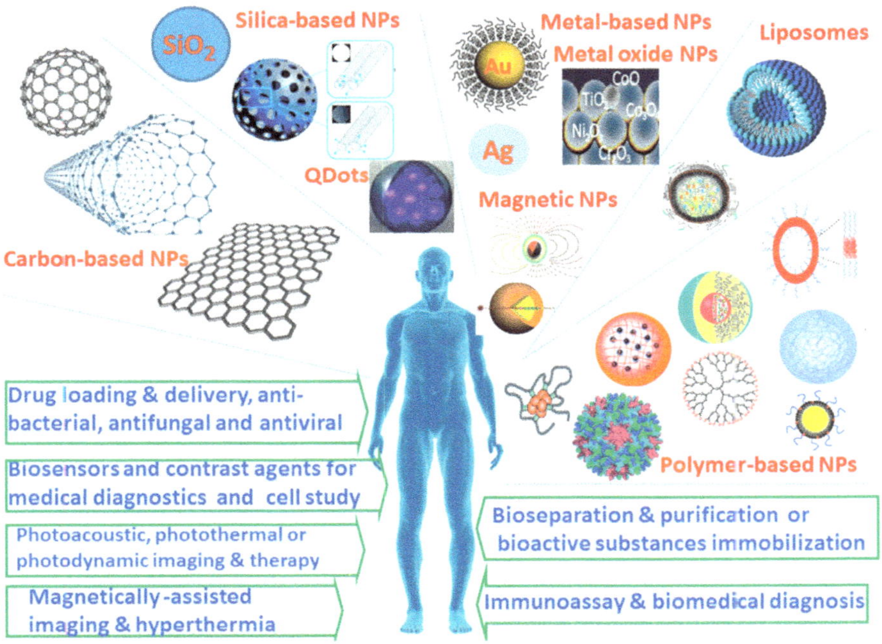

Figure 1.1. Types of typical nanoparticles and their bio-applications. Reproduced from [7]. CC BY 4.0.

by discussing the scope and importance of nanoplatforms in biomedical imaging, emphasizing their potential to revolutionize diagnostics and therapeutics. The chapter then provides a detailed examination of the fundamentals of nanotechnology in imaging applications, including the properties of nanomaterials and nanofabrication techniques.

A key focus of the chapter is on defining nanoplatforms for imaging and elucidating their characteristics, roles, advantages, and challenges in biomedical imaging. The chapter categorizes nanoplatforms into different types, such as contrast agents, nanoparticles, quantum dots (QDs), and nanosensors, and examines their specific applications and benefits in various imaging modalities. Design considerations for nanoplatforms in biomedical imaging are thoroughly discussed, encompassing biocompatibility, targeting strategies, imaging modalities, and probe stability. The chapter also delves into the applications of nanoplatforms in specific imaging techniques, such as MRI, x-ray imaging, PET, single-photon emission computed tomography (SPECT), and optical imaging, highlighting their respective advantages and limitations.

Furthermore, the chapter explores characterization techniques for imaging nanoplatforms, including size and morphology analysis, surface chemistry evaluation, and imaging performance assessment. It also addresses regulatory considerations and safety assessments for nanoplatforms in imaging applications, ensuring their safe and effective use in clinical settings. The chapter concludes with a forward-looking perspective on the future of nanoplatform-based biomedical imaging, discussing emerging trends, challenges, and opportunities in the field. It also considers the ethical and societal implications of nanoplatforms in imaging, emphasizing the need for responsible innovation and deployment of these technologies. Overall, the chapter serves as a comprehensive guide to nanoplatform-based biomedical imaging, providing researchers, practitioners, and students with a thorough understanding of this exciting and rapidly evolving field.

1.2 Fundamentals of nanotechnology in biomedical imaging

1.2.1 Nanoscale science and engineering in imaging applications

Nanoscale science and engineering are pivotal in advancing imaging applications, offering unique properties and capabilities that are revolutionizing the field [8]. At the nanometer scale, materials exhibit distinct characteristics, such as altered electrical resistance, lower melting points, accelerated chemical reactions, and modified optical behaviors. These properties open up new avenues for designing and developing innovative imaging technologies that are more efficient, sensitive, and versatile than their macroscopic counterparts. Nanoscale science involves the study and manipulation of materials at this scale, typically between 1 and 100 nm, while nanoscale engineering encompasses the design, synthesis, characterization, and application of materials and devices in this range, drawing from various disciplines, such as physics, chemistry, biology, and engineering.

The impact of nanoscale science and engineering on imaging applications is profound. One notable application is the use of nanoparticle-based contrast agents in a wide range of biomedical imaging modalities, including fluorescence imaging, MRI, CT, ultrasound, PET, and SPECT [9]. These contrast agents offer several advantages, such as enhanced stability and metabolic kinetics of drugs in the body, improved therapeutic or imaging effects on diseases, and reduced toxicity and side effects. Additionally, meta-surfaces, which enable the control of light at the nanoscale, have emerged as a promising platform for novel imaging techniques. These surfaces are smaller and less complex than conventional imaging systems, offering potential advancements in super-resolution imaging, computational holography, and other functional imaging techniques, such as polarimetric and hyper spectral imaging.

Looking ahead, the future of nanoscale science and engineering in imaging applications is promising. Scientists are continuously developing new tools and techniques to synthesize and manipulate materials at the nanoscale, expanding the possibilities for imaging technologies. For example, the ability to synthesize nanoparticles of materials like titanium dioxide (TiO_2) at the nanoscale has paved the way for more efficient and effective contrast agents across various imaging modalities [10]. These advancements hold the potential to drive significant progress in medical diagnostics and therapeutics, offering improved imaging capabilities and better patient outcomes.

Nanoscale science and engineering are pivotal in imaging applications due to the unique properties of nanoparticles (NPs) that can transform imaging techniques [11]. NPs like iron oxide NPs are particularly valuable in imaging because of their magnetic properties, low toxicity, and biodegradability, making them suitable for sensing, imaging, and therapeutic applications. The composition of NPs, such as iron oxide existing in different chemical compositions like magnetite (Fe_3O_4) or maghemite (γ-Fe_2O_3), impacts significantly on their imaging capabilities and biotransformation, which is crucial for understanding their long-term toxicity. One of the significant challenges in NP imaging is accurately determining the spatial distribution of molecules on nanoscale curved surfaces. Techniques like molecular-scale imaging or mass spectrometry are essential for this precise measurement. NPs can be engineered to serve multiple functions in imaging applications, such as combining heat mediation and drug delivery. This capability broadens the scope of biomedical applications by providing spatial and temporal control over drug release mechanisms.

1.2.2 Properties of nanomaterials for biomedical imaging

Nanomaterials used for biomedical imaging possess a diverse range of properties that make them ideal for various imaging modalities. One of the key properties is their size, typically ranging from 1 to 100 nm. This small size allows nanomaterials to penetrate tissues and cells, enabling them to be used as imaging agents for various applications. Additionally, the small size of nanomaterials contributes to their high surface area-to-volume ratio, which can enhance their reactivity and effectiveness in imaging applications.

Another important property of nanomaterials used in biomedical imaging is their high sensitivity. Nanoparticles, in particular, make excellent contrast agents due to their ability to enhance the contrast of images. This high sensitivity enables more accurate imaging and diagnosis of diseases, as well as the monitoring of therapeutic interventions. Furthermore, the unique optical or magnetic properties of certain nanomaterials make them ideal for specific imaging modalities. For example, iron oxide nanoparticles are commonly used in MRI, while fluorescent nanoparticles are used in optical imaging [12, 13]. These properties allow nanomaterials to be tailored for specific imaging applications, improving their effectiveness and versatility. Figure 1.2 presents schematics of different physicochemical properties of nanomaterials that influence their bio-applications.

Surface functionalization is another important property of nanomaterials used in biomedical imaging. Nanoparticles can be functionalized with targeting ligands on their surface, allowing them to selectively bind to specific tissues or cells [15]. This targeting ability enhances the specificity of imaging, enabling more precise and accurate diagnosis of diseases. Additionally, surface functionalization can improve the stability and biocompatibility of nanomaterials, making them safer for use in medical applications.

Biocompatibility is a critical property of nanomaterials used in biomedical imaging. Nanomaterials must be biocompatible to ensure they are well tolerated by the body and do not cause adverse reactions [16]. Biocompatible nanomaterials are essential for safe use in medical imaging, as they can be administered to patients without causing harm. Moreover, the physicochemical properties of nanomaterials, such as their reactivity, strength, electrical characteristics, optical characteristics, and magnetic

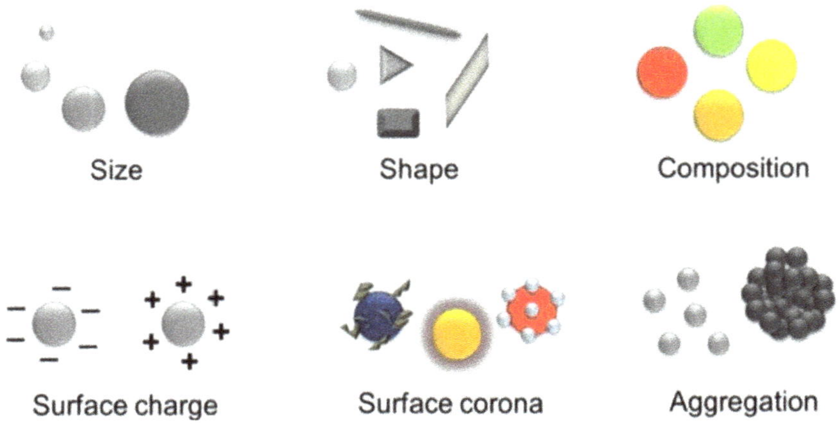

Figure 1.2. Schematic illustration of different parameters of nanomaterials that influence their bio-applications. Reproduced from [14]. CC BY 4.0.

characteristics, are enhanced due to their large surface area-to-volume ratio and the dominance of quantum effects at the nanoscale. These properties contribute to the effectiveness and versatility of nanomaterials in biomedical imaging, making them valuable tools for advancing medical diagnostics and therapeutics.

- **Composition variability:** nanomaterials exhibit diverse compositions in their cores and shells, influencing their properties and applications. This variability allows for the tailoring of nanomaterials with specific characteristics suitable for various imaging modalities, such as optical, magnetic, or multimodal imaging.
- **Magnetic properties:** nanomaterials with magnetic properties, such as iron oxide nanoparticles, are valuable for MRI, magnetic separation, and hyperthermia treatment. These properties enable enhanced imaging contrast, targeted delivery, and therapeutic interventions in biomedical applications.
- **Biocompatibility and low toxicity:** biomedical imaging nanomaterials must be biocompatible and exhibit low toxicity to ensure safety in biological systems. This property is crucial for minimizing adverse effects and enabling long-term imaging studies without harming living organisms.
- **Targeting ligands:** the incorporation of targeting ligands on nanomaterials facilitates specific interactions with biological targets, enhancing imaging specificity. These ligands contribute to targeted imaging, allowing for precise localization and visualization of specific tissues or cells *in vivo*.
- **Imaging contrast enhancement:** nanomaterials designed for imaging contrast enhancement improve the visualization of anatomical structures or molecular processes. By enhancing contrast in imaging modalities, these nanomaterials aid in accurate diagnosis, monitoring of diseases, and tracking of therapeutic responses in biological systems. Figure 1.3 provides schematics for different physical and chemical properties of nanomaterials that influence their bio-applications along with toxicological issues.

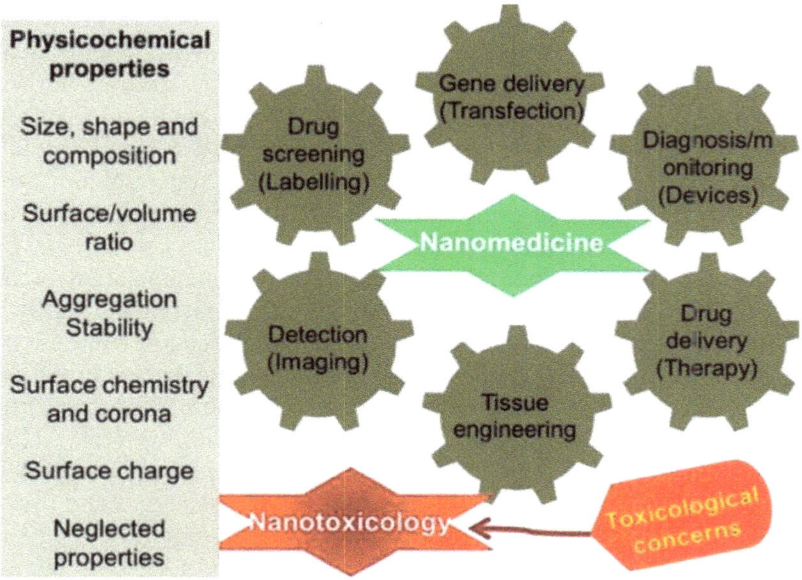

Figure 1.3. Schematics for different physical and chemical properties of nanomaterials that influence their bio-applications along with toxicological issues. Reproduced from [14]. CC BY 4.0.

1.2.3 Nanofabrication techniques for imaging nanoplatforms

Nanofabrication techniques play a critical role in the creation of nanoplatforms used in various imaging applications [17]. These techniques enable the precise control and manipulation of materials at the nanoscale, allowing for the fabrication of structures with unique properties and functionalities. Some of the key nanofabrication techniques used in imaging nanoplatforms include lithography, self-assembly, molecular beam epitaxy, sol–gel synthesis, nanoimprint lithography, focused ion beam deposition, and the atomic layer deposition-enabled nano-molding process [18–22].

Lithography is a widely used technique in nanofabrication that involves creating a desired pattern in a resist layer on top of a substrate [23]. Various deposition and etching processes are then used to transfer this pattern from the resist layer to the material below. Lithography allows for the creation of nanoscale patterns with high precision and resolution, making it ideal for fabricating nanoplatforms used in imaging applications.

Self-assembly is a bottom-up nanofabrication technique that involves the spontaneous assembly of molecules or particles into a desired structure based on binding forces that occur between them when in close proximity [24]. This technique is often used to create complex nanostructures with high precision and efficiency. Self-assembly is particularly useful for fabricating nanoplatforms with specific functionalities, such as targeting ligands or imaging agents.

Molecular beam epitaxy is a method used to deposit highly controlled thin films of particles onto a substrate [25]. This technique allows for the precise control of the thickness and composition of the deposited films, making it ideal for creating nanoplatforms with tailored properties for imaging applications. Sol–gel synthesis is another technique used to create nanoplatforms, which involves the transition of a system from a liquid 'sol' into a solid 'gel' phase [26]. This process allows for the fabrication of nanoplatforms with uniform properties and controlled structures.

Nanoimprint lithography is a simple and cost-effective method for fabricating nanometer-scale patterns [27]. It offers high throughput and resolution, making it suitable for producing nanoplatforms used in imaging applications. Focused ion beam deposition is a technique that uses a focused beam of ions to deposit or remove material at the nanoscale. This technique allows for the precise manipulation of materials, making it useful for creating complex nanostructures for imaging nanoplatforms.

The atomic layer deposition-enabled nano-molding process is a unique technique used to create high-aspect-ratio nano-pillars from materials such as titanium dioxide (TiO_2) [28]. This technique enables the fabrication of nanoplatforms with specific structural features that enhance their imaging properties. Overall, these nanofabrication techniques are essential for the development of advanced nanoplatforms for biomedical imaging, offering precise control over the structure and properties of the fabricated materials.

These nanofabrication techniques are often combined and used in conjunction with traditional microfabrication techniques to create a wide variety of nanostructured devices for biomedical imaging. For example, lithography can be used to pattern surfaces with nanoscale features, while self-assembly can be employed to create complex three-dimensional nanostructures. Molecular beam epitaxy and sol–gel synthesis are used to deposit thin films and create nanomaterials with specific properties, respectively.

Nanoimprint lithography, with its high resolution and low cost, is particularly useful for mass production of nanoplatforms for imaging applications. Focused ion beam deposition enables precise manipulation of materials at the nanoscale, allowing for the fabrication of custom-designed nanoplatforms. The atomic layer deposition-enabled nano-molding process provides a unique method for creating nano-pillars with specific properties, such as enhanced optical or magnetic characteristics, which are beneficial for imaging applications.

Overall, nanofabrication techniques are essential for advancing biomedical imaging by enabling the creation of nanoplatforms with tailored properties for specific imaging modalities [1, 29]. These techniques continue to evolve, offering new possibilities for creating novel nanoplatforms that can further enhance the capabilities of biomedical imaging and contribute to improved diagnostics and therapeutics. As researchers further refine these techniques and explore new materials and approaches, the field of nanoplatform-based biomedical imaging is expected to continue to grow and make significant contributions to healthcare.

1.3 Nanoplatforms for biomedical imaging

1.3.1 Definition and characteristics of nanoplatforms for imaging

1.3.1.1 Definition

Nanoplatforms for imaging represent a class of microscopic structures engineered specifically for application in biomedical imaging techniques. Ranging in size from

1 to 100 nm, these platforms are meticulously designed to interact with biological systems at the cellular and molecular levels. Composed of diverse materials such as polymers, metal oxides, lipids, or biomolecules, nanoplatforms can be tailored to fulfill specific requirements across a spectrum of imaging modalities, offering a versatile toolkit for diagnostic and therapeutic endeavors.

1.3.1.2 Characteristics

- **Nanoscale advantage:** the diminutive scale of nanoplatforms affords them unique advantages over traditional imaging methods. Their minuscule size enables penetration into tissues and cells with unparalleled precision, facilitating detailed imaging and analysis at the molecular level.
- **Tailorable functionalities:** nanoplatforms boast tailorable characteristics that render them highly adaptable to diverse imaging applications. Through strategic modification, they can be endowed with various functionalities, including targeting ligands that bind specifically to disease biomarkers, imaging agents that interact with specific modalities to generate signals, and even therapeutic agents for combined imaging and treatment—a concept known as 'theranostics.'
- **Biocompatibility:** crucially, nanoplatforms are engineered to exhibit excellent biocompatibility, ensuring compatibility with the biological milieu and minimizing the risk of adverse reactions. This essential characteristic enhances their suitability for clinical translation and minimizes potential harm to the patient.
- **Stability:** nanoplatforms must maintain stability in complex biological environments and during circulation within the body to ensure effective delivery and functionality. Robust stability is vital for sustaining imaging efficacy and therapeutic outcomes over extended periods.
- **Multimodality:** many nanoplatforms are designed to integrate multiple imaging functionalities, enabling simultaneous acquisition of information from different modalities. This multimodal approach enhances diagnostic accuracy and provides a comprehensive assessment of pathological conditions, facilitating informed clinical decision-making.

In essence, nanoplatforms for imaging represent a cutting-edge frontier in biomedical technology, offering unparalleled precision, versatility, and adaptability in visualizing and diagnosing diseases. With their tailorable functionalities and remarkable biocompatibility, these microscopic marvels hold immense promise for revolutionizing healthcare by enabling earlier detection, more accurate diagnosis, and targeted therapeutic interventions. Figure 1.4 presents a schematic representation of different types of hybrid nanoplatforms employed for bio-applications.

1.3.2 Role of nanoplatforms in biomedical imaging

Nanoplatforms play a pivotal role in the realm of biomedical imaging, offering a myriad of advantages over traditional methods and significantly impacting diagnostics and therapeutics [31]. These platforms are meticulously designed to interact

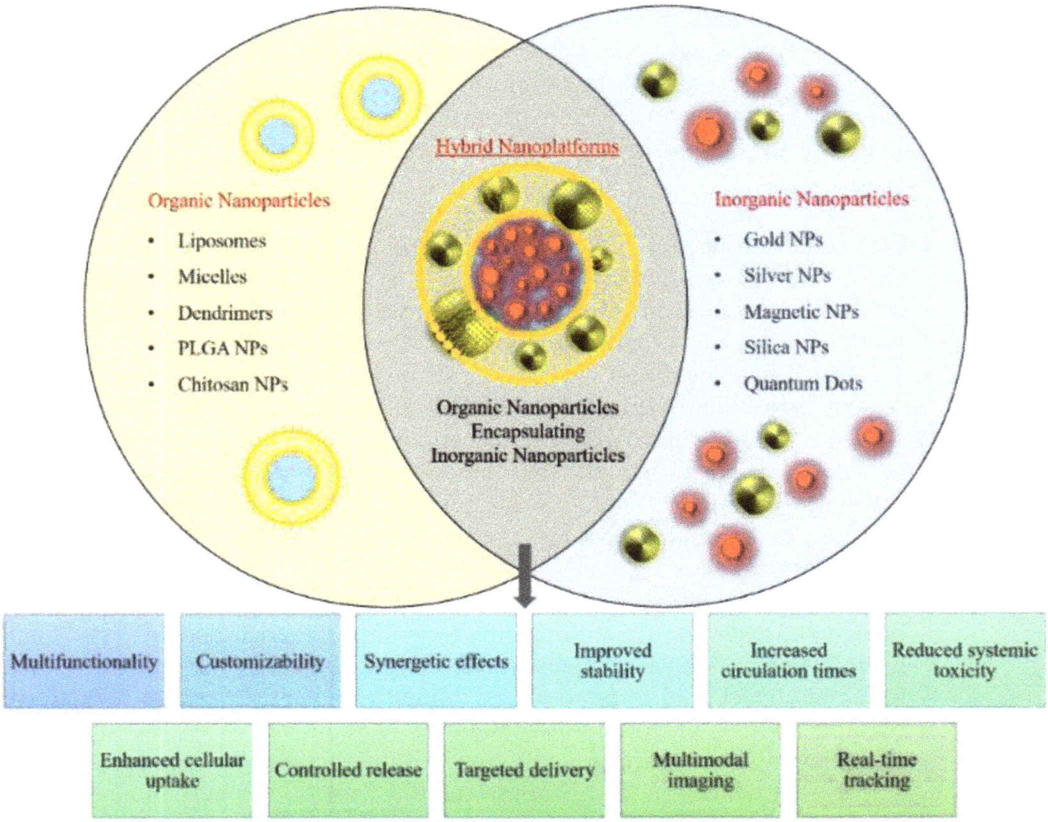

Figure 1.4. Schematics of different types of hybrid nanoplatforms for bio-applications. Reproduced from [30]. CC BY 4.0.

with biological systems at the cellular and molecular levels, enabling enhanced imaging capabilities and targeted therapies. One of their key contributions lies in serving as contrast agents across various imaging modalities, including fluorescence imaging, MRI, CT, ultrasound (US), PET, and SPECT. By enhancing image contrast, nanoplatforms enable clearer visualization of tissues and organs, aiding in the accurate diagnosis and monitoring of diseases [32].

Another critical role of nanoplatforms in biomedical imaging is their ability to facilitate targeted drug delivery. Through functionalization with targeting ligands, these platforms can be directed to specific tissues or cells, improving the specificity of both imaging and therapeutic interventions. This targeted approach enhances treatment efficacy while minimizing off-target effects, highlighting the versatility and precision of nanoplatforms in biomedical applications.

Additionally, certain nanomaterials used as photothermal and photoacoustic agents absorb light and convert it into heat or sound, enabling imaging and therapy. Nanoplatforms can also act as radiation dose enhancers, improving the effectiveness of radiation therapy. These functionalities underscore the multifaceted nature of nanoplatforms, making them valuable tools for advancing imaging techniques and therapeutic strategies.

Moreover, nanoplatforms exhibit excellent biocompatibility, ensuring minimal adverse reactions in the body. This characteristic is crucial for their safe use in medical applications, further highlighting their suitability for clinical translation and patient care. Furthermore, their stability in biological environments and during circulation within the body ensures effective delivery and functionality, contributing to their efficacy in imaging and therapy.

Nanoplatforms are also characterized by their versatility, as they can be tailored to integrate multiple imaging functionalities within a single platform. This multimodal approach allows for simultaneous data acquisition from various imaging modalities, providing a more comprehensive assessment of pathological conditions. Additionally, some nanoplatforms are developed as theranostic agents, combining diagnostic and therapeutic functionalities. This integrated approach enables real-time monitoring of treatment effectiveness and personalized treatment strategies, marking a significant advancement in personalized medicine. Nanoplatforms represent a revolutionary advancement in biomedical imaging, offering enhanced sensitivity, improved resolution, multimodal functionality, and theranostic potential. These platforms hold immense promise for revolutionizing healthcare by enabling earlier disease detection, more accurate diagnosis, and targeted therapeutic interventions, ultimately improving patient outcomes and quality of life.

1.3.3 Advantages and challenges of nanoplatforms in biomedical imaging

Nanoplatforms in biomedical imaging offer a range of advantages but also face several challenges that must be addressed for their safe and effective use.

1.3.3.1 Advantages

- **Enhanced sensitivity and specificity:** nanoplatforms can be equipped with targeting ligands that bind specifically to disease biomarkers [33]. This leads to improved detection of small and early-stage lesions and reduces background noise, enabling clearer and more accurate images. This can facilitate earlier diagnosis and intervention for better treatment outcomes.
- **Improved resolution:** due to their small size, nanoplatforms can penetrate deep into tissues, allowing visualization of structures at the cellular and even subcellular level [29]. This capability provides high-resolution images, enabling detailed observation of cellular processes and abnormalities for improved diagnosis.
- **Multimodality:** certain nanoplatforms integrate multiple imaging modalities into a single platform, allowing for simultaneous information gathering from different modalities. This approach provides a more comprehensive picture of the disease state without requiring multiple scans, leading to improved diagnosis and treatment planning.

- **Theranostics:** some nanoplatforms combine imaging and therapeutic functionalities, enabling real-time monitoring of treatment effectiveness and targeted delivery of therapeutic agents [34]. This integration facilitates personalized treatment strategies and reduces side effects by delivering drugs directly to the diseased area.
- **Enhanced contrast:** nanoparticles often serve as contrast agents in imaging, enhancing the contrast of the images and making it easier to distinguish between different tissues. This improves the accuracy of imaging and can lead to more precise diagnoses.

1.3.3.2 Challenges

- **Biocompatibility and toxicity:** ensuring the safety of nanoplatforms is crucial, as some nanoparticles may be potentially toxic or difficult to clear from the body. Careful design and testing are necessary to minimize any potential harmful effects and ensure patient safety.
- **Targeting specificity and efficiency:** achieving specific and efficient targeting remains challenging, as off-target effects and delivery barriers can hinder the effectiveness of nanoplatforms. Overcoming these challenges requires further research to optimize targeting strategies and improve delivery mechanisms.
- **Cost and regulatory issues:** developing and manufacturing nanoplatforms can be expensive, posing challenges in terms of accessibility and affordability for patients. Navigating the regulatory approval process for clinical translation also requires significant resources and expertise.
- **Limited long-term data:** as a relatively new technology, long-term data on the safety and efficacy of nanoplatforms are scarce. More research and clinical trials are needed to establish their long-term effects and ensure patient safety. Unforeseen consequences of long-term use may arise, necessitating further investigation to address potential risks.

While nanoplatforms offer tremendous potential for revolutionizing biomedical imaging, addressing the existing challenges is crucial for their safe and effective clinical translation [35]. Continued research and development efforts are essential to overcome these hurdles and unlock the full potential of this technology in improving healthcare. Figure 1.5 shows the immunological effects and bio-application of nano-imaging materials.

1.4 Types of nanoplatforms for biomedical imaging

1.4.1 Contrast agents for molecular imaging

Nanoplatform contrast agents are playing an increasingly crucial role in molecular imaging, offering unique properties that enhance the capabilities of various imaging modalities [37]. Functionalized silica nanoplatforms, inorganic nanoparticles, and nanoparticle-based contrast agents are among the key players in this field, each with its distinct advantages and applications. Functionalized silica nanoplatforms, for example, are used as bimodal contrast agents for MRI and optical imaging [38]. By

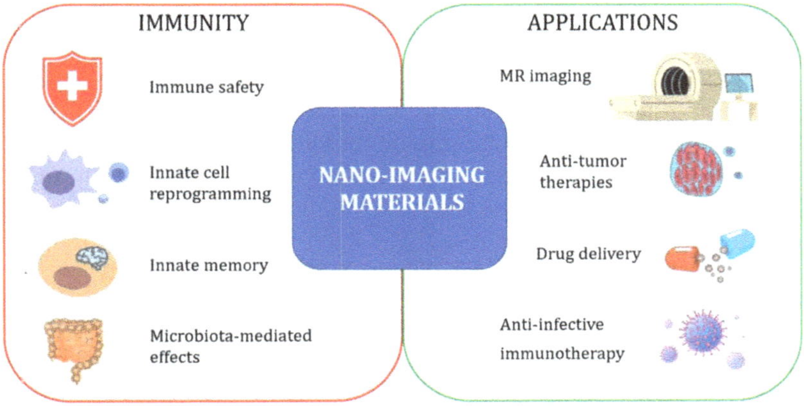

Figure 1.5. Immunological effects and bio-application of nano-imaging materials. Reproduced from [36]. CC BY 4.0.

encapsulating clinically used Gd^{3+} chelate within silica nanoparticles and grafting near-infrared-emitting probes on their surface, these nanoplatforms offer both paramagnetic and optical properties, making them versatile for different imaging needs [39].

Inorganic nanoparticles, such as semiconductor QDs, iron oxide nanoparticles, and gold nanoparticles, have been developed as contrast agents for molecular imaging [40]. Their unique properties, including strong x-ray attenuation, magnetic properties, and fluorescence, make them valuable tools for diagnostics and targeted imaging. Nanoparticle-based contrast agents offer several advantages, including improved *in vivo* detection and potentially enhanced targeting efficiencies. By engineering longer circulation times, designed clearance pathways, and multimeric binding capacities, these agents show promise for more effective and targeted imaging approaches.

Superparamagnetic iron oxide nanoparticles (SPIOs) are commonly used for MRI, especially in tumor imaging, liver and spleen imaging, and cardiovascular imaging [41]. Gadolinium-based nanoparticles, despite concerns about potential deposition in the brain, offer high relaxivity for strong signal enhancement, driving ongoing research for safer alternatives. For CT imaging, gold nanoparticles and iodinated nanoparticles are explored as contrast agents. Gold nanoparticles provide high x-ray attenuation and can be functionalized for targeted imaging, while iodinated nanoparticles offer potential benefits of improved targeting and reduced side effects compared to traditional small molecule contrast agents.

In PET imaging, radiolabeled nanoparticles and nanoparticle probes labeled with radionuclides are used for imaging specific biomarkers associated with diseases [42]. These approaches offer advantages such as longer half-lives and improved signal-to-noise ratio, enhancing the sensitivity and accuracy of PET imaging. In optical imaging, QDs and upconversion nanoparticles are used for their unique light-emitting properties [43]. QDs emit light of specific colors upon excitation, enabling precise and sensitive imaging. Upconversion nanoparticles convert near-infrared light to visible light, allowing for deeper tissue penetration and imaging of biological structures.

Overall, nanoplatform contrast agents offer a range of advantages for molecular imaging, including enhanced sensitivity, improved resolution, multimodality, and theranostic potential [44]. Despite facing challenges such as biocompatibility, targeting specificity, cost, and regulatory issues, continued research and development efforts are essential to harness the full potential of nanoplatforms in improving healthcare.

1.4.2 Nanoparticles for imaging enhancement

Nanoparticles are revolutionizing the field of bioimaging, offering tremendous potential for enhanced sensitivity, specificity, resolution, and even therapeutic capabilities [45]. Here is a detailed breakdown of their diverse applications:

a. **Enhanced sensitivity and specificity:**

   Traditional imaging techniques often struggle to detect small or early-stage lesions due to limitations in sensitivity and specificity. Nanoparticles overcome these challenges by:

   - **Targeting:** nanoparticles can be conjugated with targeting ligands, molecules that specifically bind to biomarkers associated with a particular disease, like cancer cells. This targeted approach allows the platform to accumulate in the area of interest, generating stronger signals for detection and reducing background noise.
   - **Multi-valency:** due to their small size, nanoparticles have a large surface area, allowing them to be equipped with multiple targeting ligands. This multi-valency increases the binding affinity and overall signal for better detection.

   Examples:

   - **Gold nanoparticles conjugated with HER2 antibodies:** used for x-ray imaging (CT scan) detection of tumors expressing the HER2 protein, a biomarker for breast cancer [46, 47].
   - **Magnetic nanoparticles conjugated with folate:** targeted towards folate receptors, often overexpressed in cancer cells, for MRI imaging of tumors [48].

b. **Improved resolution:**

   Conventional imaging techniques have limitations in resolving structures at the cellular and sub-cellular levels. Nanoparticles offer advantages in this aspect:

   - **Size:** due to their small size, nanoparticles can penetrate deep into tissues and reach microscopic structures. This allows for high-resolution imaging at the cellular and even sub-cellular level.
   - **Fluorescence properties:** some nanoparticles, like QDs, emit light of specific colors when exposed to specific wavelengths. This allows researchers to visualize various cellular components with high resolution and distinguish them from surrounding tissue.

Examples:

- **QDs for fluorescence microscopy:** used to visualize cellular components like proteins, organelles, and even specific molecules within cells [49].
- **Superparamagnetic iron oxide nanoparticles (SPIOs) for MRI:** used to image cellular and even sub-cellular structures in the brain and other organs [41].

c. **Multimodality:**

Traditional methods often require multiple scans using different techniques to obtain a comprehensive picture of disease. Nanoplatforms can address this limitation by:

- **Combining functionalities:** certain nanoplatforms can be designed to integrate multiple imaging modalities within a single platform. This allows for simultaneous information gathering from various modalities, such as MRI and fluorescence, providing a more complete picture of the disease state.

Example:

- **Iron oxide nanoparticles with fluorescent labels:** utilized for dual-modality imaging, combining MRI for anatomical information and fluorescence imaging for specific molecular information in the same scan [50].

d. **Theranostics:**

Nanoplatforms can be developed as theranostic agents, combining imaging and therapeutic functionalities within a single platform:

- **Dual functionality:** these platforms can be used to image tumors via modalities like optical imaging and simultaneously deliver therapeutic drugs directly to the tumor site.
- **Real-time monitoring:** theranostic platforms allow for real-time monitoring of treatment effectiveness by observing changes in the images, enabling adjustments to therapy as needed.

Example:

- **Liposomes loaded with imaging agents and chemotherapeutic drugs:** used for visualizing tumors via optical imaging and delivering chemotherapy drugs directly to the cancer cells [51].

1.4.2.1 Challenges and future directions

Despite the exciting potential of these platforms, several challenges remain:

- **Biocompatibility and toxicity:** ensuring the safety of these platforms is crucial, as some nanoparticles may pose potential toxicity risks.
- **Targeting specificity and efficiency:** achieving efficient and specific targeting to avoid off-target effects and maximize efficacy requires further research.
- **Cost and regulatory hurdles:** developing and ensuring regulatory approval for clinical use of these platforms can be expensive and time-consuming.

However, research continues to address these challenges and unlock the full potential of nanoplatforms for bioimaging. Advances in nanomaterial design, targeting strategies, and manufacturing processes pave the way for the future of personalized medicine, earlier disease detection, and improved treatment outcomes.

1.4.3 QDs for fluorescence imaging

QDs have emerged as powerful tools in the field of fluorescence bioimaging, offering unique advantages over traditional organic fluorophores [52, 53]. Here is a closer look at their applications and the reasons behind their growing popularity.

1.4.3.1 Advantages of QDs for bioimaging

QDs offer tunable emissions, unlike traditional fluorophores with fixed emission spectra. By adjusting the size of the QD, its emission wavelength can be precisely controlled, allowing for multiplexing and reduced spectral overlap [54]. This feature expands the scope of information gathered and enhances the accuracy of image analysis.

Moreover, QDs exhibit superior brightness compared to traditional fluorophores, allowing for the detection of even faint signals. Additionally, they demonstrate outstanding photostability, resisting photo-bleaching better than organic dyes. This characteristic enables longer imaging sessions and improves image quality.

Furthermore, QDs can be engineered with biocompatible coatings to minimize potential toxicity and immune response within the body [55]. Their surfaces can also be conjugated with targeting molecules like antibodies or peptides, enabling specific binding to targeted biomarkers of disease. This specificity enhances the sensitivity and accuracy of imaging.

1.4.3.2 Applications of QDs in bioimaging

QDs find applications in various areas of bioimaging:

- **Cellular and sub-cellular imaging: QDs** can visualize various cellular components and processes due to their size and ability to be internalized by cells. Specific labeling with targeting molecules allows for imaging of specific organelles or proteins within the cell.
- ***In vivo* imaging:** by incorporating QDs into nanoparticles, they can be injected into living organisms for targeted *in vivo* imaging. This enables researchers to study diseases and track therapeutic effectiveness within the body, providing valuable insights for diagnosis and treatment monitoring.
- **Biosensing and bioassays:** QDs can be utilized in biosensing applications by incorporating them into biocompatible platforms or sensors. These platforms can detect specific biomolecules like biomarkers, pathogens, or environmental toxins, offering sensitive and reliable detection methods.

1.4.3.3 Challenges and future directions

Despite their advantages, QDs face challenges:

- **Biocompatibility concerns:** ensuring long-term biocompatibility and minimizing potential toxicity remain crucial focuses in QD development.
- **Cost and complexity:** the production of QDs can be complex and expensive, limiting their wider accessibility in research and clinical settings.
- **Long-term effects and environmental impact:** further research is needed to understand the long-term effects of QDs on the body and their potential environmental impact.

Despite these challenges, ongoing advances in QD technology hold immense promise for revolutionizing bioimaging. Their unique properties and versatile applications continue to pave the way for significant breakthroughs in various fields, from basic biological research to clinical diagnostics and therapeutic monitoring.

1.4.4 Nanosensors for *in vivo* imaging

Nanosensors, microscopic sensors built from nanomaterials, offer a revolutionary approach to *in vivo* imaging [56]. Harnessing their unique size, properties, and functionalities can provide valuable insights into biological processes at the cellular and molecular level within living organisms. Here is a detailed look at their potential applications.

1.4.4.1 Advantages of nanosensors for in vivo *imaging*

Nanosensors can be designed with targeting moieties that bind specifically to particular biomolecules of interest, such as disease markers, enzymes, or metabolites. This targeted approach allows for sensitive detection of even low concentrations of these molecules, leading to early disease diagnosis and monitoring of treatment effectiveness.

Moreover, unlike traditional imaging methods that provide snapshots, some nanosensors can offer real-time information about changes in biological processes within the body. This allows for continuous monitoring of disease progression and therapeutic response, enabling dynamic adjustments to treatment strategies.

Certain nanosensors can be designed to integrate multiple imaging modalities within a single platform. This enables the gathering of comprehensive information from different imaging techniques, providing a more complete picture of the biological system under study.

Some nanosensors can be developed for theranostic applications, combining imaging and therapeutic functionalities. This allows for visualization of the targeted area to guide treatment delivery, monitoring of therapeutic response in real time, and targeted delivery of therapeutic agents directly to the area of interest, minimizing side effects.

1.4.4.2 Examples of nanosensors for in vivo *imaging*

Fluorescent nanosensors can be designed to bind specific biological targets and emit light upon interaction, allowing for visualization through fluorescence imaging techniques [57]. MRI nanosensors can be used as contrast agents to enhance the signal in MRI scans, enabling detailed imaging of specific tissues or organs. Electrochemical nanosensors can detect changes in electrical signals within the body, providing information about cellular processes and potential abnormalities.

1.4.4.3 Challenges and future directions

Ensuring the safety of nanosensors for *in vivo* use is crucial. Careful design and testing are needed to minimize potential toxicity and immune response. Achieving high targeting efficiency and specificity remains a challenge. Overcoming biological barriers and minimizing off-target effects requires further research. Developing nanosensors that can be efficiently cleared from the body after their function is complete is crucial to avoid long-term accumulation and potential risks. The development and manufacture of nanosensors can be expensive, and navigating regulatory approvals for clinical use is a complex process.

Despite these challenges, the potential of nanosensors for *in vivo* imaging is immense. Continued research efforts hold great promise for early diagnosis and improved treatment outcomes for various diseases [58]. Personalized medicine approaches based on individual patient needs and the development of new therapeutic strategies guided by real-time information from nanosensors are also promising areas of advancement. As researchers continue to refine and develop nanosensors, they are poised to revolutionize *in vivo* imaging and advance our understanding of health and disease at the most fundamental level.

1.4.5 Comparison and evaluation of different nanoplatforms for biomedical imaging

1.4.5.1 Contrast agents for molecular imaging

- **Strengths:** contrast agents for molecular imaging offer enhanced sensitivity and specificity for targeted imaging of specific molecules. They encompass a wide variety of platforms available for different imaging modalities, such as MRI, CT, and PET. These agents have established clinical applications in various diagnostic procedures, enabling the visualization, quantification, and characterization of biological processes at the cellular and molecular levels.
- **Limitations:** despite their strengths, contrast agents have limitations. They typically have limited functionality beyond imaging, restricting their application in therapeutic interventions. There are also potential concerns regarding the long-term safety and side effects of some contrast agents, necessitating further research and development in this area.
- **Applications:** contrast agents for molecular imaging find applications in the diagnosis of various diseases like cancer, cardiovascular diseases, and neurological disorders. They are also used for monitoring treatment response and disease progression, providing valuable insights into the effectiveness of therapeutic interventions.

1.4.5.2 Nanoparticles for imaging enhancement

- **Strengths:** nanoparticles for imaging enhancement offer versatile platforms with diverse functionalities beyond imaging, including drug delivery and theranostics. They provide improved resolution and deeper tissue penetration compared to traditional imaging methods. Additionally, they have the potential for multimodal imaging capabilities, allowing for the integration of multiple imaging modalities within a single platform.
- **Limitations:** despite their versatility, nanoparticles for imaging enhancement have limitations. They encompass a broader category encompassing various specific platforms, each with its own limitations and challenges. Concerns

regarding biocompatibility and the potential toxicity of some nanoparticles remain, requiring careful consideration in their design and development.

- **Applications:** nanoparticles for imaging enhancement find applications in enhancing the sensitivity and specificity of various imaging modalities. They enable theranostic applications for combined imaging and treatment, offering personalized medicine approaches based on individual patient needs. Additionally, they improve drug delivery by targeting specific tissues or cells, minimizing off-target effects.

1.4.5.3 QDs for fluorescence imaging

- **Strengths:** QDs offer tunable emission spectra, allowing for multiplexing and reduced spectral overlap, enabling imaging of multiple targets simultaneously. They provide superior brightness and photostability compared to traditional fluorophores. Additionally, they have the potential for biocompatible coatings and targeted imaging capabilities, enhancing their utility in biomedical imaging.
- **Limitations:** despite their strengths, QDs have limitations. They are costly and complex to produce compared to traditional fluorophores, limiting their widespread adoption. There are also concerns regarding potential long-term toxicity and environmental impact, necessitating further investigation into their safety profile.
- **Applications:** QDs find applications in cellular and sub-cellular imaging for studying biological processes, as well as *in vivo* imaging for disease diagnosis and monitoring. They are also used in biosensing applications for detecting specific biomolecules, offering sensitive and reliable detection methods.

1.4.5.4 Nanosensors for in vivo *imaging*

- **Strengths:** nanosensors offer high potential for sensitive and specific detection of biomolecules and monitoring of biological processes in real time. They provide the possibility for theranostic applications combining imaging and therapeutic functionalities. Additionally, they have the potential for gathering information from multiple modalities within a single platform, enhancing their utility in biomedical imaging.
- **Limitations:** despite their strengths, nanosensors have limitations. Many platforms are still in the early stages of development, with ongoing research needed to address challenges such as biocompatibility, targeting efficiency, and clearance from the body. Additionally, the high cost and complex development process of nanosensors pose challenges for their widespread adoption.
- **Applications:** nanosensors find applications in early disease diagnosis and monitoring of treatment response. They enable personalized medicine approaches based on real-time information, offering tailored treatment strategies for individual patients. Additionally, they facilitate the development of new therapeutic strategies guided by nano-sensor data, leading to improved healthcare outcomes.

- **Overall evaluation:** all four nanoplatforms offer unique advantages and hold immense potential for revolutionizing various aspects of biomedical imaging. While contrast agents are the most established and have diverse clinical applications, nanoparticles for imaging enhancement offer broader functionalities and potential for theranostics. QDs excel in brightness and photostability, while nanosensors hold promise for real-time monitoring and theranostic applications. Further research and development efforts are crucial to unlock the full potential of these technologies and address their respective limitations.

1.5 Design considerations for nanoplatforms in biomedical imaging

Biocompatibility and safety are paramount considerations for the use of imaging nanoplatforms in biomedical applications [59]. Various biocompatible nanoplatforms, such as manganese-based hollow nanoplatforms and near-infrared-II hollow nanoplatforms, have been studied extensively for their potential in the diagnosis and therapy of deep tumors. These nanoplatforms offer diversified diagnostic and therapeutic capabilities, and their magnetic properties are known to cause little damage to tissue. Conventional organic dyes and inorganic fluorescent contrast agents have been hindered in bioimaging and biomedical applications due to their intrinsic drawbacks, including toxicity and poor biocompatibility. Therefore, there is a pressing need to develop innovative classes of nanomaterials and fluorescent contrast agents with high photostability, remarkable safety, and significant biocompatibility for biomedical and clinical applications. Despite the promising prospects, further investigations and comprehensive evaluations are needed to address the challenges in this important field of science.

1.5.1 Biocompatibility and safety of imaging nanoplatforms

Biocompatibility and safety are crucial considerations for the use of imaging nanoplatforms in biomedical applications [60]. These platforms, which encompass a range of technologies from contrast agents to nanosensors, interact with biological systems, necessitating thorough assessment to ensure they do not cause harm. Biocompatibility refers to the ability of a material to interact with living organisms without eliciting an adverse response. It encompasses factors such as cytotoxicity, immunogenicity, and biodistribution. For imaging nanoplatforms, biocompatibility is essential to ensure they do not harm cells or tissues, do not trigger immune responses, and are efficiently distributed and cleared from the body. Safety considerations for imaging nanoplatforms include acute and chronic toxicity, as well as their potential environmental impact [61]. Acute toxicity assessments are crucial to understand immediate harm from exposure, while chronic toxicity studies evaluate long-term effects such as carcinogenicity and genotoxicity. Additionally, the environmental impact of these platforms, including their potential accumulation in ecosystems, needs to be carefully evaluated.

Strategies to enhance biocompatibility and safety include careful material selection, surface engineering to minimize toxicity and improve targeting specificity, and optimization of size and shape to influence biological interactions. Rigorous testing, including comprehensive *in vitro* and *in vivo* studies, is essential to assess biocompatibility and potential risks before clinical translation. Challenges in ensuring the biocompatibility and safety of imaging nanoplatforms include the complexity of nanomaterials, limited long-term safety data, and the need for clear regulatory pathways [61]. Continued research and development efforts, focused on addressing these challenges, are essential to ensure the safe and responsible use of imaging nanoplatforms for biomedical applications.

1.6 Conclusions

Nanomaterials have made significant strides in biomedical imaging, offering unparalleled capabilities for detection, diagnosis, and treatment monitoring [62]. The future of nanomaterial-based bioimaging holds immense promise, with several exciting perspectives on the horizon:

- **Multimodal imaging integration:**
  Future developments will likely focus on integrating multiple imaging modalities into a single nanomaterial platform. This will enable complementary information acquisition, enhancing diagnostic accuracy and providing a more comprehensive understanding of biological processes.
- **Smart nanoprobes with stimuli-responsive properties:**
  Nanomaterials capable of responding to specific stimuli within the biological environment, such as pH, temperature, or enzyme activity, will enable dynamic imaging with enhanced specificity and sensitivity. These smart nanoprobes could be engineered to trigger imaging signal activation in response to disease-specific biomarkers, facilitating early detection and precise localization of pathological sites.
- ***In Vivo* imaging with high spatial and temporal resolution:**
  Advances in nanomaterial design and imaging techniques will likely lead to the development of non-invasive *in vivo* imaging modalities with unprecedented spatial and temporal resolution. This will enable real-time monitoring of dynamic biological processes at the cellular and sub-cellular levels, providing invaluable insights into disease progression and treatment response.
- **Theranostic nanoparticles for personalized medicine:**
  Theranostic nanoparticles capable of simultaneous imaging and therapy will play a central role in personalized medicine approaches. These multifunctional nanomaterials will enable real-time monitoring of treatment efficacy and facilitate timely adjustments to therapeutic regimens based on individual patient responses, ultimately improving clinical outcomes.
- **Nanomaterials for targeted drug delivery and image-guided therapy:**
  Nanomaterials engineered for targeted drug delivery and image-guided therapy will continue to revolutionize the field of precision medicine. By combining imaging capabilities with therapeutic functionalities, these nanoplatforms will enable precise drug delivery to diseased tissues while

minimizing off-target effects, thus maximizing therapeutic efficacy and minimizing systemic toxicity.

- **Biodegradable and clearance-friendly nanomaterials:**
  The development of biodegradable nanomaterials with efficient clearance pathways will be crucial for minimizing long-term toxicity and improving the safety profile of nanomaterial-based imaging agents. Biocompatible nanomaterials capable of undergoing controlled degradation and elimination from the body will enable repeated imaging studies without accumulation-related side effects.
- **Emerging nanomaterials for novel imaging modalities:**
  Ongoing research into novel nanomaterials, such as carbon-based nanoparticles, metal–organic frameworks, and two-dimensional materials, holds promise for the development of next-generation imaging modalities with unique properties and functionalities. These emerging nanomaterials will expand the capabilities of bioimaging and open up new avenues for scientific exploration and clinical translation.
- **Point-of-care and resource-limited settings applications:**
  Streamlined fabrication processes and the development of portable imaging devices will facilitate the deployment of nanomaterial-based bioimaging technologies in point-of-care settings and resource-limited environments. This will democratize access to advanced diagnostic tools, improve healthcare delivery, and empower healthcare providers to make informed clinical decisions in real time. In summary, the future of nanomaterial-based bioimaging is characterized by rapid technological advancements, interdisciplinary collaboration, and a strong emphasis on personalized, precise, and non-invasive diagnostic and therapeutic approaches. These innovations hold the potential to transform healthcare delivery, improve patient outcomes, and address unmet medical needs across diverse disease areas. Addressing the arising challenges requires interdisciplinary collaborations among scientists, engineers, clinicians, and regulatory bodies to harness the full potential of nanomaterials for biomedical imaging while ensuring their safety and efficacy in clinical settings.

References

[1] Kateb B, Chiu K, Black K L, Yamamoto V, Khalsa B, Ljubimova J Y, Ding H, Patil R, Portilla-Arias J A and Modo M 2011 Nanoplatforms for constructing new approaches to cancer treatment, imaging, and drug delivery: what should be the policy? *Neuroimage* **54** S106–24

[2] Siddique S and Chow J C 2020 Application of nanomaterials in biomedical imaging and cancer therapy *Nanomaterials* **10** 1700

[3] Chen X 2011 *Nanoplatform-Based Molecular Imaging* (New York: Wiley)

[4] Chen Z-Y, Wang Y-X, Lin Y, Zhang J-S, Yang F, Zhou Q-L and Liao Y-Y 2014 Advance of molecular imaging technology and targeted imaging agent in imaging and therapy *BioMed Res. Int.* **2014** 819324

[5] Han X, Xu K, Taratula O and Farsad K 2019 Applications of nanoparticles in biomedical imaging *Nanoscale* **11** 799–819

[6] Yao J, Yang M and Duan Y 2014 Chemistry, biology, and medicine of fluorescent nanomaterials and related systems: new insights into biosensing, bioimaging, genomics, diagnostics, and therapy *Chem. Rev.* **114** 6130–78

[7] Zhao F, Yao D, Guo R, Deng L, Dong A and Zhang J 2015 Composites of polymer hydrogels and nanoparticulate systems for biomedical and pharmaceutical applications *Nanomaterials* **5** 2054–130

[8] National Research Council, Division on Earth and Life Studies, Board on Chemical Sciences and Technology, Committee on Revealing Chemistry through Advanced Chemical Imaging 2006 *Visualizing Chemistry: The Progress and Promise of Advanced Chemical Imaging* (National Academies Press)

[9] Hahn M A, Singh A K, Sharma P, Brown S C and Moudgil B M 2011 Nanoparticles as contrast agents for in-vivo bioimaging: current status and future perspectives *Anal. Bioanal. Chem.* **399** 3–27

[10] Pourmadadi M, Rajabzadeh-Khosroshahi M, Eshaghi M M, Rahmani E, Motasadizadeh H, Arshad R, Rahdar A and Pandey S 2023 TiO_2-based nanocomposites for cancer diagnosis and therapy: a comprehensive review *J. Drug Deliv. Sci. Technol.* **82** 104370

[11] Mahmoudi M, Serpooshan V and Laurent S 2011 Engineered nanoparticles for biomolecular imaging *Nanoscale* **3** 3007–26

[12] Shi D, Sadat M, Dunn A W and Mast D B 2015 Photo-fluorescent and magnetic properties of iron oxide nanoparticles for biomedical applications *Nanoscale* **7** 8209–32

[13] Thomas R, Park I-K and Jeong Y Y 2013 Magnetic iron oxide nanoparticles for multimodal imaging and therapy of cancer *Int. J. Mol. Sci.* **14** 15910–30

[14] Navya P and Daima H K 2016 Rational engineering of physicochemical properties of nanomaterials for biomedical applications with nanotoxicological perspectives *Nano Converg.* **3** 1–14

[15] Wang M and Thanou M 2010 Targeting nanoparticles to cancer *Pharmacol. Res.* **62** 90–9

[16] Lotfipour F, Shahi S, Farjami A, Salatin S, Mahmoudian M and Dizaj S M 2021 Safety and toxicity issues of therapeutically used nanoparticles from the oral route *BioMed Res. Int.* **2021** 9322282

[17] Gratton S E, Williams S S, Napier M E, Pohlhaus P D, Zhou Z, Wiles K B, Maynor B W, Shen C, Olafsen T and Samulski E T 2008 The pursuit of a scalable nanofabrication platform for use in material and life science applications *Acc. Chem. Res.* **41** 1685–95

[18] Nguyen T-D and Tran T-H 2014 Multicomponent nanoarchitectures for the design of optical sensing and diagnostic tools *RSC Adv.* **4** 916–42

[19] Sowmiya P, Dhas T S, Inbakandan D, Anandakumar N, Nalini S, Suganya K U, Remya R, Karthick V and Kumar C V 2023 Optically active organic and inorganic nanomaterials for biological imaging applications: a review *Micron* **172** 103486

[20] Chung C and Yam V 2011 Induced self-assembly and Förster resonance energy transfer *Communications* **47** 2898–900

[21] Topete Camacho A 2013 Development of hybrid nanoplatforms for theranostic applications *Dissertation* Universidade de Santiago de Compostela

[22] Hong E, Liu L, Bai L, Xia C, Gao L, Zhang L and Wang B 2019 Control synthesis, subtle surface modification of rare-earth-doped upconversion nanoparticles and their applications in cancer diagnosis and treatment *Mater. Sci. Eng.* C **105** 110097

[23] Pimpin A and Srituravanich W 2012 Review on micro-and nanolithography techniques and their applications *Eng. J.* **16** 37–56

[24] Thiruvengadathan R, Korampally V, Ghosh A, Chanda N, Gangopadhyay K and Gangopadhyay S 2013 Nanomaterial processing using self-assembly-bottom-up chemical and biological approaches *Rep. Prog. Phys.* **76** 066501

[25] Herman M A and Sitter H 2012 *Molecular Beam Epitaxy: Fundamentals and Current Status* (Berlin: Springer Science & Business Media)

[26] Singh L P, Bhattacharyya S K, Kumar R, Mishra G, Sharma U, Singh G and Ahalawat S 2014 Sol–gel processing of silica nanoparticles and their applications *Adv. Colloid Interface Sci.* **214** 17–37

[27] Wu D, Rajput N S and Luo X 2016 Nanoimprint lithography-the past, the present and the future *Curr. Nanosci.* **12** 712–24

[28] Ito S, Kasuya M, Kurihara K and Nakagawa M 2017 Nanometer-resolved fluidity of an oleophilic monomer between silica surfaces modified with fluorinated monolayers for nanoimprinting *ACS Appl. Mater. Interfaces* **9** 6591–8

[29] Kunjachan S, Ehling J, Storm G, Kiessling F and Lammers T 2015 Noninvasive imaging of nanomedicines and nanotheranostics: principles, progress, and prospects *Chem. Rev.* **115** 10907–37

[30] Yanar F, Carugo D and Zhang X 2023 Hybrid nanoplatforms comprising organic nano-compartments encapsulating inorganic nanoparticles for enhanced drug delivery and bioimaging applications *Molecules* **28** 5694

[31] Jones E F, He J, Vanbrocklin H F, Franc B L and Seo Y 2008 Nanoprobes for medical diagnosis: current status of nanotechnology in molecular imaging *Curr. Nanosci.* **4** 17–29

[32] Wu H, Wang M D, Liang L, Xing H, Zhang C W, Shen F, Huang D S and Yang T 2021 Nanotechnology for hepatocellular carcinoma: from surveillance, diagnosis to management *Small* **17** 2005236

[33] Azizi M, Dianat-Moghadam H, Salehi R, Farshbaf M, Iyengar D, Sau S, Iyer A K, Valizadeh H, Mehrmohammadi M and Hamblin M R 2020 Interactions between tumor biology and targeted nanoplatforms for imaging applications *Adv. Funct. Mater.* **30** 1910402

[34] Siafaka P I, Okur N Ü, Karantas I D, Okur M E and Gündoğdu E A 2021 Current update on nanoplatforms as therapeutic and diagnostic tools: a review for the materials used as nanotheranostics and imaging modalities *Asian J. Pharm. Sci.* **16** 24–46

[35] Singh D, Dilnawaz F and Sahoo S K 2020 Challenges of moving theranostic nanomedicine into the clinic *Future Medicine* **15** 111–4

[36] Li Y, Zhang P, Tang B Z and Boraschi D 2022 Immunological effects of nano-imaging materials *Front. Immunol.* **13** 886415

[37] Cai W and Chen X 2007 Nanoplatforms for targeted molecular imaging in living subjects *Small* **3** 1840–54

[38] Garifo S, Stanicki D, Boutry S, Larbanoix L, Ternad I, Muller R N and Laurent S 2021 Functionalized silica nanoplatform as a bimodal contrast agent for MRI and optical imaging *Nanoscale* **13** 16509–24

[39] Li D 2020 Design and synthesis of multifunctional nanoparticles for multi-modal imaging and theranostics applications *PhD Thesis* University of Technology, Sydney

[40] Cho E C, Glaus C, Chen J, Welch M J and Xia Y 2010 Inorganic nanoparticle-based contrast agents for molecular imaging *Trends Mol. Med.* **16** 561–73

[41] Ittrich H, Peldschus K, Raabe N, Kaul M and Adam G 2013 Superparamagnetic iron oxide nanoparticles in biomedicine: applications and developments in diagnostics and therapy *RöFo-Fortschritte auf dem Gebiet der Röntgenstrahlen und der bildgebenden Verfahren* (Stuttgart-Feuerbach: Georg Thieme Verlag KG) pp 1149–66

[42] Sun X, Cai W and Chen X 2015 Positron emission tomography imaging using radiolabeled inorganic nanomaterials *Acc. Chem. Res.* **48** 286–94

[43] Kosaka N, McCann T E, Mitsunaga M, Choyke P L and Kobayashi H 2010 Real-time optical imaging using quantum dot and related nanocrystals *Nanomedicine* **5** 765–76

[44] Hellebust A and Richards-Kortum R 2012 Advances in molecular imaging: targeted optical contrast agents for cancer diagnostics *Nanomedicine* **7** 429–45

[45] Kairdolf B A, Qian X and Nie S 2017 Bioconjugated nanoparticles for biosensing, *in vivo* imaging, and medical diagnostics *Anal. Chem.* **89** 1015–31

[46] Nakagawa T, Gonda K, Kamei T, Cong L, Hamada Y, Kitamura N, Tada H, Ishida T, Aimiya T and Furusawa N 2016 X-ray computed tomography imaging of a tumor with high sensitivity using gold nanoparticles conjugated to a cancer-specific antibody via polyethylene glycol chains on their surface *Sci. Technol. Adv. Mater.* **17** 387–97

[47] Hainfeld J F, O'Connor M J, Dilmanian F, Slatkin D N, Adams D J and Smilowitz H M 2011 Micro-CT enables microlocalisation and quantification of Her2-targeted gold nanoparticles within tumour regions *Br. J. Radiol.* **84** 526–33

[48] Heydari Sheikh Hossein H, Jabbari I, Zarepour A, Zarrabi A, Ashrafizadeh M, Taherian A and Makvandi P 2020 Functionalization of magnetic nanoparticles by folate as potential MRI contrast agent for breast cancer diagnostics *Molecules* **25** 4053

[49] Deerinck T J 2008 The application of fluorescent quantum dots to confocal, multiphoton, and electron microscopic imaging *Toxicol. Pathol.* **36** 112–6

[50] Shkilnyy A, Munnier E, Hervé K, Soucé M, Benoit R, Cohen-Jonathan S, Limelette P, Saboungi M-L, Dubois P and Chourpa I 2010 Synthesis and evaluation of novel biocompatible super-paramagnetic iron oxide nanoparticles as magnetic anticancer drug carrier and fluorescence active label *J. Phys. Chem.* C **114** 5850–8

[51] Petersen A L, Hansen A E, Gabizon A and Andresen T L 2012 Liposome imaging agents in personalized medicine *Adv. Drug Deliv. Rev.* **64** 1417–35

[52] Pandey S and Bodas D 2020 High-quality quantum dots for multiplexed bioimaging: a critical review *Adv. Colloid Interface Sci.* **278** 102137

[53] Zrazhevskiy P, Sena M and Gao X 2010 Designing multifunctional quantum dots for bioimaging, detection, and drug delivery *Chem. Soc. Rev.* **39** 4326–54

[54] Petryayeva E, Algar W R and Medintz I L 2013 Quantum dots in bioanalysis: a review of applications across various platforms for fluorescence spectroscopy and imaging *Appl. Spectrosc.* **67** 215–52

[55] Liang Y, Zhang T and Tang M 2022 Toxicity of quantum dots on target organs and immune system *J. Appl. Toxicol.* **42** 17–40

[56] Adam T and Gopinath S C 2022 Nanosensors: recent perspectives on attainments and future promise of downstream applications *Process Biochem.* **117** 153–73

[57] Shamsipur M, Barati A and Nematifar Z 2019 Fluorescent pH nanosensors: design strategies and applications *J. Photochem. Photobiol.*, C **39** 76–141

[58] Elmore L W, Greer S F, Daniels E C, Saxe C C, Melner M H, Krawiec G M, Cance W G and Phelps W C 2021 Blueprint for cancer research: critical gaps and opportunities *CA: Cancer J. Clin.* **71** 107–39

[59] Ibarra-Ruiz A M, Rodríguez Burbano D C and Capobianco J A 2016 Photoluminescent nanoplatforms in biomedical applications *Adv. Phys.: X* **1** 194–225
[60] Jiao M, Zhang P, Meng J, Li Y, Liu C, Luo X and Gao M 2018 Recent advancements in biocompatible inorganic nanoparticles towards biomedical applications *Biomater. Sci.* **6** 726–45
[61] Damasco J A, Ravi S, Perez J D, Hagaman D E and Melancon M P 2020 Understanding nanoparticle toxicity to direct a safe-by-design approach in cancer nanomedicine *Nanomaterials* **10** 2186
[62] Chen G, Roy I, Yang C and Prasad P N 2016 Nanochemistry and nanomedicine for nanoparticle-based diagnostics and therapy *Chem. Rev.* **116** 2826–85

Chapter 2

Fundamentals of nanoplatform-based imaging for cancer diagnosis

Gaurav Ranjan, Srijani Dasgupta, Abhay Kumar Yadav, Priyashree Sunita and Shakti Prasad Pattanayak

Nanoplatform-based imaging for cancer diagnosis is an emerging and promising approach that utilizes nanoscale materials to enhance imaging sensitivity and accuracy for detecting cancerous tissues. This innovative technique combines the unique properties of nanomaterials with various imaging modalities to provide valuable information for cancer diagnosis. The fundamentals of nanoplatform-based imaging for cancer diagnosis encompass key aspects such as nanomaterial selection, imaging modalities, targeting strategies, contrast enhancement, multimodal imaging, the theranostic approach, biocompatibility, and safety. Nanomaterials play a crucial role in nanoplatform-based imaging, and their careful selection is essential for successful cancer diagnosis. Materials with high biocompatibility, stability, and efficient contrast agent properties, such as quantum dots, gold nanoparticles, and iron oxide nanoparticles, are commonly used. The choice of imaging modality is equally important and includes fluorescence imaging, computed tomography (CT), magnetic resonance imaging (MRI), and photoacoustic imaging (PAI). Multimodal imaging, achieved by integrating multiple modalities, enhances diagnostic accuracy and provides comprehensive information about cancer lesions. To achieve better targeting specificity, nanoplatforms can be functionalized with targeting ligands, enabling selective accumulation in cancer cells. This targeted approach enhances contrast and improves the accuracy of cancer detection. Surface modifications and engineering further enhance nanoplatforms' contrast enhancement capabilities. This precise and personalized treatment approach shows great promise for improved cancer management. Biocompatibility and safety are paramount considerations in nanoplatform-based imaging. Extensive preclinical studies are necessary to ensure the safe use of nanomaterials in humans without causing adverse effects. In conclusion, nanoplatform-based imaging for cancer diagnosis holds immense potential in advancing the

doi:10.1088/978-0-7503-5864-4ch2

field of oncology. By enhancing imaging sensitivity and providing precise diagnostic information, nanoplatforms offer new avenues for personalized medicine and improved patient outcomes. As this field continues to progress, nanoplatforms may become an integral component of routine cancer diagnosis and therapeutic strategies, revolutionizing cancer management and patient care.

2.1 Introduction

Nanoscience breakthroughs have revolutionized various scientific disciplines, enabling the advancement of nanotechnologies that greatly simplify our lives today. This expanding realm of research encompasses structures, devices, and systems that possess unique properties and functions, owing to the precise arrangement of their atoms on a scale ranging from 1 to 100 nm. The field garnered significant attention and generated controversy in the early 2000s, coinciding with the development of commercial applications for nanotechnology. Nanotechnologies have made significant contributions to diverse scientific domains, such as physics, materials science, chemistry, biology, computer science, and engineering. Notably, recent years have witnessed promising advancements in the application of nanotechnologies to improve human health, particularly in the realm of cancer treatment. To gain a comprehensive understanding of nanotechnology, it is beneficial to examine the timeline of discoveries that have shaped our current knowledge in this field. This chapter serves to illustrate the progress and fundamental principles of nanoscience and nanotechnology, spanning both historical and modern milestones in these areas. In recent decades, there has been significant research focus on the development of nanotechnology utilizing nanoparticles (NPs) as carriers for both small and large molecules. The formulation of NPs has involved the use of various polymers. This chapter aims to highlight the most notable advancements in the field of nanotechnology. The term 'nano' finds its origins in the Latin word *nanus* and its Greek etonym *nanos*, denoting 'dwarf.' When referring to scale, it represents one billionth of a particular unit. A nanometer, abbreviated as 1 nm, is equivalent to one billionth of a meter (1 nm $= 10^{-9}$ m). While the term nanotechnology has long been commonly used in scientific fields such as electronics, physics, and engineering, its exploration in biomedical and pharmaceutical domains is still ongoing. Nanotechnology represents a multidisciplinary field, bringing together basic sciences and applied disciplines like biophysics, molecular biology, and bioengineering. Size reduction, a fundamental process in pharmacy, offers significant advantages in nano-sizing, including increased surface area, enhanced solubility, and accelerated dissolution rate and oral bioavailability, rapid onset of action, and reduced required dosage. In the realm of medicine and physiology, these nanomaterials and devices can be designed precisely to interact with biological systems, providing a level of functional specificity that was previously unattainable. It is important to note that nanotechnology is not a single emerging scientific discipline, but rather a convergence of traditional sciences such as chemistry, physics, material science, and biology, bringing together the collective expertise necessary to develop these innovative technologies.

2.1.1 Nanoscience and nanotechnology

2.1.1.1 Definition of nanoscience and nanotechnology

Nanoscience and nanotechnology can be distinguished based on their respective definitions. Nanoscience encompasses the study and exploration of molecules and structures within the range of 1–100 nm. On the other hand, nanotechnology pertains to the practical applications, such as devices, that make use of nanoscience [1]. To provide a sense of scale, it is worth noting that a single human hair is approximately 60 000 nm thick, while the radius of a DNA double helix measures about 2 nm (figure 2.1) [2].

The roots of nanoscience can be traced back to the ancient Greeks, particularly during the 5th century BCE, when scholars contemplated whether matter was continuous and infinitely divisible, or composed of small, indivisible, and indestructible particles known as atoms. Nanotechnology, regarded as one of the most promising technologies in the 21st century, encompasses the conversion of nanoscience principles into practical applications through the observation, measurement, manipulation, assembly, control, and engineering of matter at the nanometer scale. According to the National Nanotechnology Initiative (NNI) in the USA, nanotechnology is defined as the scientific, engineering, and technological endeavors led at the nanoscale. At this scale, unique phenomena emerge, leading to novel applications across diverse fields, including chemistry, physics, biology, medicine, engineering, and electronics.

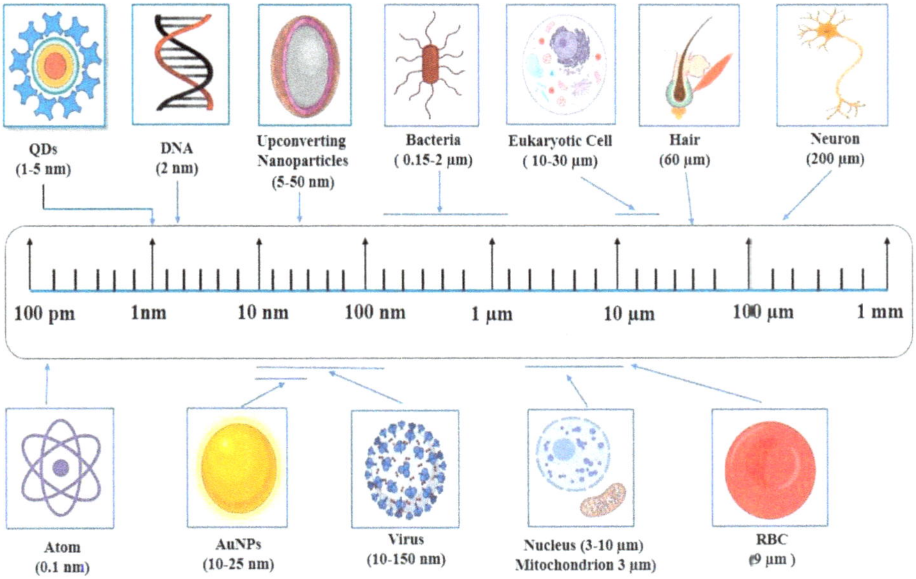

Figure 2.1. Size comparison among nanomaterials.

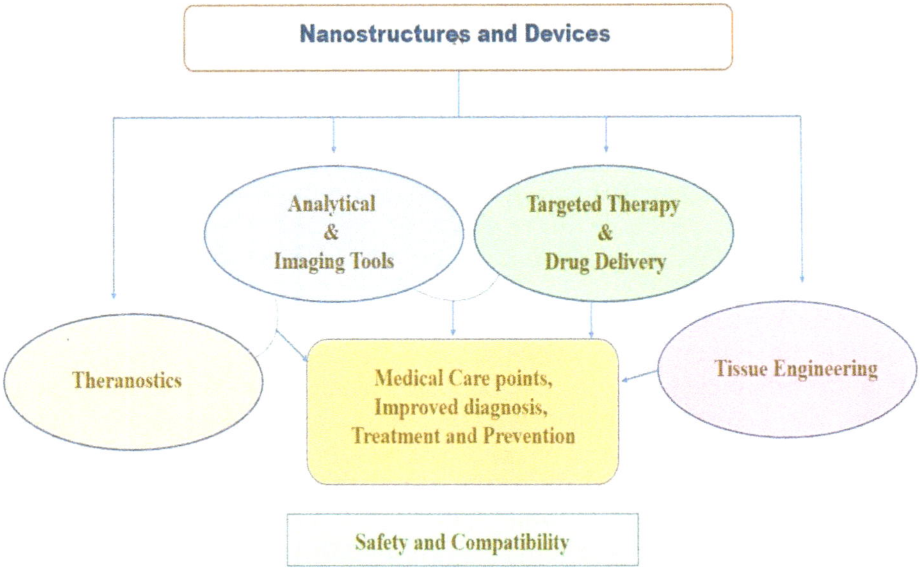

Figure 2.2. Application and goals of nanomedicine in different sphere of healthcare research.

Nanotechnology acts as a connector between the physical and biological sciences, employing nanostructures and nanophases across multiple scientific domains, with a particular focus on nanomedicine and drug delivery systems. These NPs are of great interest in these fields [3, 4]. Nanomaterials, defined as materials ranging in size from 1 to 100 nm, play a crucial role in nanomedicine, including applications in drug delivery, biosensors, microarray techniques, microfluidics, and tissue engineering [5]. Nanotechnology utilizes therapeutic substances on a nanoscale to craft nanomedicines, propelling progress in fields such as biomedicine, nanobiotechnology, the transportation of drugs, biosensors, and the construction of tissues through the application of NPs [6]. NPs, designed at the atomic or molecular level, typically exist as small nanospheres, allowing them greater mobility within the human body when compared to larger materials. Their nanoscale size offers distinctive structural, biochemical, mechanical, magnetic, and electrical properties. Nanomedicines have gained recognition due to their ability to serve in drug delivery, encapsulating agents or binding with therapeutic agents and distributing them precisely to target cells with controlled and sustained release [7, 8]. Nanomedicine is an evolving field that applies the information and methods of nanoscience in biology, medicine, disease prevention, and treatment. Due to their small size and specific characteristics, nanodimensional materials hold great promise for advancing research, innovation, and practical solutions in diverse domains (figure 2.2).

2.1.1.2 Classification of NPs

Classification of NPs is primarily based on their size, morphology, and chemical characteristics, leading to various well-known classes of NPs as outlined here.

(A) **Carbon-based NPs**

Among carbon-based NPs, two major classes stand out: fullerenes and carbon nanotubes (CNTs). Fullerenes are nanomaterials characterized by globular hollow structures, representing various allotropic forms of carbon. Carbon-based NPs have garnered significant viable interest because to their remarkable properties, including high strength, unique arrangement, electron affinity, and electrical conductivity [9]. Fullerenes contain organized pentagonal and hexagonal carbon rings, with each C remaining in an sp^2 hybridized state. Figure 2.3 displays some well-known fullerenes, such as C60 and C70, with diameters of 7.114 and 7.648 nm, respectively.

CNTs exhibit an elongated, tubular structure with diameters ranging from 1 to 2 nm [10]. Depending on their diameter, they can be classified as metallic or semiconducting [11]. Structurally, CNTs resemble graphite sheets rolled upon themselves (figure 2.4). These rolled sheets can have single, double, or multiple walls, leading to their designations as single-walled (SWNTs), double-walled (DWNTs), or multi-walled carbon nanotubes (MWNTs), respectively. Typically, the synthesis techniques entail placing carbon precursors, especially individual carbon atoms that are

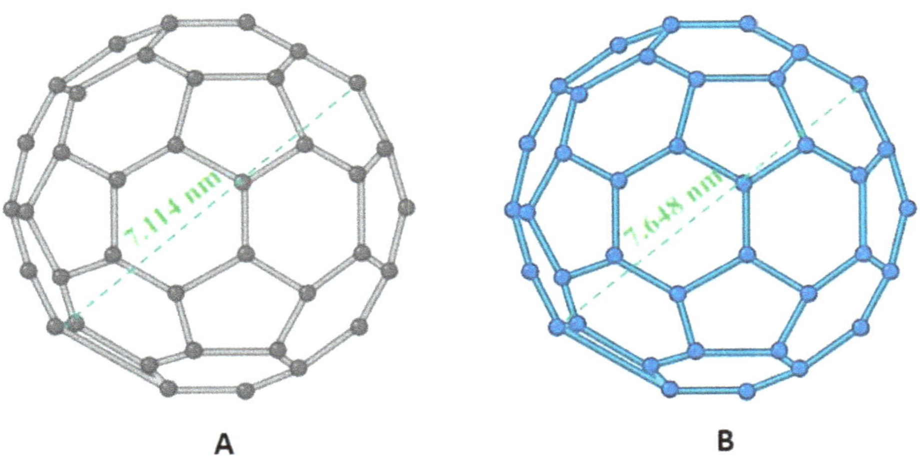

Figure 2.3. Different form of fullerenes (A) C_{60} and (B) C_{70}.

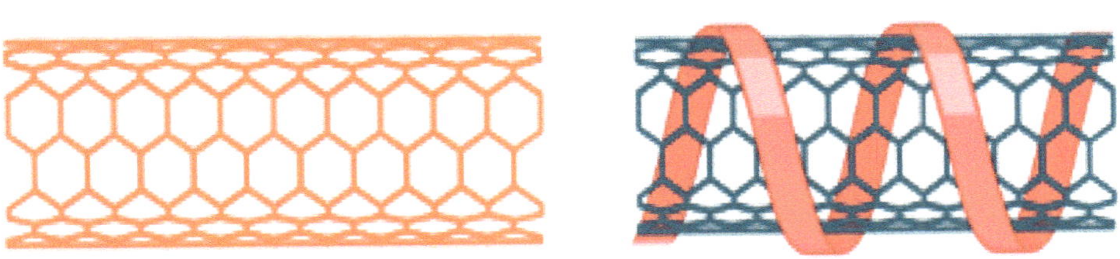

Figure 2.4. Single-walled and multi-walled carbon nanotubes.

vaporized from graphite through methods such as lasers or electric arcs, onto metal particles. Lately, the process of chemical vapor deposition (CVD) has been utilized in their creation [12].

Owing to their distinctive physical, chemical, and mechanical properties, CNTs find applications not only in their pristine form but also as nanocomposites in various commercial fields. They are utilized as fillers in composites [13, 14] and serve as effective adsorbents for environmental cleanup [15] and as substrates to support a wide range of inorganic and organic catalysts [15].

(B) **Metallic NPs**

Comprising only metal precursors, metal NPs display unique optoelectronic attributes primarily linked to the widely recognized localized surface plasmon resonance (LSPR) traits. Notably, NPs of alkaline and noble metals such as Cu, Ag, and Au display a wide absorption band within the visible range of the electromagnetic solar spectrum. Metallic NPs have garnered significant interest in various industrial applications due to their distinct physical and chemical properties compared to bulk metals. These NPs possess a range of advantageous characteristics, including enhanced mechanical strength, high surface area, lower melting points, unique optical properties, and magnetic attributes. In addition, metallic NPs have been found to exhibit exceptional catalytic performance, as they are selective, highly active, and have long lifetimes in many chemical reactions. The unique optical properties of gold, silver, lead, and platinum NPs stem from the resonant oscillation of their free electrons when exposed to light. This phenomenon is known as LSPR (figure 2.5).

Unique properties of metallic NPs

- **Surface atoms:** the percentage of surface atoms in a cluster can be understood by examining the structure of full-shell clusters, which consists of atoms arranged according to specific magic numbers. These magic numbers represent the count of either protons or neutrons, forming complete shells within the atomic nucleus. The concept of magic numbers originated from studies on rare gas clusters. As the clusters increase in size, the proportion of surface atoms decreases. Central atoms are encompassed by a greater number of atoms, and the atoms in the inner shell are surrounded by atoms in the outer shell. When clusters remain separate from one another, they are referred to as dispersed clusters, whereas if these clusters combine, they are known as aggregated clusters. When both dispersed and aggregated clusters contain an equal number of atoms, the dispersed clusters exhibit a higher surface area than the aggregated ones. The surface area of the reactant affects the rates of chemical reactions. Therefore, reactants consisting of dispersed clusters are expected to have higher reactivity compared to aggregated clusters.

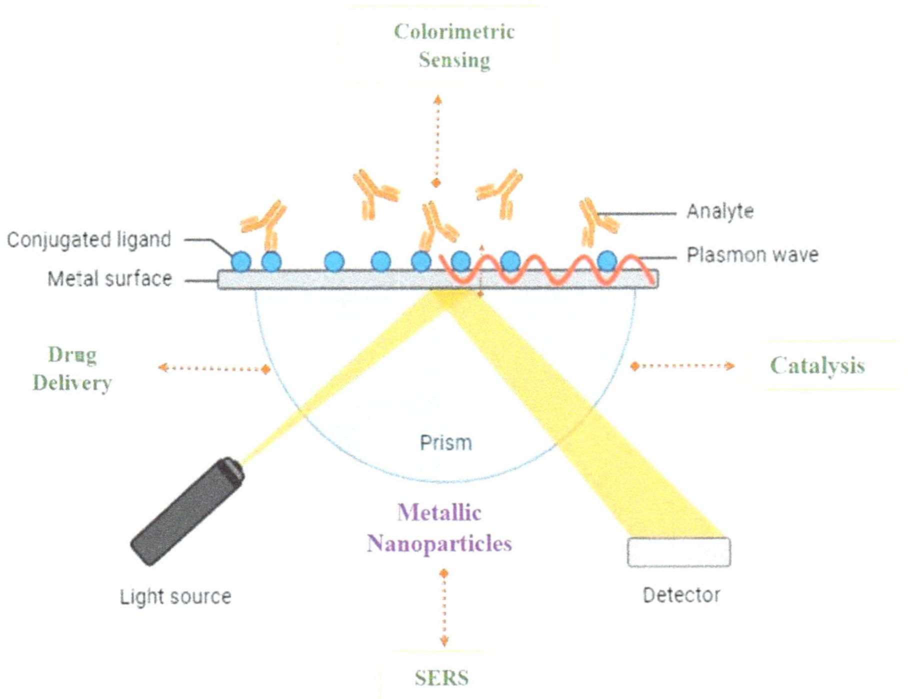

Figure 2.5. Surface plasmon resonance labeled metallic nanoparticles.

- **Quantum dots:** quantum dots are minute particles found within the nanometer range, comprising thousands of atoms. These semiconductor materials can be made from silicon or germanium. The band theory in semiconductors explains the behavior of quantum dots. Specifically, the band gap represents the energy difference between the valence band (top) and conduction band (bottom). Semiconductors possess a band structure where a partially occupied band is separated from an unoccupied conduction band by a band gap. When considering interacting molecular orbitals, the primary orbitals at play are the HOMO (highest occupied molecular orbital) of one molecule and the LUMO (lowest unoccupied molecular orbital) of another molecule. These specific HOMO and LUMO orbitals are termed frontier orbitals, as they are situated at the outermost electron boundaries of the molecules. As a result, they play a crucial role in strong interactions between molecules. The energy of metal NPs can be accurately described using quantum mechanics.

(C) **Ceramic NPs**

These inorganic nonmetallic solids are created through heating and subsequent cooling processes, adopting amorphous, polycrystalline, dense,

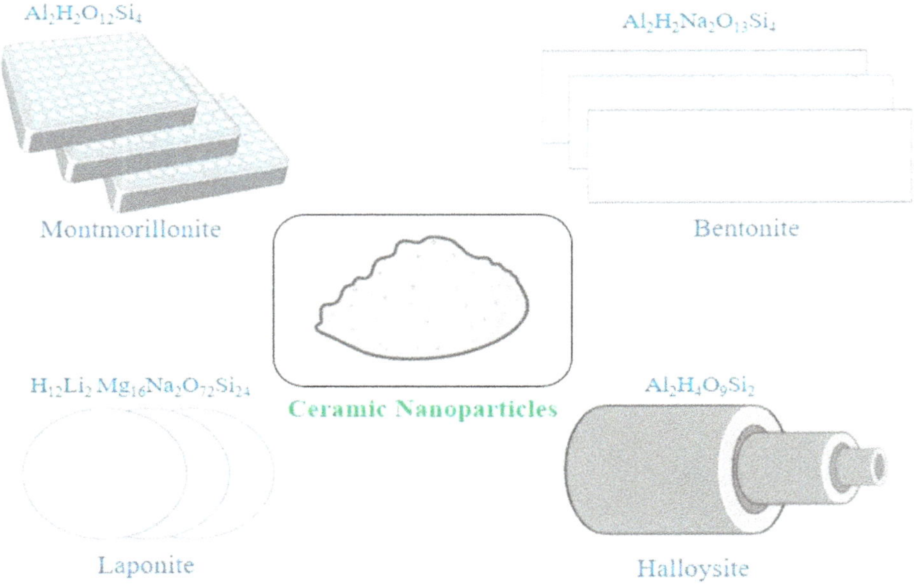

Figure 2.6. Types of ceramic nanoparticle along with their morphology.

porous, or hollow structures [17]. Consequently, these NPs are attracting significant research interest for their utilization in diverse fields, including catalysis, photocatalysis, dye photodegradation, and imaging applications [16] (figure 2.6).

(D) **Semiconductor NPs**

Semiconductor materials exhibit properties that lie between metals and nonmetals, making them highly versatile with various applications in the literature [17]. Semiconductor NPs possess wide band gaps, allowing for significant modifications in their properties through band gap tuning. This characteristic makes them crucial materials in areas such as photocatalysis, photo optics, and electronic devices [18]. For instance, a variety of semiconductor NPs have shown exceptional efficiency in water splitting applications due to their suitable band gap and band edge positions [19].

(E) **Polymeric NPs**

Polymeric NPs are organic-based NPs commonly referred to as polymer nanoparticles (PNPs) in the literature. They mostly exist in nanospheres or nanocapsular shapes [20]. Nanospheres are matrix particles with a solid overall mass, and other molecules are adsorbed at the outer boundary of the spherical surface. On the other hand, nanocapsules completely encapsulate the solid mass within the particle [21]. PNPs are easily functionalized, making them highly versatile and finding numerous applications [22]. Polymeric NPs exhibit variations in their physical properties, including

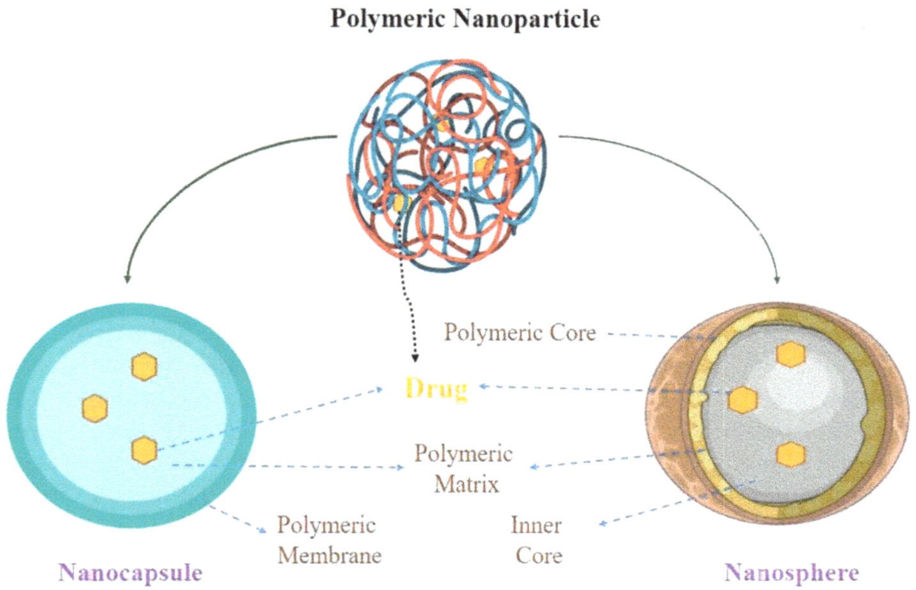

Figure 2.7. Schematic illustration depicting the structure of nanocapsules and nanospheres, where the arrow indicates the presence of drug or bioactive substances encapsulated within the nanoparticles.

composition, concentration, size, shape, surface properties, crystallinity, and dispersion state. A thorough examination of these attributes is accomplished using an array of techniques, including electron microscopy, dynamic light scattering (DLS) or photon correlation spectroscopy (PCS), near-infrared (NIR) spectroscopy, electrophoresis, and chromatography, all of which are frequently employed for this purpose [23, 24].

Accurate characterization of polymeric NPs is crucial not only for their applicability but also for assessing nanotoxicology and exposure in workplaces, which are essential to understand their health and safety hazards and to regulate manufacturing processes [25] (figure 2.7).

(F) **Lipid-based NPs**

Comprising lipid components, lipid-based nanoparticles (NPs) find widespread use across various biomedical domains. Ordinarily, these lipid NPs assume a spherical morphology, varying in diameter from 10 to 1000 nm. Much like their polymeric counterparts, lipid NPs exhibit a compact lipid core and an encompassing matrix housing soluble lipophilic substances. The outer shell of these NPs is upheld by surfactants or emulsifying agents [26]. Lipid nanotechnology is a specialized field that focuses on the design and synthesis of lipid NPs for various applications, including drug carriers and delivery and RNA release in cancer therapy [27, 28].

2.1.1.3 Synthesis of NPs

The synthesis of NPs can be accomplished using diverse methods, which are generally categorized into two main classes: the bottom-up approach and the top-down approach [29], as depicted in figure 2.8. These approaches are further subdivided into various subclasses based on the specific operations, reaction conditions, and adopted protocols. Top-down approaches involve the division of bulk materials to create nanostructured materials. Some of the top-down methods utilized are mechanical milling, laser ablation, thin film separation, etching, sputtering, and electro-explosion. Extending from techniques used for producing particles at the micron scale, top-down synthesis methods are inherently simpler. They involve the removal, division, or downsizing of bulk materials, or the adaptation of bulk manufacturing processes to create specific structures with desired properties. Nonetheless, a key challenge within the top-down approach revolves around the imperfections in surface configurations. To illustrate, nanowires fashioned through lithography might lack smoothness and could harbor multiple impurities and structural flaws on their exteriors. Illustrative techniques encompass high-energy wet ball milling, electron beam lithography, manipulation via atomic force, gas-phase condensation, and aerosol spray, among others. The alternative approach, known as the bottom-up method, holds the potential for creating less waste and achieving greater cost-effectiveness. In the bottom-up approach, materials

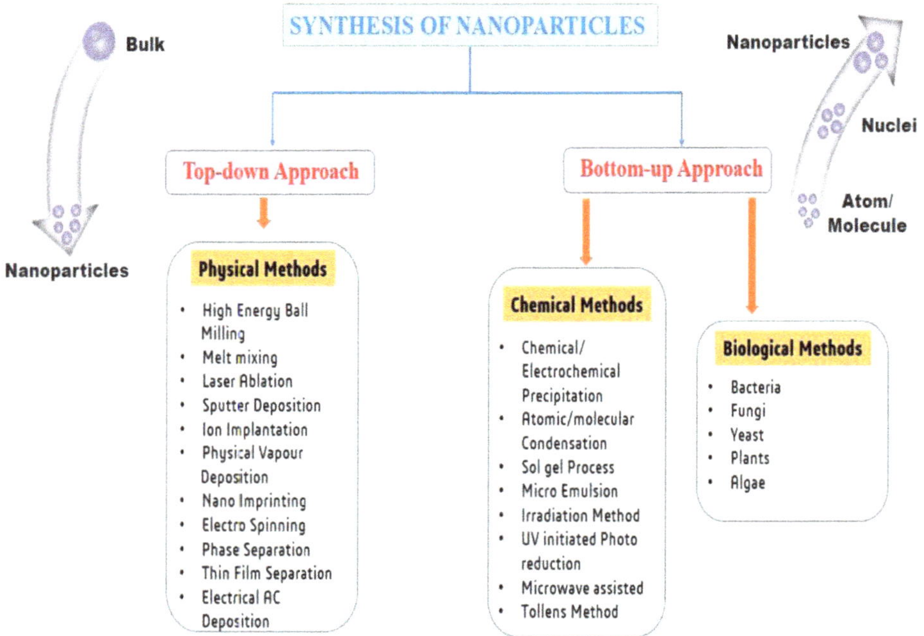

Figure 2.8. Schematic representation illustrating the top-down and bottom-up approaches for the synthesis of nanoscale materials.

are built up from the atomic, molecular, or cluster level, allowing for precise control of the final structure.

Many of these techniques are currently under development or are in the early stages of being employed for commercial production of nanopowders. Notable bottom-up techniques, such as the organometallic chemical route, the reverse-micelle route, sol–gel synthesis, colloidal precipitation, hydrothermal synthesis, template-assisted sol–gel, and electrodeposition, have been reported for the preparation of luminescent NPs. These methods offer promising pathways towards efficient and controlled NP synthesis.

2.1.2 Nanotechnology and nanomedicine

Nanomedicine, a rapidly growing field that combines nanoscience, nanoengineering, and nanotechnology with life sciences, has produced fascinating outcomes for the medical community and society at large [30]. Within the realm of nanomedicine, there exist numerous platforms, but the focus lies primarily on nanotechnology-based drug delivery systems and imaging nano-agents [31]. One particularly intriguing area is theranostic nanomedicine, which involves the utilization of nanosized theranostics capable of targeted delivery, controlled release, and enhanced transport efficiency via endocytosis, responsive systems to external stimuli, and the integration of various therapeutic approaches such as multimodal diagnosis and therapy [32]. The term 'theranostics' refers to systems that can serve both as therapeutic agents and imaging agents [33]. Nanotheranostics are strategies based on carriers that are either submicron or nano-sized. These carriers encompass a range of materials, including polymeric NPs, dendrimers, liposomes, carbon-based nanomaterials, metal or inorganic nanocarriers, and hybrid systems that combine polymers and nanocarriers [34–38]. Carbon-based nanomaterials, such as CNTs either in their pure form or adorned with other substances, graphene oxide, fullerenes, and carbon quantum dots, have found applications in detecting drugs in biological samples or facilitating imaging procedures [39–41]. Moreover, Prussian blue cubes, characterized by their octahedral structure of metal hexacyanoferrates, have been engineered as diagnostic tools due to their magnetic and conductive properties [44]. An optimal nanotheranostic agent should exhibit prolonged circulation within the body, controlled release behavior, precise targeting, deep tissue penetration, imaging functionalities, and a favorable target-to-background ratio [45]. The advantage of nanotheranostics lies in their capability to concentrate diagnostic and therapeutic agents at specific disease sites, thereby minimizing unwanted side effects. Their extended duration in the bloodstream is attributed to their nanoscale dimensions. Particularly for tumor diagnosis and treatment, NPs within nanotheranostics can effectively exit blood vessels and accumulate in tumor tissues due to limited lymphatic drainage, unlike multifunctional small molecules or modified macromolecules [42, 43] (figure 2.9).

Currently, nanomedicine has sparked new and promising possibilities in diagnosing and treating various diseases. However, it remains crucial to develop novel tools with enhanced imaging capabilities that can enable early disease detection. The use of efficient imaging agents for early-stage cancer detection would greatly benefit the

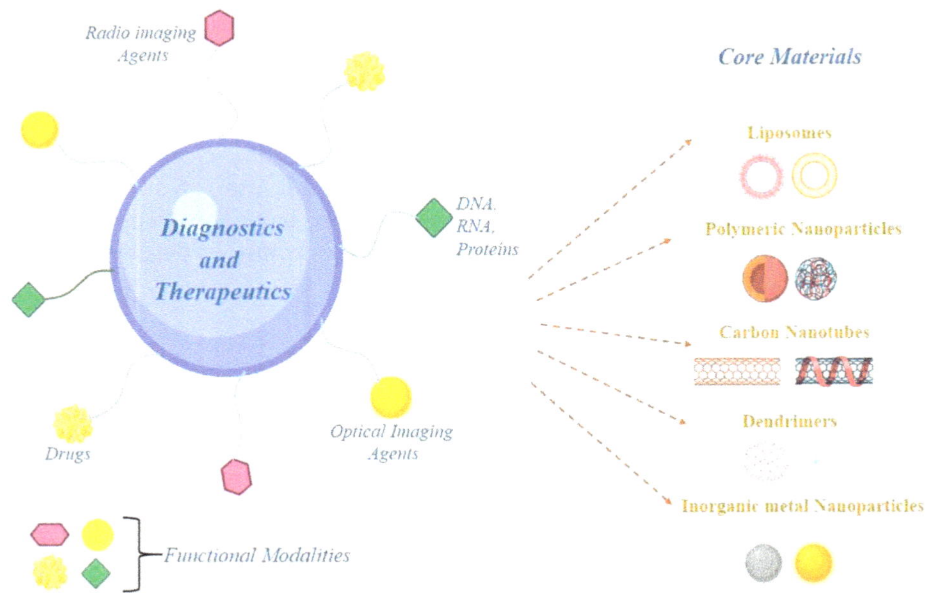

Figure 2.9. Schematic illustration of nanotheranostics demonstrating their capability for simultaneous release and imaging.

medical community. Moreover, nanotherapeutics play a vital role in treating severe illnesses [44]. Nevertheless, most reported NPs are primarily evaluated through animal models, with limited clinical studies conducted. Previously, nanotheranostics were predominantly focused on cancer applications, but now they have expanded to encompass neurological disorders and cardiovascular diseases (CVD). Encouraging findings have gradually led to the preclinical application of theranostics in CVD [45–47].

Nuclear medicine imaging has emerged as an advanced diagnostic tool, involving the introduction of radionuclides into the body and the detection of emitted gamma rays to generate detailed images, providing insights into the distribution and physiological characteristics of organs and tissues [48]. Several nanoimaging agents have been developed, serving dual purposes as both diagnostic and therapeutic tools. However, some of these nanomaterials exhibit limited distribution and cell penetration, necessitating improvements in their pharmacokinetics. Numerous novel strategies have been employed to enhance their pharmacokinetics and biodistribution [49].

In recent years, the applications of nanotheranostics or NP-based theranostics have made significant progress. Summarizing the current developments in nanotheranostics could aid medical professionals in advancing this field further. Furthermore, analyzing the current utilization of imaging modalities and nanotheranostics has the potential to drive evolution in the field of nanomedicine.

2.1.3 Nanomedicine in cancer imaging

Cancer, a highly lethal disease, is projected to become the leading cause of death and a significant obstacle to increasing life expectancy in the coming decades. According to a report from the International Agency for Research on Cancer, there were approximately 18.1 million new cases and 9.6 million deaths from cancer worldwide in 2018 [50]. Furthermore, the number of new cases is expected to continue rising over the next 20 years [50, 51]. While conventional cancer treatments such as surgery, chemotherapy, and radiotherapy have been widely employed in clinical settings, they have limitations in completely eradicating tumors and often result in severe side effects. In addition to improving the efficacy of current therapies, researchers are actively exploring alternative approaches to cancer imaging and therapy that are safe, effective, and cost-efficient.

Phototherapies, which encompass photodynamic therapy (PDT) and photothermal therapy (PTT), are emerging as promising interventions for tumor eradication while preserving organ function, offering great potential for clinical cancer therapy. These phototherapies involve the use of non-toxic agents that can be activated by light irradiation, selectively killing cancer cells without inducing severe side effects. By carefully designing phototherapeutic agents and precisely controlling light illumination at the site of lesions, such as tumor tissues, phototherapies achieve dual selectivity, reducing the systemic toxicity associated with traditional chemotherapy and radiotherapy [52, 53]. Moreover, the rapid advancements in nanotechnology over the past decade have led to the emergence of phototheranostic nanomedicine, which combines phototherapies with nanotechnology to enhance therapeutic efficacy.

An example of NP-based therapy involves combining cancer diagnosis and treatment modalities. The first generation of NP-based therapy featured lipid systems like liposomes and micelles, which have received approval from the United States Food and Drug Administration (FDA). These lipid systems may contain inorganic NPs like gold or magnetic NPs, leading to increased use in drug delivery, imaging, and therapeutic applications. Nanostructures have been found to protect drugs in the gastrointestinal region and aid the delivery of poorly water-soluble drugs to their target sites, resulting in higher oral bioavailability through typical uptake mechanisms of absorptive endocytosis (figure 2.10).

Nanotechnology encompasses two key conditions. Firstly, it revolves around manipulating structures at the nanometer scale, focusing on controlling their shape and size. Secondly, nanotechnology involves leveraging the unique properties that arise due to the nanoscale, thereby addressing the challenge of effectively working with small entities [54]. Nanoscience is an interdisciplinary field that combines physics, materials science, and biology, focusing on the manipulation of materials at the atomic and molecular scales. On the other hand, nanotechnology involves the ability to observe, measure, manipulate, assemble, control, and manufacture matter at the nanometer scale. While there are reports available that discuss the history of nanoscience and technology, none provide a comprehensive summary of the entire development of these fields up to the present era, including the progressive events. Therefore, there is a crucial need to summarize the key events in nanoscience and technology in order to gain a complete understanding of their advancement within this domain.

Notably, this chapter focuses on the progress made in the field of phototherapy-synergized cancer immunotherapy, given the increasing interest in clinical immunotherapy. Finally, the challenges and future prospects of phototheranostic

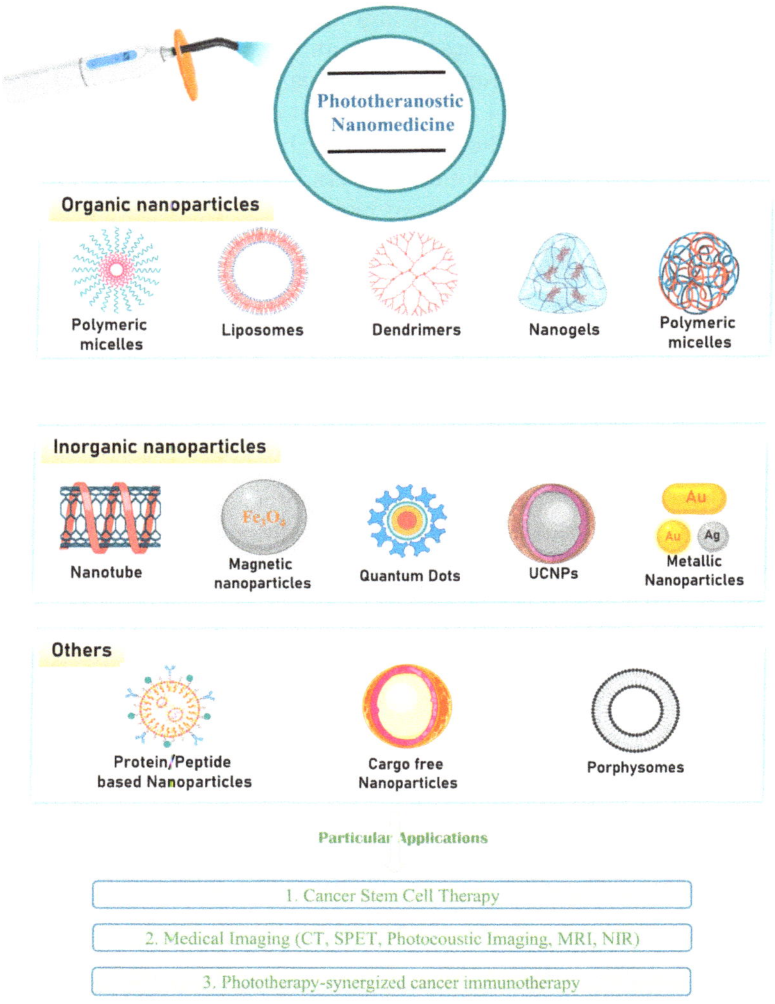

Figure 2.10. Overview of different categories and specific applications of phototheranostic nanomedicine.

nanomedicine for advanced cancer treatment are discussed. Diverse nanomaterials possess unique functionalities not observed in bulk materials, opening up innovative possibilities in biomedical applications. Over the past two decades, nanomedicine has emerged as a prominent research field within nanotechnology, encompassing various applications. Cancer, currently the second leading cause of death, continues to increase in prevalence each year [55]. Conventional therapies have made limited progress in treating cancer patients effectively, highlighting the urgent need for disruptive innovations. Cancer nanomedicine, harnessing the distinctive properties of nanomaterials, holds great potential in early cancer diagnosis, imaging, and treatment. NPs, characterized by their small size, large surface area, aqueous solubility, and multifunctionality, have revolutionized biomedical applications.

These NPs possess novel properties that enable novel interactions with complex cellular functions. This rapidly advancing interdisciplinary field focuses on developing multifunctional nanostructures and approaches to target, diagnose, and treat devastating cancers. Extensive efforts have led to FDA approval of liposomes and lipid-based NPs for enhanced delivery and bioavailability of drugs like doxorubicin [56, 57]. Furthermore, the utilization of micelles and nanocomplexes has led to enhancements in the pharmacokinetics and biodistribution of hydrophobic drug compounds [62]. Notably, carboxy methyl dextran-coated iron oxide NPs have obtained clearance for their use in iron supplementation within medications and are currently undergoing examination as contrast agents for magnetic resonance imaging (MRI) [58, 59]. Approximately 100 nanomedicine products have been successfully commercialized, while numerous other nanomaterials are currently undergoing approximately 800 clinical trials [60].

During preclinical assessments, a multitude of nanomaterials have exhibited exceptionally favorable characteristics for applications in cancer imaging and therapeutic interventions. Nevertheless, the scope of potential clinical utilization has primarily centered on a constrained selection of nanomaterials, specifically those composed of iron (Fe), silicon (Si), gold (Au), polysaccharide polymers, and natural products. Notably, iron oxide NPs, which share an elemental composition with blood, have been utilized for cellular hyperthermia and MR imaging contrast [61, 62]. The superparamagnetic properties of nanoscale iron oxide particles have found diverse applications in medicine. The magnetic properties and functions of these NPs can be finely tuned for specific purposes by adjusting their size and structure. In recent times, unique gold nanostructures displaying anisotropic and intricate characteristics, including hyper-branched or dendritic formations, have showcased their merits by offering a greater abundance of active sites and surface atoms per given area in contrast to their spherical NP counterparts [68]. Diverse metallic NPs possessing distinct shapes and distinct light absorption attributes produce substantial heat advantageous for localized ablation treatments. Additionally, high-density metallic NPs facilitate contrast effects in CT imaging [63]. Magnetic disk-shaped particles coated with gold, exhibiting a magnetic spin vortex, can directly eliminate cancer cells through magneto-mechanical stimulation under an external magnetic field [64]. Temperature-sensitive polymeric micelles deliver drug molecules efficiently at specific temperatures [65]. Clusters of magnetic particles amplify the properties of MRI and also function as conveyors for delivering drugs through nanopores [72]. Mesoporous silica NPs have prominently exhibited their capacity as effective carriers for drugs [66, 67]. NPs designed for upconversion have been created to achieve enduring luminescence and to serve in various imaging capacities spanning preoperative, intraoperative, and postoperative scenarios [75]. These emerging nanomedicines, hinging on innovative NPs, offer a hopeful strategy for the proficient treatment of cancer.

2.1.4 Bio-engineering targeted nanostructures for cancer imaging

The primary objective of targeted cancer therapy is threefold: (a) to directly administer a potent anticancer drug to the tumor site, (b) to enhance drug absorption by cancerous cells, and (c) to minimize drug absorption by noncancerous cells. The overall strategy for designing targeted cancer therapies involves creating drug delivery systems that exploit the unique characteristics of tumor cells and tissues. Researchers in targeted delivery have concentrated on understanding the specific traits of the tumor microenvironment, such as leaky vasculature, overexpressed cell surface receptors, intratumoral pH variations, and features of the cell uptake process, such as endosomal pH. Recent progress in the realms of micro- and nanotechnology has led to the development of micro- and NPs, including entities such as liposomes and micelles, which are designed to encapsulate and proficiently transport therapeutic drugs [68]. Recent advances in cancer research, in conjunction with breakthroughs in biomaterials and nanotechnology, have opened up new possibilities for targeted anticancer drug delivery and personalized treatment approaches tailored to specific cancer types. This multidisciplinary approach combining cancer biology, biomaterials, and nanotechnology holds the potential to improve treatment outcomes while minimizing harmful side effects. Designing an effective targeted therapy entails optimizing therapeutic particles, cancer cell targeting, and drug release mechanisms. Both passive and active targeting mechanisms can be employed to enhance targeted delivery. By modifying the physical properties of particles, toxicity to noncancerous cells can be reduced, and circulation time can be increased. Utilizing targeting moieties, such as ligands that bind to receptors overexpressed on cancerous cells, allows for enhanced cellular uptake, thereby improving treatment efficacy. Additionally, environmentally responsive polymers can be utilized to achieve controlled drug release under specific conditions. The current state of targeted cancer therapies under development, with a focus on the design and optimization of individual components crucial for achieving effective cancer treatment, has been explored. The integration of cancer biology, biomaterials, and nanotechnology offers promising opportunities to revolutionize cancer therapy and pave the way for personalized and more effective treatment approaches. A novel opportunity in interventional oncology, a subspecialty of interventional radiology, involves the targeted diagnosis and treatment of cancer using minimally invasive procedures under image guidance (figure 2.11). Techniques like x-ray, ultrasound, computed tomography (CT), or MRI aid in guiding miniaturized instruments, enabling precise treatment of solid tumors in various organs. Recent advances in medical imaging and image guidance have paved the way for minimally invasive image-guided therapies that bypass the toxicities associated with chemotherapy and radiation, resulting in fewer complications, faster recovery, and reduced costs [69, 70].

Commonly employed procedures include transcatheter-directed therapies (e.g. transcatheter arterial embolization and chemoembolization) with intratumoral or intra-arterial delivery, and percutaneous or endoscopic ablative therapies (e.g. radiofrequency ablation and cryo-ablation) that destroy lesions through percutaneous needle placement. Medical imaging plays pivotal roles in these image-guided therapies, encompassing pre-procedure planning, intra procedural targeting and monitoring, intra procedural control, and post-procedure assessment. Contrast agents are often utilized to enhance visualization of target sites in pre-, intra-, and post-procedural therapies where unenhanced scans may not offer sufficient visibility.

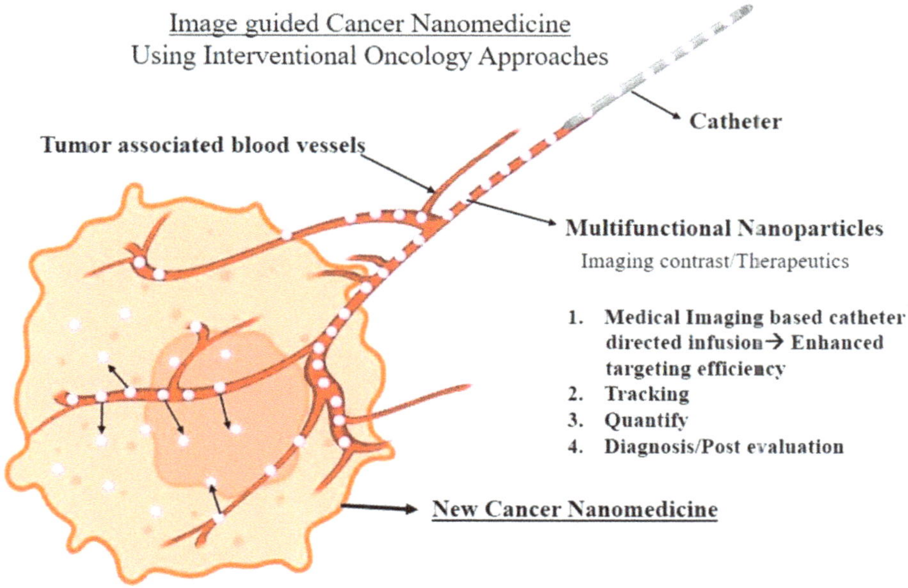

Figure 2.11. Precision-targeted cancer nanotherapy: revolutionizing treatment through image-guided infusion.

Incorporating traditional interventional therapies such as radiofrequency/cryo/chemical tumor ablation, focal laser ablation, and tumor (chemo-) embolization, with multifunctional NP-based nanomedicine has become a promising approach. Preclinical studies of various image-guided cancer nanomedicine approaches have shown encouraging results (table 2.1).

NPs with advanced functionalities offer enhanced imaging contrast during image-guided therapeutic procedures, along with targeted and triggered therapeutics for tumors. This harmonious interplay introduces a novel prospect for nanomedicine, surmounting past obstacles related to limited tumor targeting and apprehension about toxicity during clinical adaptation. The evolving notion of 'image-guided cancer nanomedicine,' fused with interventional oncology, guarantees restrained systemic dispersion, uniform deployment at specified locales, and potent localized conveyance of nanomedicine, thus enhancing the efficacy of forefront nanotherapeutic approaches. Furthermore, image-guided nanomedicine delivery holds significant potential in future clinical practice. It enables precise localization of nanomedicine in tumor regions, minimizing systemic toxicity. Additionally, it allows real-time monitoring and confirmation of proper nanomedicine delivery to the disease site through local infusion and tracking. Non-invasive quantification of the injected NPs assists in determining the post-infusion amount, and long-term monitoring of NP distribution aids in diagnosis and post-evaluation.

This proposed image-guided cancer nanomedicine approach paves the way for patient-specific dosimetry and tumor-specific cancer treatments, providing superior therapeutic effects personalized to individual patients [71, 84]. Moreover, the

Table 2.1. Advanced image-guided cancer nanomedicine treatment approaches.

Treatment approach	Type of cancer	Nanoparticles	Imaging	References
Image-guided surgery	Breast cancer and hepatocellular carcinoma Liver cancer	Eu_2O_3 NP Upconversion NPs	Radio fluorescence MRI/luminescence	[71, 72]
Image-guided immunomodulation	Liver cancer	Fe_2O_3 nanotubes	MRI	[73]
Image-guided delivery	Brain cancer Prostate cancer	Hybrid Fe_2O_3 oxide/Au silica NPs	MRI/CT MRI/fluorescence	[74, 75]
Image-guided photothermal therapy	Ovarian cancer	Nanoporphyrin	MRI, NIR fluorescence imaging, PET	[76]
Image-guided photodynamic therapy	Pancreatic cancer Prostate cancer Colorectal cancer	Fluorescence MRI MRI	Branched gold NPs Gold NPs Hybrid gold/iron oxide NPs	[77–79]
Image-guided radiation	Lung cancer	Gadolinium/bismuth	CT/MRI	[80]
Image-guided drug delivery	Pancreatic tumors Peritoneal tumors Liver carcinoma	Fe_2O_3 NPs	MRI MRI MRI/CT	[61, 81–83]

integration of nanomedicine techniques into interventional oncology promises exceptional therapeutic efficacy [85]. Significantly, the realm of image-guided cancer nanomedicine encompasses innovative medical imaging methods, NPs, molecular components, and a spectrum of therapeutic agents such as siRNA, mRNA, gene editing tools, and immune checkpoint inhibitors, alongside established drugs and therapeutics. Progressing in this domain mandates robust collaboration among multifaceted teams comprising clinicians, fundamental researchers, and experts in nanoscience, all working in unison to accomplish effective translation to clinical applications.

2.2 General principles for theranostic nanoplatforms

Theranostics is a term initially coined to describe a novel approach that integrates diagnostics and therapeutics, aiming to achieve comprehensive diagnosis, molecular imaging, and personalized treatment plans [86]. In recent times, there has been a growing interest in merging this innovative approach with nanotechnologies, leading to the development of theranostic nanoplatforms and methodologies [87]. As cancer is a highly diverse and adaptive disease, a wide range of treatment options must be considered based on individual patient characteristics and disease progression. The integration of theranostic NPs offers the potential to provide patients with diverse treatment options tailored to their specific needs, ultimately leading to improved prognoses. Moreover, theranostic NPs can play a crucial role in monitoring therapeutic effectiveness post-treatment, enabling clinicians to make timely and personalized therapeutic decisions. This chapter presents a comprehensive assessment of theranostic nanoplatforms used in cancer theranostics, encompassing magnetic NPs, CNTs, gold nanostructures, polymeric NPs, and silica NPs. While much research focuses on NP-based diagnostic or therapeutic systems for cancer treatment, there is a dearth of literature covering theranostic NPs that can simultaneously image and treat cancer. Therefore, this chapter primarily concentrates on NP systems that seamlessly integrate tumor imaging and therapy in a unified approach.

The chapter offers comprehensive perspectives on the theranostic potential of a range of nanoplatforms, classified according to distinct nanomaterial types including polymers, gold, carbon, magnetic, and silica nanomaterials. The discussed applications include three main aspects:

(1) Diagnostics for assessing intracellular localization and *in vivo* biodistribution;
(2) Therapeutics for effective cancer treatment;
(3) Theranostics for monitoring biological responses and evaluating therapeutic efficacy post-treatment.

This comprehensive examination sheds light on the potential and versatility of nanoplatforms in advancing cancer theranostics [88]. Theranostic systems based on NPs utilize a wide array of nanoplatforms, such as magnetic NPs, CNTs, gold nanostructures, polymeric NPs, and silica NPs. Interestingly, certain NPs, like gold nanoshells/nanorods or carbon nanotubes, possess a unique ability to absorb light energy and emit specific diagnostic/therapeutic signals, such as ultrasound, heat, Raman, or fluorescence signals, making them inherently capable of acting as theranostic NPs independently. Nevertheless, in the majority of instances, nanoplatforms undergo supplementary modifications with added diagnostic and therapeutic components, enabling their role as all-encompassing theranostic NPs. This is realized by chemically or physically incorporating radionuclides, MRI agents, or optical imaging agents onto the nanoplatforms, facilitating meticulous imaging and precise diagnosis. Simultaneously, anticancer agents, spanning hydrophobic chemical drugs, peptides, proteins, and genetic drugs, are either enclosed within the NPs or linked to them through chemical conjugation, thereby facilitating targeted and effective therapeutic dispensation (table 2.2).

Table 2.2. Illustration of nanoplatforms, imaging modalities, and treatment approaches of theranostic nanoparticles. Abbreviations: MRI: magnetic resonance imaging; CMT: chemotherapy; BT: biotherapeutics; PET: positron emission tomography; OI: optical imaging; USI: ultrasound imaging; PTT: photothermal therapy; HTT: hyper thermal therapy; MWD: microwave detection; NIRFI: near-infrared fluorescence imaging; PDI: photodynamic imaging; DFI: dark field imaging; PLI: photoluminescence imaging.

Nanoplatforms	Imaging modalities	Treatment approach	References
		Inorganic nanoplatforms	
Magnetic NPs	MRI, optical imaging (NIRFI)	CMT (doxorubicin, cisplatin, methotrexate) BT (pDNA, siRNA)	[89, 90]
Gold NPs	Optical imaging (PLI)	Photothermal therapy (PTT)	[91]
Silica NPs	Optical imaging (PDI, NIRFI)	Photodynamic therapy, CMT (doxorubicin), BT (protein, siRNA)	[92]
Gold nanoshell	MRI, optical imaging (DFI), USI	Photothermal therapy	[93]
Gold nanorod	Optical imaging (DFI)	Photothermal therapy	[94]
		Organic nanoplatforms	
Liposome	MRI	BT (siRNA, peptide)	[95]
Polymeric micelle	USI, MRI	CMT (doxorubicin, platinum anticancer drug)	[96]
Carbon nanotube	OI (PLI), RS, MWD	HTT, PTT, CMT (platinum anticancer drug)	[97]
Polymeric NP	MRI, optical imaging (PDI, NIRFI), PET	Photodynamic therapy, CMT (paclitaxel, camptothecin, cisplatin, docetaxel), BT (pDNA, siRNA, protein)	[98, 99]
Nanoemulsion	MRI, optical imaging (NIRFI)	CMT (prednisolone acetate valerate)	[100]
Polymersome	MRI	CMT (doxorubicin)	[101]

In particular, NPs have demonstrated the ability to target tumors through passive and/or active targeting mechanisms. The abnormal leaky vasculature and inadequate lymphatic drainage in tumor tissues enable passive accumulation of NP platforms within the tumor, collectively known as the enhanced permeation and retention (EPR) effect. Additionally, when NPs are modified with tumor-targeting moieties like antibodies, nucleic acids, proteins, or other ligands, they can recognize, bind to, and internalize into tumor cells through receptor-mediated endocytosis. This dual targeting approach enhances the specificity and efficacy of NP-based therapies for cancer treatment.

2.2.1 Functional compounds and construction strategies

The field of NP-based imaging and therapy has progressed independently, but recent advances have led to the emergence of NP-based theranostics, where nanoplatforms can simultaneously deliver therapeutic and imaging functions. This represents an extension of traditional theranostics, with a greater emphasis on 'co-delivery' during treatment. The integration of imaging and therapy allows for real-time monitoring and assessment of treatment efficacy. Many nanomaterials inherently possess imaging capabilities and can easily be transformed into theranostic agents by incorporating therapeutic functions. Both imaging and therapy require efficient accumulation in diseased areas, bringing these research domains closer together.

Various targeting strategies can be employed to suit specific targets, such as identifying biomarkers overexpressed in cancer cells and using them as binding vectors for probes or carriers to achieve tumor homing. Nanoplatforms take advantage of their unique scale to exploit the EPR effect for tumor targeting. Care must be taken with the surfaces of the NPs to avoid immune recognition and ensure sufficient circulation time for effective targeting. While NP-based imaging and therapy are still progressing towards clinical trials, NP-based theranostics are in their early stages of development. Advances in nanotechnology and the demand for personalized medicine have made NP-based theranostics a research hotspot. This chapter aims to summarize the progress made in this field so far, focusing on theranostic agents categorized by their core nanomaterials. The techniques used to link nanoplatforms with functional entities have been well developed. While many of the described nanoplatforms have existing imaging functions and have been widely studied for imaging applications, the chapter primarily focuses on their potential as theranostic agents, with an emphasis on surface coating and coupling chemistry that influence transport, delivery, and cargo release.

2.2.1.1 Iron oxide nanoparticle-based theranostic agents

Method of preparation and study of surface chemistry of iron oxide nanoparticles

Iron oxide nanoparticles (IONPs) constitute nanoscale crystals constructed from either magnetite or hematite. Despite harboring surface irregularities and spin canting phenomena, IONPs generally manifest noteworthy saturation magnetization (M_s) values at ambient temperatures, particularly when synthesized using pyrolysis methodologies that yield high crystalline quality. Unlike their bulk counterparts, IONPs with sizes <20 nm exhibit superparamagnetic behavior, wherein they display no magnetic properties in the absence of an external magnetic field but can be magnetized when exposed to one. This behavior arises from the small size of the NPs, where thermal energy is sufficient to overcome the anisotropy energy of each individual magnet, resulting in random fluctuations of magnetizations that, on a macroscopic scale, lead to a net coercivity and magnetic moment of zero. The preparation and surface chemistry of IONPs are critical factors that influence their properties and applications in various fields, including medicine, environmental remediation, and electronics. The synthesis of IONPs can be achieved through several methods, such as co-precipitation, thermal decomposition, sol–gel, and hydrothermal methods. These techniques allow for the control of particle size, shape, and crystallinity, which are essential for tailoring their properties to specific applications. Surface chemistry plays a vital role in determining the stability, biocompatibility, and functionality of IONPs. As-prepared IONPs often have a bare surface, which can lead to agglomeration and potential toxicity. To address these issues, surface functionalization is commonly employed. Surface functionalization involves the coating of IONPs with various organic molecules, polymers, or inorganic materials, which enhances their dispersibility, stability, and biocompatibility.

The most common surface coatings include biocompatible polymers like polyethylene glycol (PEG), dextran, or chitosan, which confer excellent stability and minimize immune responses. In some cases, bioactive molecules, such as antibodies or peptides, are conjugated to the surface of IONPs to target specific cells or tissues, making them ideal for applications in targeted drug delivery or imaging. Furthermore, surface modification of IONPs can also be achieved by introducing specific functional groups, such as carboxyl, amine, or hydroxyl, which enable the attachment of additional ligands or molecules for various purposes. The preparation and surface chemistry of IONPs are crucial for tailoring their properties and improving their biocompatibility, stability, and functionality. These advancements open up numerous opportunities for the development of novel and versatile IONP-based technologies with promising applications in diverse fields.

Due to their remarkable magnetic properties, inherent biocompatibility, and cost-effectiveness, IONPs have become a preferred material for numerous bioapplications, including contrast probes for MRI. Their elevated magnetic moments facilitate a decrease in T2 relaxation time, resulting in signal dampening within T2- or T2*-weighted mappings. When customized with precise targeting capabilities, these modified signals can proficiently indicate anomalous biological processes.

The synthesis of IONPs has been extensively recorded. Conventionally, these NPs are synthesized in aqueous mediums through the co-precipitation of Fe (II) and Fe (III) precursor compounds. In order to maintain colloidal stability, hydrophilic polymers, such as poly vinyl pyrrolidone (PVP), dendrimers, polyaniline, and dextran, are introduced during the particle formation process. This addition serves to coat the surface of the nanocrystals, preventing their aggregation and ensuring stability. Dextran and its derivatives have undergone extensive investigation and have even progressed to clinical trials as contrast agents for MRI. An illustrative example is Feridex particles from AMAG Pharmaceuticals, which have received

FDA approval for identifying lesions in the liver and spleen. Moreover, the equivalent Combidex is presently in the midst of phase III clinical trials aimed at facilitating lymph node imaging. The presence of a polymer coating not only augments colloidal stability but also furnishes imperative chemical groups for the linkage of functional entities. For instance, they have developed polyaspartic acid (PASP)-coated IONPs and coupled them with RGD and ^{64}Cu-DOTA for positron emission tomography (PET)/MRI dual imaging. Lee *et al* have successfully converted dextran-IONPs aminated with epichlorohydrin and ammonia, making them readily conjugatable with a wide range of bio species.

Recently, high-temperature decomposition has emerged as a promising strategy for NP preparation. Unlike traditional methods using aqueous solutions, pyrolysis synthesis occurs in organic solvents upon high-temperature treatment. Due to highly concentrated surfactant ligands, this controlled process results in IONPs with superior crystallinity and higher magnetism than those obtained through conventional methods. Importantly, pyrolysis allows accurate control of product size, down to one nanometer, which is significant for achieving controllable T2 contrast effects since particle size and magnetic properties are closely related. A limitation of IONPs synthesized through pyrolysis is the presence of a dense alkyl coating, rendering them insoluble in water. Consequently, significant endeavors have been directed towards the development of surface modification techniques aimed at imparting conjugation capability and water solubility to these particles.

These surface modification techniques can be broadly divided into two categories: ligand exchange and ligand addition. The former involves using high-affinity, hydrophilic ligands to replace the original hydrophobic coating, while the latter employs amphiphilic materials to form a bilayer structure with the existing alkyl coating. IONPs with suitable coatings offer a convenient means of coupling drug molecules. For example, the Zhang group linked the anticancer drug methotrexate (MTX) onto an aminated IONP surface. Experiments conducted *in vitro* unveiled that, upon cellular uptake, the particles amassed within lysosomes, subsequently releasing the drug due to the acidic environment and the existence of proteases. Notably, Hwu *et al* achieved a successful conjugation of paclitaxel (PTX) to IONP surfaces via a phosphodiester moiety at the (C-2′)–OH position [102]. The particles exhibited effective PTX release when exposed to phosphodiesterase. Utilizing meso-2,3-dimercaptosuccinic acid (DMSA), the Cheon research team made alterations to IONPs, subsequently grafting cross-linked Herceptin antibody molecules onto the NP surface. In this approach, Herceptin served as a targeting element, distinct from its therapeutic role [103].

Beyond covalent attachment, drug compounds can also be co-encapsulated alongside IONPs within polymeric matrices. To illustrate, Jain *et al* integrated doxorubicin (DOX) and PTX, alongside oleic acid-coated IONPs, into pluronic-stabilized NPs [110]. Meanwhile, Yu *et al* accomplished DOX incorporation within anti-biofouling polymer-coated IONPs. Such DOX-loaded nanoconjugates exhibited enhanced pharmacokinetics and therapeutic impacts in a xenograft model of Lewis lung carcinoma, owing to the particles' inherent anti-biofouling trait. Furthermore, protein molecules have been explored as potential drug carriers.

Researchers adopted a two-step coating approach to produce human serum albumin (HSA)-coated IONPs, potentially capable of housing various lipophilic pharmaceutical agents to generate multifunctional theranostic entities. Hollow iron oxide nanostructures have been pursued to load small molecules via physical absorption. The Hyeon group reported a 'wrap–bake–peel' treatment to achieve hollow IONPs with DOX loading and sustained release under physiological conditions [104]. The Sun group produced porous IONPs by controlled oxidation and acid etching of Fe particles, leading to selective affinity to ErbB2/Neu-positive breast cancer cells and sustained cytotoxicity upon cisplatin release from the particle carriers. NP-based delivery has emerged as a crucial avenue for gene therapy, where DNAs/RNAs serve as therapeutics to regulate abnormal gene expression. NP carriers play a significant role in facilitating gene delivery to target cells and achieving intracellular release for therapeutic effects. Medarova and colleagues achieved siRNA delivery using thiolated siRNA coupled to aminated dextran particles with a membrane translocation peptide and NIR dye. The therapeutic potential of the nanoconjugate was demonstrated in a human colorectal carcinoma xenograft model, resulting in a significant drop in survivin transcript levels and increased tumor-associated apoptosis and necrosis. In the mentioned study, the accumulation of particles in the tumor was achieved through the EPR effect. Additionally, biovectors can be added to nanoplatforms to achieve site-specific delivery. For instance, the Cheon group coupled siRNA and a PEGylated cyclic Arg-Gly-Asp (RGD) peptide onto magnetic NPs. In an experiment using MDA-MB-435 and A549 cells, which have high and negative integrin $\alpha\nu\beta3$ expression, respectively, GFP siRNA-loaded NPs were used. The particle internalization rates varied between the two cell lines due to RGD–integrin interaction, leading to a substantial difference in gene regulation efficacy. While the particles alone or coupled with RGD showed no effect on knocking down GFP expression in A549 cells, a significant and concentration-dependent decrease in GFP expression was observed in MDA-MB-435 cells.

Leveraging the magnetic attributes of IONPs, their aggregation can be induced by an external magnetic field, a strategy exploited to bolster the efficiency of drug delivery. Corresponding investigations encompassing both animal and human subjects have been undertaken. For instance, in a trial encompassing seven patients afflicted with metastatic breast cancer, IONPs laden with epirubicin (measuring 100 nm in diameter and accounting for 0.5% of the estimated blood volume) were administered via infusion, concomitant with the application of a magnetic field encircling the tumor. For certain patients, the magnetic field effectively steered the ferrofluid toward the tumor, culminating in tumor regression. In a recent endeavor, Namiki *et al* conducted a comprehensive screening of cationic lipid-coated IONPs and unveiled a formulation termed LipoMag, which surpassed the performance of the commercial PolyMag in transfection and gene knockdown across all 13 tested cell lines. The researchers additionally fine-tuned the siRNA sequence to achieve diminished cytokine induction without compromising the knockdown efficacy. This altered siRNA was loaded onto NPs, and their therapeutic efficacy was assessed in two gastric cancer models. Remarkably, the treatment group exhibited a notable 50% reduction in tumor volume following a 28-day regimen, accompanied by other desirable outcomes such as angiogenesis inhibition and apoptosis induction. Importantly, the gene knockdown effect was distinctly evident solely during the application of magnetic fields at the tumor sites, as the lipid particles alone did not serve as effective delivery vehicles (figures 2.12 and 2.13).

Due to its capacity for addressing hyperthermia, IONPs hold the potential to fulfill a dual function in both imaging and therapy. This phenomenon relies on IONPs acting as antennae when subjected to an external alternating magnetic field (AMF), converting electromagnetic energy into heat. This characteristic holds significant promise in tumor therapy, particularly for tumor cells that are more sensitive to elevated temperatures than normal cells. For instance, in one study, phospholipid-coated IONPs were injected into a subcutaneous tumor model in F344 rats and exposed to an AMF. The combination of AMF and IONPs elevated the tumor temperature above 43 °C, leading to tumor regression. However, no such effect was observed in the control group without IONPs.

In another example, IONPs were chemically coupled with the Fab fragment of an anti-human MN antigen-specific antibody and administered systemically to tumor-bearing mice. The particles exhibited high tumor uptake, likely due to the interaction between the antibody and the antigen, and effectively induced tumor hyperthermia when exposed to an AMF. In a different study, $CoFe_2O_4$ NPs loaded with Zn-Pc, a

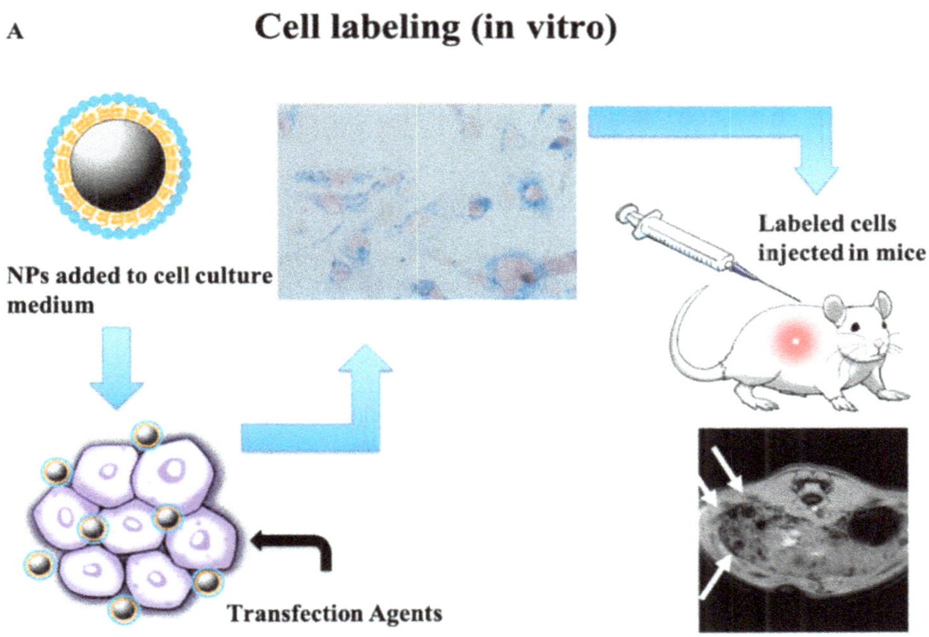

Figure 2.12. *In vitro* cell labeling using iron oxide NPs. (a) The *in vitro* labeling involved the addition of NPs to the cell culture medium, preferably in the presence of transfection agents. Subsequent tests on cell viability and iron content were performed before transplanting the labeled cells into living organisms. Reproduced from [105]. CC BY 4.0.

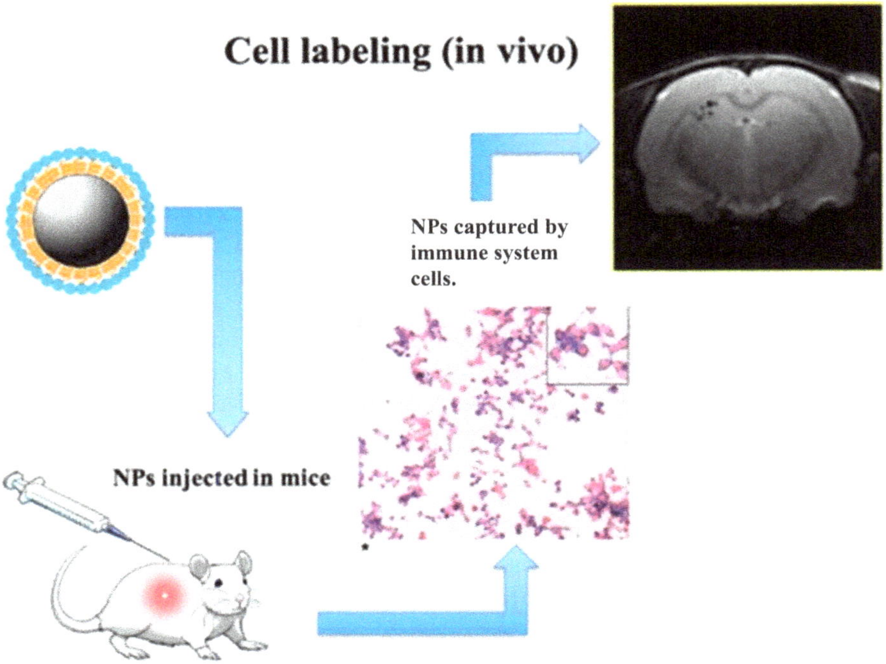

Figure 2.13. *In vivo* cell labeling using iron oxide nanoparticles (IONPs). For *in vivo* labeling, the experimental protocol included the injection of NPs into the bloodstream, where they were captured by immune system cells. MRI was employed to visualize regions of immune cell accumulation. Reproduced from [105]. CC BY 4.0. The histological image is from [106]. Originally published by and used with permission from Dove Medical Press Ltd.

photodynamic therapeutic (PDT) agent, demonstrated even better hyperthermia effects than IONPs. Combining PDT with magneto hyperthermia showed promising results *in vitro* with J774-A1 macrophage cells, displaying a synergistic combined toxicity. However, further research is needed to fully understand the potential synergy of such a combinational *in vivo* therapy.

2.2.1.2 Theranostic agents based on quantum dots

Method of preparation and study of surface chemistry of quantum dots

Quantum dots (QDs) are nanoscale crystals crafted from semiconductor materials, featuring distinct optical characteristics that distinguish them from organic dyes or fluorescent proteins. Particularly noteworthy is their heightened brightness, enhanced photo and chemical stability, and possession of a tightly confined emission spectrum. One of the distinctive features of QDs is their ability to finely adjust their optical properties by altering their size and composition. Early generations of QDs, made from materials like CdSe, CdTe, and PbS, spanned most of the visible spectrum, but their use in *in vivo* applications was limited due to the limited tissue penetration of visible light. To overcome this, NIR-emitting QDs have been developed, including those composed of CdTe/CdSe, Cd3P2, InAs/ZnSe, and InAs/InP/ZnSe. Inorganic coatings, such as ZnS, are often added to enhance the photoluminescent quantum efficiencies of the QDs.

The synthesis process for QDs is similar to that for IONPs. It involves heating appropriate organometallic precursors in high-boiling-point organic solvents to initiate particle formation, with surfactants like trioctylphosphine (TOP) and trioctylphosphine oxide (TOPO) controlling particle growth. As-synthesized QDs are alkylated and not water-soluble. To make them water-soluble, thiolated species are commonly added to form disulfide linkages with the QD core or ZnS shell. Various thiolated molecules, such as mercaptoacetic acid, mercaptopropionic acid, and glutathione, have been used for this purpose. Recent research has demonstrated the use of cysteine modification, rendering QDs water-soluble with smaller hydrodynamic sizes, facilitating renal clearance rather than RES organ accumulation. Efforts have also been made to enhance linkage strength with polydentate ligands or explore strong Zn (II)–His interactions with proteins/peptides.

In addition to ligand-exchange techniques, researchers have explored ligand addition-based surface modifications using amphiphilic compounds like phospholipids and amphiphilic saccharides. This approach was utilized in a study where a triblock copolymer was used to modify QDs, conjugated with a prostate-specific membrane antigen (PSMA) targeting antibody. The resulting nanoconjugates accumulated in the tumor area in prostate cancer-bearing mice, attributed to both the EPR effect and specific antibody–antigen interactions. QDs have the potential to function as gene delivery vehicles when modified with positively charged polymers like liopofectamine. For instance, researchers have encapsulated QDs in poly (maleic-anhydride-alt-1-decene) and modified them with dimethyl amino propyl amine to render them positively charged. These modified QDs showed better delivery efficiency and reduced toxicity compared to traditional delivery agents like PEI. Covalent coupling of siRNA to QDs has also been explored, with promising results in gene silencing efficiency.

In addition to gene delivery, QDs have significant potential in PDT, either as photosensitizers themselves or as carriers for PDT agents. QDs can generate reactive oxygen intermediates when photoactivated, causing cell damage. They offer advantages such as better chemical stability and water solubility compared to small molecule-based photosensitizers. QDs have been investigated as carriers for PDT agents like Ir-complex, phthalocyanine, and meso-tetra (4-sulfonatophenyl) porphine-di-hydrochloride (TSPP), where QDs act as drug carriers and energy hubs for activating PDT functions.

The unique physicochemical properties of QDs, such as broad absorption spectra, size-dependent narrow and stable emission spectra, photo stability, and the ability to carry additional agents like targeting ligands and therapeutic drugs, make them ideal candidates for biomedical applications. Moreover, the multiplexing and fluorescence resonance energy transfer (FRET) capabilities of QDs offer unexplored possibilities for developing QD-based theranostic agents. However, it is crucial to understand the metabolism of QDs in the body and address heavy metal-related toxicity issues for safe and effective use in biomedical applications.

2.2.1.3 Theranostic agents based on silica NPs

Method of preparation for and study of surface chemistry of silica NPs

Silica is extensively acknowledged as a secure substance and has found application as a surgical implant. Its synthesis enables meticulous regulation of the size and structure of silica NPs. While silica NPs lack innate imaging attributes, they excel as a versatile framework for effortless integration of diverse imaging and therapeutic functionalities, positioning them as a prime contender for theranostic endeavors.

The synthesis of silica NPs can be achieved by subjecting tetraethyl orthosilicate (TEOS) to hydrolysis and condensation processes. To introduce functional units onto these particles, amino propyl trimethoxy silane (APS) or mercaptopropyl methoxy silane (MPS) are conventionally employed as co-precursors. These co-precursors amalgamate with the TEOS structure, imparting amine or thiol groups onto the particle surface. During particle formation, functional molecules can be readily integrated into the nanosystem by pre-complexing them with APS/MPS. This technique has been applied to incorporate organic dyes and Gd–DTPA complexes into the silica particle matrix, yielding agents exhibiting optical or magnetic activities. In addition to small molecules, NPs like IONPs, gold NPs, and QDs can be easily encapsulated into silica matrices, as reported in numerous studies. Furthermore, it is possible to encapsulate multiple functionalities within a single silica particle simultaneously. For instance, Nie *et al* developed a hybrid silica NP encapsulating both IONPs and QDs, retaining both magnetic and optical properties. Similarly, Koole *et al* presented a dual-function core–shell–shell (CSS) NP, where silica NPs were loaded with both QDs and Gd complexes. Silica NPs offer an easy and effective method for incorporating drug molecules during their formation. Roy *et al* successfully integrated the hydrophobic photosensitizing anticancer drug, 2-devinyl-2-(1-hexyloxyethyl) pyropheophorbide (HPPH), into silica matrices. The HPPH displayed enhanced fluorescence within the silica matrices, and when exposed to laser irradiation, efficiently eradicated cancer cells through PDT. In a recent advance, the same research group co-encapsulated HPPH and a two-photon absorbing dye, 9,10-bis[4′-(4″-aminostyryl) styryl]anthracene (BDSA), within silica NPs. This innovative combination enabled BDSA to efficiently upconvert NIR light and transfer the energy to activate HPPH's PDT function [107].

A significant breakthrough in silica NP preparation is the ability to create mesoporous structures with precise pore size control. These nanostructures, featuring numerous empty channels and a large surface area (>900 m_2 g^{-1}), hold great promise for drug delivery as they can serve as excellent reservoirs for small molecules. Various chemical and physical methods have been reported to achieve these mesoporous nanostructures. Typically, n-alkyl tri-alkoxy silane or other surfactants are incorporated into the matrices during particle formation, which are subsequently removed via post-synthesis solvent extraction or calcinations to yield the mesoporous structure. Mesoporous silica NPs possess the capability to effectively encapsulate small molecule pharmaceuticals through uncomplicated physical interactions. Cutting-edge methodologies have been devised to seal these mesopores subsequent to drug encapsulation, thwarting untimely drug discharge. As an illustration, mesoporous silica NPs were laden with PTX and subsequently sealed with photosensitive gold NPs, which can be unsealed to release the encapsulated molecules upon exposure to light irradiation.

In a recent investigation, Park and colleagues introduced luminescent porous silicon nanoparticles (LPSiNPs) produced through physical methodologies. The procedure entailed high-frequency etching of single-crystal silicon wafers, detachment of the porous silicon film, ultra sonication, filtration using a 0.22 μM membrane, and initiation of luminescence within an aqueous solution. The observed luminescence was a result of quantum confinement effects and localized defects at the Si–SiO_2 interface. Subsequently, these luminescent porous NPs were loaded with DOX, and their drug release and impact on cell viability were assessed through *in vitro* experiments. A captivating attribute of these silica NPs lies in their capability to undergo self-destruction within the body, followed by renal clearance within a relatively brief timeframe. This quality serves to mitigate the potential harm to normal organs, minimizing the associated risks [108].

2.2.1.4 Theranostic agents based on gold NPs

Method of preparation for and study of the surface chemistry of gold NPs

Gold nanoparticles (Au NPs) possess unique features and have been studied extensively for various imaging applications, including CT, photo acoustics, and surface-enhanced Raman spectroscopy (SERS). The synthesis of Au NPs is well established, enabling precise control of their shapes, such as spheres, cubes, rods, cages, and wires. This morphology control is crucial as it impacts significantly on the physical properties of the NPs, influencing their role as imaging probes. For example, spherical Au NPs with a size of 10 nm exhibit characteristic surface plasmonic absorption at approximately 520 nm. As the particle size increases, there is a slight red-shift in the absorption spectrum, with maximum absorption for 48.3 and 99.4 nm Au NPs occurring at 533 and 575 nm, respectively. By changing the NP shape to rod-like, the absorption can be shifted to the NIR region (650–900 nm), making them suitable as probes for photoacoustic imaging or mediators in photothermal therapeutics.

The robust binding offered by thiol–Au interactions makes this a prevalent choice for the surface alteration of gold nanostructures. Bifunctional compounds are frequently utilized, with one thiol end affixed to the particle surface, exposing carboxyl or amine ends for linkage with functional components. Alternatively, biomolecules can be pre-modified with thiol groups and subsequently incorporated into the particles as intact entities. Monodentatethiol ligands are generally considered sufficient for stable ligand anchoring of Au, offering higher loading capacity compared to multidentate species. In nanorod synthesis, cetrimonium bromide (CTAB) is widely used to promote longitudinal growth, leading to most thiol–Au interaction occurring at the ends of the nanorods. To improve loading efficiency, a layer-by-layer deposition approach can be utilized, capitalizing on the highly positively charged CTAB coating to load alternatively charged species onto the particle surface. Through this approach, substantial functional molecules such as antibodies can be directly anchored onto the exterior layer of the particle surface via electrostatic interactions. As mentioned earlier, Au–thiol chemistry is frequently harnessed to incorporate functional components onto Au NPs, leading to the successful loading of several therapeutic agents through this means. For example, PTX was modified at its C-7 position and covalently coupled to 4-mercaptophenol-modified Au NPs, resulting in conjugates with improved therapeutic effects compared to MTX alone, both *in vitro* and *in vivo*. Similarly, protein-based pharmaceutics, such as tumor necrosis factor (TNF), have been coupled to PEGylated Au NPs, leading to conjugates with enhanced therapeutic efficacy and reduced toxicity compared to native TNF.

Besides thiol–Au interactions, other methods of anchoring pharmaceutics to Au NPs have also been explored. One study utilized chitosan as a reducing agent and coating material to create highly positively charged chitosan–Au NPs capable of efficiently loading insulin via electrostatic interaction (53%). These insulin-loaded Au NP conjugates were tested in a diabetic model and showed significant reductions in blood glucose levels after administration. Additionally, PDT agents, such as Pc4 and zinc-Pc, were directly adsorbed onto PEGylated Au NPs, demonstrating efficient drug delivery with a considerably shorter delivery time compared to free drugs.

Furthermore, Au NPs have been modified into polyelectrolytes for gene delivery applications. Alkylated quaternary ammonium-functionalized Au NPs have been utilized to load plasmid DNA, offering protection against enzymatic digestion and controlled release upon GSH activation. Branched PEI has also been employed to confer gene loading capacity to Au NPs, leading to significantly enhanced transfection potency compared to the parent polymer. Therapeutic genes can be loaded onto Au NPs through covalent linking as well. Thiolated antisense DNA oligos were efficiently loaded onto Au NPs and demonstrated high translocation rates and effective gene knockdown in cellular studies.

The unique surface plasmon resonance feature of Au NPs makes them promising materials for photothermal therapy. By concentrating Au NPs in tumor areas and irradiating them with laser light, they can convert light into heat and selectively destroy adjacent cancerous cells while minimizing damage to normal tissue. Various gold nanostructures, such as nanorods, nanocages, and nanoshells, have been explored to shift the absorption to the NIR region, facilitating photothermal applications. For instance, PEG-coated Au nanocages were shown to accumulate in a xenograft model and achieve efficient tumor surface temperature increase upon NIR light exposure. Gold nanoshells coupled with α-melanocyte-stimulating hormone (MSH) analog demonstrated successful ablation of melanoma in response to laser illumination and reduced tumor metabolic activity upon photothermal therapy. Au nanoshells were also used as light-controllable siRNA carriers, exhibiting light-inducible siRNA release and subsequent downregulation of the target gene NF-κB P65 both *in vitro* and *in vivo*. Combining photothermal therapy with chemotherapy further improved the therapeutic index, enhancing the sensitivity to chemotherapy treatment. Due to their unique characteristics, such as strong surface plasmon absorption, stability, biosafety, and ease of modification, Au NPs have been extensively explored as promising materials for creating functional agents in imaging and therapy applications. However, a major drawback is high production cost, which may limit their widescale clinical use despite their promising potential. Another noteworthy concern is the stability of thiol–Au chemistry when exposed to reducing environments like glutathione (GSH), which is abundant in living organisms. As research progresses towards *in vivo* applications, the development of alternative chemistry that ensures more stable Au NP conjugates becomes crucial and highly advantageous.

2.2.1.5 Theranostic agents based carbon nanotubes

Method of preparation and study of surface chemistry of carbon nanotubes

CNTs have exhibited potential in applications such as Raman and photoacoustic imaging, and have been under scrutiny as drug carriers by multiple research teams. Yet, the graphite-like composition of CNTs bestows them with inertness and resistance to a majority of conjugation methodologies. To address this hurdle, scientists have delved into employing highly oxidative conditions to instigate defects on the surface of CNTs, thereby generating attachment points for conjugation.

For instance, subjecting single-walled nanotubes (SWNTs) to refluxing 2.5 M HNO_3 for specific periods followed by sonication results in water-soluble SWNTs due to the generation of multiple carboxyl groups on the nanotube surface. These carboxyl groups enable covalent conjugation of molecules through amide bonds. Another approach involves anchoring azomethineylide and its derivatives to the CNT surface through 1,3-dipolar cycloaddition, allowing the conjugation of various functional molecules like organic dyes, peptides, and antibiotics.

The hydrophobic and aromatic attributes of CNTs additionally promote the non-covalent tethering of molecules. Amphiphilic substances such as sodium dodecyl sulfate (SDS), triton-*X*-100, CTAB, sodium dodecyl benzene sulfonate (SDBS), and sodium dodecane sulfonic acid (SDSA) have been utilized to disperse CNTs in aqueous environments. Interestingly, SDBS has shown greater efficiency than SDS in producing CNT suspensions due to the aromatic ring in SDBS that interacts with the CNT surface, reducing the energy required for dispersion. Aromatic compounds such as 1-pyrenebutanoic acid succinimidyl ester, PS-b-PAA, and 1-pyrenepropyl-amine hydrochloride have also been successful in modifying CNTs. In recent efforts, DNA oligos have been utilized for CNT modification, with multiple bases forming π–π interactions with the graphite surface, resulting in a helical wrapping of the DNA around the CNT and exposing sugar–phosphate backbones to the solution.

Among the various ligands explored for functionalizing CNTs, PEGylated phospholipids have garnered significant attention due to their effectiveness and biocompatibility. In a study by the Schipper group, mice were intravenously administered phospholipid-coated CNTs for four months, with careful monitoring. Although some CNTs accumulated in the liver and spleen without degradation, there was no evidence of toxicity observed from the survival, clinical, and laboratory parameters, as well as necropsy and tissue histology studies. While the safety of CNTs for *in vivo* applications remains a topic of debate, these studies suggest that inconsistent observations in CNT toxicity studies might be attributed to the coating materials rather than the CNTs themselves. The cellular uptake of CNTs has sparked extensive research on their potential applications in drug delivery. However, the exact mechanisms underlying this efficient cell penetration remain unclear. It has been observed that CNTs can be internalized via different routes, depending on their surface coatings. Both endocytosis and passive diffusion have been reported as responsible for CNT uptake [109].

In prior investigations, MTX was linked to CNTs via 1,3-dipolar cycloaddition, while CNTs with multiple amine termini were employed for DNA plasmid loading and delivery. Nonetheless, the covalent amide linkage in the MTX scenario failed to facilitate intracellular drug release, as evidenced by the fact that the therapeutic effectiveness of the conjugates did not surpass that of standalone MTX. The research conducted by the Dai group delved into phospholipid–CNT conjugates for the dual purposes of imaging and therapy. They successfully coupled siRNA to CNTs via a disulfide bond, which underwent enzymatic breakage in the endolysosome, leading to high transfection efficiency and better RNAi induction than lipofectamine. They also used PEGylated CNTs to deliver either Pt(IV) prodrug or PTX, resulting in improved pharmacokinetics and therapeutic effects. The PTX-loaded CNTs demonstrated enhanced tumor homing and superior tumor suppression compared to Taxol.

Aromatic stacking was utilized for DOX loading onto SWNTs, with high efficiency and pH-dependent drug release in acidic endolysosomes and tumor microenvironments, showing promising therapeutic efficacy and reduced toxicity in lymphoma xenografts. The strong optical absorbance of CNTs in the NIR region makes them promising in photothermal therapy. NIR irradiation of CNTs internalized in cells triggers endosomal rupture and cell death. Studies in carcinoma models and xenografts have shown successful tumor eradication with combined treatments of PEGylated SWNTs and NIR irradiation. CNTs possess unique physical and surface features and are significant players in nanomedicine. They can also serve as platforms for other NPs like IONPs or Au NPs to enhance their functionalities. However, concerns about their non-biodegradability and potential chronic damage remain. Establishing a standardized protocol for large-scale production of pure CNTs is essential for their clinical translation.

2.2.2 Tumor diagnosis and bioavailability of nanoplatforms

In the field of biomedicine, *in vivo* imaging plays a crucial role, enabling real-time monitoring and accurate localization of lesions, which is essential for effective treatment and prognostic detection. This is especially significant in cancer treatment, where advanced imaging technologies can provide vital information for treatment strategies and personalized therapies in the early stages of tumor development, improving diagnosis and treatment outcomes. The most common imaging methods include fluorescence imaging, CT, MRI, and PAI, all of which contribute to real-time monitoring during tumor treatment, enhancing treatment precision.

Nanomaterials have become widely utilized carriers in biomedicine due to their controllable size, excellent biocompatibility, and unique physical and chemical properties, allowing them to accumulate at tumor sites. Recent advancements in nanoscience and nanotechnology have transformed nanomaterials into versatile platforms for imaging and treating various cancers. These cancer treatment nanoplatforms encompass nanogels, dendrimers, micro bubbles, CNTs, graphene, SiO_2 NPs, and nanoscale metal–organic framework (NMOF) materials. For effective cancer treatment, the ideal approach is to integrate imaging components and anticancer drugs into nanoplatforms, enabling precise treatment guided by imaging techniques. However, relying solely on a single imaging modality for guiding cancer treatment may not yield satisfactory accuracy and imaging effects. As a result, researchers often combine multiple imaging methods for multimodal imaging-guided precision treatment (figure 2.14).

In the field of biomedicine, emerging biocompatible nanoplatforms have shown great promise in both diagnosis and therapy. These nanoplatforms offer versatile applications and functionalities, making them valuable tools in the fight against diseases, especially cancer.

For diagnosis, several imaging techniques have been utilized in conjunction with nanoplatforms. PAI is a notable technique that uses laser-induced ultrasound waves to produce high-resolution images. CT employs x-rays to create detailed cross-sectional images, while MRI uses powerful magnets and radio waves for excellent soft tissue visualization. Additionally, PAI combines optical and ultrasound

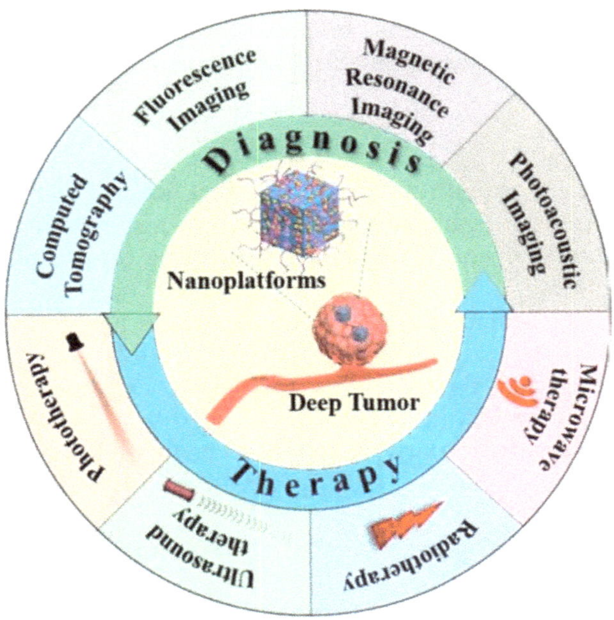

Figure 2.14. An outline of emergent biocompatible theranostic nanoplatforms. The diagnostic methods include computed tomography, magnetic resonance imaging, fluorescence imaging, and photoacoustic imaging. The treatment methods include phototherapy, ultrasound imaging, radiation therapy, and magnetic hyperthermia therapy. Reproduced from [110]. CC BY 4.0.

methods to enable deeper tissue penetration and better contrast in imaging. In terms of therapy, biocompatible nanoplatforms offer various treatment methods. Phototherapy, for instance, utilizes light-absorbing agents to generate localized heat, resulting in photothermal therapy (PTT) or photodynamic therapy (PDT) to destroy cancer cells selectively. Ultrasound therapy employs focused ultrasound waves to target and treat tumors precisely. Radiation therapy (RT) utilizes ionizing radiation to damage cancer cells' DNA, halting their growth. Moreover, magnetic hyperthermia therapy (MWT) employs magnetic NPs to generate heat when exposed to an alternating magnetic field, thus selectively destroying cancer cells. These emerging biocompatible nanoplatforms hold immense potential in advancing personalized medicine, offering precise and effective diagnosis and therapy, ultimately leading to improved patient outcomes and better healthcare practices. Four tumor diagnosis techniques, namely fluorescence imaging, CT, MRI, and PAI, offer distinct advantages and limitations.

A. **Fluorescence imaging**

Advantages:

- High sensitivity for detecting fluorescently labeled biomarkers;
- Real-time imaging capabilities for dynamic monitoring;
- Non-ionizing radiation, making it safe for repeated use;
- Suitable for molecular imaging and tracking specific cellular processes.

Limitations:

- Limited tissue penetration depth due to light scattering;
- Low spatial resolution compared to other modalities;
- Autofluorescence from surrounding tissues may interfere with signal detection.

B. **CT**

Advantages:

- Excellent spatial resolution, providing detailed anatomical images;
- Widespread availability and relatively short imaging acquisition time;
- Suitable for bone imaging and identifying calcifications in tumors.

Limitations:

- Ionizing radiation exposure can be a concern, especially with repeated scans;
- Limited soft tissue contrast, leading to challenges in distinguishing between certain tumor types;
- Less sensitive to early-stage tumors compared to other modalities.

C. **MRI**

Advantages:

- Excellent soft tissue contrast, allowing for detailed visualization of tumor morphology;
- Multi-parametric imaging capabilities (e.g. T1, T2, diffusion-weighted imaging) for functional insights;
- Non-ionizing radiation, making it safer for certain populations (e.g. pregnant women).

Limitations:
- Longer imaging acquisition time compared to CT and FI;
- Costly equipment and examination, resulting in higher inspection costs;
- Limited sensitivity to molecular and cellular changes in early tumor stages.

D. **PAI**

Advantages:
- High spatial resolution, providing detailed morphological information;
- Deep tissue penetration, combining the benefits of both optical and ultrasound imaging;
- Potential for functional imaging by using specific contrast agents.

Limitations:
- Expensive equipment and higher imaging costs;
- Limited depth compared to CT and MRI for imaging deep-seated tumors;
- Still relatively under development compared to well-established modalities.

Each tumor diagnosis technique has its strengths and weaknesses (table 2.3). Fluorescence imaging excels in molecular imaging and real-time monitoring, while CT provides high spatial resolution but may have radiation concerns. MRI offers excellent soft tissue contrast and multi-parametric imaging, but imaging acquisition

Table 2.3. Comparative study of different tumor treatment methods.

Diagnostic method	Advantages	Limitations
CT	This imaging technique offers high image resolution, leading to accurate diagnosis results and high diagnostic efficiency	The imaging equipment can be costly, leading to high inspection expenses, and limitations in achieving high resolution for soft tissue imaging
MRI	The imaging method is non-invasive and capable of deep tissue penetration	Low sensitivity
FI	Operation is simple, extensive range of marking substances and very high sensitivity	The signal-to-noise ratio and spatial resolution are relatively low, and there is significant background noise
PAI	This imaging techniques offer deeper penetration, improved spatial resolution, and heightened sensitivity, enabling more precise and detailed imaging results	The main challenges with the current imaging methods are the limited imaging area and extended imaging acquisition time

can be time-consuming and expensive. PAI combines optical and ultrasound advantages, but is still in the early stages of development and may have higher costs. A comprehensive approach, considering the specific clinical scenario, is often required for accurate tumor diagnosis and treatment planning.

2.3 Construction strategies of theranostic nanoplatforms

2.3.1 Nanoplatform models with single-modal imaging functionality

Monomodal imaging refers to the utilization of a single imaging technique for cancer diagnosis and therapy, guided by imaging [111]. This involves using nanoplatforms as contrast agents or carriers to load materials with contrast agent functions. The enrichment of the contrast agent in the tumor microenvironment significantly enhances imaging sensitivity. Common monomodal imaging techniques for cancer diagnosis include fluorescence imaging, CT, MRI, and PAI [112].

Fluorescence imaging employs fluorescent imaging molecules or contrast agents to generate fluorescent signals at the target or enhance signals between tumors and surrounding tissues. While fluorescence imaging offers simple operation and wide marking capabilities, its clinical application is limited by relatively low spatial resolution, strong background noise, and low signal-to-noise ratio [113]. Nanoplatforms show promise as *in vivo* contrast agents for fluorescence imaging, and various photosensitive materials like photosensitive dyes, NMOF nanomaterials, and fluorescent quantum dots have been developed for this purpose. Nanoplatforms can encapsulate photosensitive dyes to enhance fluorescence imaging, improving tumor imaging and providing better guidance for surgical removal of tumors. However, fluorescence imaging's shallow penetration depth of light restricts its application in deep tumors. Despite these limitations, researchers are exploring the potential of nanoplatforms to improve fluorescence imaging's capabilities and expand its clinical utility.

CT, a widely used diagnostic tool, employs x-rays with high energy and penetration for imaging purposes. It holds a dominant position among other imaging methods due to its significant advantages in providing high image resolution, accurate diagnosis results, and efficient diagnostics [114]. CT is well suited for detecting neoplasms in various body parts, localizing small tumor regions, and assessing tumor distribution, infiltration, and metastasis, as well as enabling *in vivo* detection under CT guidance. However, the expensive equipment and high inspection costs associated with CT limit its application for routine diagnosis, especially in specific areas [115].

To address this limitation, researchers are developing nanoplatforms with high x-ray absorption capabilities to serve as contrast agents, aiming to significantly enhance the resolution and diagnostic accuracy of CT examinations for certain organs. For instance, Liu and colleagues introduced a tantalum-based multifunctional nanoplatform (PEG–TaS_2 NSs) composed of tantalum sulfide (TaS_2) nanoflakes with excellent biocompatibility. Thanks to the high x-ray attenuation coefficient of tantalum, PEG–TaS_2 NSs can efficiently function as CT imaging contrast agents. *In vitro* imaging experiments demonstrated a linear relationship between the concentration of PEG–TaS_2 NSs and the Hounsfield unit (HU) value, validating their potential for enhancing CT imaging performance. To further evaluate the potential of *in vivo* imaging, researchers performed time-dependent whole-body CT imaging by intravenously injecting PEG–TaS_2 NSs into mice with prostate cancer PC3 tumor cells. The results demonstrated that the cardiac CT signal of PEG–TaS_2 NSs remained significantly stronger even 2 h after injection, indicating an extended circulation time for PEG–TaS_2 NSs. This characteristic makes PEG–TaS_2 NSs a promising and effective platform for combined cancer treatment under CT imaging guidance. Additionally, other nanoplatforms like IL@ZrO_2, MnSe@Bi_2Se_3–PEG, C–Fe_3O_4 quantum dots, and more, are also considered excellent candidates for tumor therapy guided by enhanced CT imaging [116].

MRI is an essential tool in molecular imaging and clinical diagnosis due to its non-invasiveness, low toxicity, high spatial resolution, and deep tissue penetration [117]. It finds widespread use in tumor diagnosis, such as cancer, Alzheimer's disease, liver disease, and enteropathy. However, MRI's spatial resolution is inferior to CT, and patients with cardiac pacemakers or metal foreign bodies cannot be examined using MRI. Furthermore, MRI is relatively expensive, requires longer scanning times, and may produce more artifacts compared to CT. To enhance MRI sensitivity, contrast agents are often used to differentiate tumors from normal tissues. These contrast agents include positive (T1-weighted) and negative (T2-weighted) agents. T2-weighted contrast agents produce dark images, similar to bleeding, metal deposition, or calcification, leading to potential false-positive diagnoses. Additionally, T2-weighted agents can form susceptibility artifacts, resulting in unclear display images. As a consequence, the primary limitation of MRI lies in its relatively low sensitivity with contrast agents. Researchers have worked on developing various contrast agents using Fe-, Mn-, and Gd-based nanoplatforms to improve MRI detection capabilities. For instance, hybrid core–shell vesicles (HCSVs) have been synthesized to increase Fe^{2+} in an exogenous circularly polarized magnetic field, which subsequently causes a change in MRI-R2* signal, useful for monitoring Fenton reaction and tracking HCSVs. Another example is the T1-weighted MRI contrast agent UMFNP-CREKA, which combines ultrafine manganese ferrite nanoparticles (UMFNPs) with tumor-targeted pentapeptide CREKA, enabling the detection of metastases with an unprecedented minimum detection limit of 0.39 mm in *in vivo* T1-weighted MRI experiments. This substantially extends the detection limit of previously reported MRI probes [118].

2.3.2 Nanoplatform models with the multimodal imaging functionality

The ideal platform for tumor diagnosis and therapy should offer excellent therapeutic efficacy and reliable assessment of tumor characteristics [119]. Conventional imaging diagnostic techniques include fluorescence imaging, CT, MRI, and PAI. However, each method has limitations and cannot provide complete information. For instance, *in vivo* fluorescence imaging has high sensitivity but low spatial resolution, while CT provides high spatial resolution and tomographic information but lacks sensitivity for soft tissue contrast. MRI offers superior soft tissue imaging resolution but lower sensitivity compared to CT. PAI can only image small areas due to moderate laser energy. To overcome the limitations of monomodal imaging, scientists have turned their attention to multimodal imaging. Multimodal imaging combines the complementary information from multiple imaging methods, allowing for more accurate and detailed disease diagnosis. Early tumor diagnosis significantly improves the cure rate, and multimodal imaging enhances accuracy and reduces the risk of misdiagnosis. Thus, researchers have integrated multiple imaging functions into a single nanoplatform to promote the application of multimodal imaging and enable more precise disease diagnosis, particularly in cancer cases.

The NIR-II biological window has distinct advantages over the NIR-I window, including lower absorption and scatter by skin tissue, deeper tissue penetration, and suitability for guiding fluorescence imaging and PAI. For instance, Guo and colleagues developed organic contrast agents (CP NPs) with dual NIR-II fluorescence and PAI capabilities (NIR-II fluorescence imaging/PAI). These CP NPs have excellent biocompatibility and light stability, and high temporal resolution, enabling real-time monitoring of deep cerebrovascular and blood flow in the micron range. When combined with focused ultrasound to open the blood–brain barrier, the dual-function NIR-II fluorescence imaging/PAI provides unprecedented clarity in locating microscopic brain tumors (<2 mm in diameter) through the intact scalp and skull (high signal background ratio of 7.2). Consequently, the NIR-II fluorescence imaging/PAI holds great promise in offering powerful performance, including good temporal and spatial resolution, deep tissue penetration, and large signal-to-background ratio for accurate brain diagnosis.

Multimodal imaging plays a significant role in guiding tumor diagnosis and therapy, enabling more precise and effective cancer treatment. For example, Fe_3O_4@Au supraparticles (SPs) have been designed as multimodal imaging agents, offering excellent capabilities for CT imaging and MRI with good biocompatibility both *in vivo* and *in vitro*. CT experiments demonstrated visible signals at the tumor site 12 h after intravenous injection of Fe_3O_4@Au SPs, becoming stronger after 24 h, making them an ideal contrast agent for *in vivo* CT imaging. Due to their magnetic properties, Fe_3O_4@Au SPs can also be used for T2-weighted MRI, showing clear dark signals in the tumor area 24 h after injection. Additionally, Fe_3O_4@Au SPs possess PAI functionality, which becomes more apparent over time in Hela solid tumors. With highly integrated multimodal imaging capabilities, Fe_3O_4@Au SPs hold great promise for diagnosing and treating clinical deep tumors. In summary, imaging technology significantly influences diagnosis and therapy as it enables clear differentiation of lesions from surrounding tissues. The effectiveness of imaging largely depends on the selectivity and sensitivity of contrast agents. Thus, developing efficient nanoplatforms as imaging contrast agents is crucial. Nanoplatforms can combine diagnosis and therapy, enhancing the effectiveness of tumor treatments [120].

2.4 Nanomedicine in cancer therapy

Chemotherapy is currently one of the most established and extensively utilized techniques for treating tumors in clinical settings. Nonetheless, it faces several challenges during its application. These include the absence of precise targeting, significant adverse effects caused by traditional chemotherapy drugs, and the limited solubility of key frontline medications like doxorubicin and paclitaxel. These factors together add to the intricate nature of cancer treatment in clinical scenarios. Utilizing nanomaterials in the development and administration of the aforementioned chemotherapy drugs holds the potential to enhance the precision and effectiveness of chemotherapy while also enhancing its safety. Nanomaterials have proved their potential over the years. For more than 20 years, progress in comprehending the biology of cancer has translated into advancements in cancer treatment at a gradual pace.

Despite these efforts, projections indicate that the number of new cancer cases worldwide is anticipated to rise from 14 million in 2012 to potentially 22 million within the next 20 years. A primary factor behind this challenge is the inability to deliver cancer-fighting substances specifically to the tumor tissue. Often, exposing the entire system to these anticancer agents leads to severe toxic effects that restrict the dosage that can be administered. This emphasizes the critical importance of targeted delivery methods to overcome the current limitations in cancer treatment.

2.4.1 Nanocarriers in cancer therapy

Recent advances in the field of nanotechnology hold the promise of revolutionizing how drugs are delivered, aiming to simultaneously amplify the effectiveness of anticancer medications while minimizing their adverse effects. Nanocarriers possess distinct attributes, including their tiny size, large surface area relative to volume, and favorable physical and chemical traits. These features grant them the ability to finely influence how drugs are distributed and how they interact within the body. This potential adjustment to both the movement and impact of drugs can ultimately amplify their effectiveness while also reducing their negative impact, a concept encapsulated within the term 'therapeutic index' [121]. Incorporating drugs into nanocarriers offers several advantages, including enhancing the drug's stability within the body, prolonging its circulation time in the bloodstream, and enabling controlled release of the drug. Consequently, nanomedicine formulations have the capacity to influence how drugs are distributed in the body, encouraging them to accumulate more preferentially at the tumor location. This phenomenon is termed the EPR. A diverse array of nanomaterials derived from various sources such as organic, inorganic, lipid, protein, or carbohydrate compounds, as well as synthetic polymers, have been harnessed in the creation of innovative cancer treatments. These materials are employed to develop novel therapeutic approaches that take advantage of the unique properties of nanoscale structures [122]. Over the last few decades, there has been significant focus on studying nanocarriers for their potential as delivery systems for drugs (figure 2.15).

These nanocarriers encompass a range of developed technologies, such as solid lipid nanoparticles (SLNPs), polymer micelles, dendrimers, polymer nanoparticles (PNPs), liposomes and other similar hydrogels, NPs based on viruses (vNPs), gold NPs, CNTs, quantum dots, mesoporous silica nanoparticles (MSNPs) and various hybrid nanocarriers that combine organic and inorganic components [123]. These

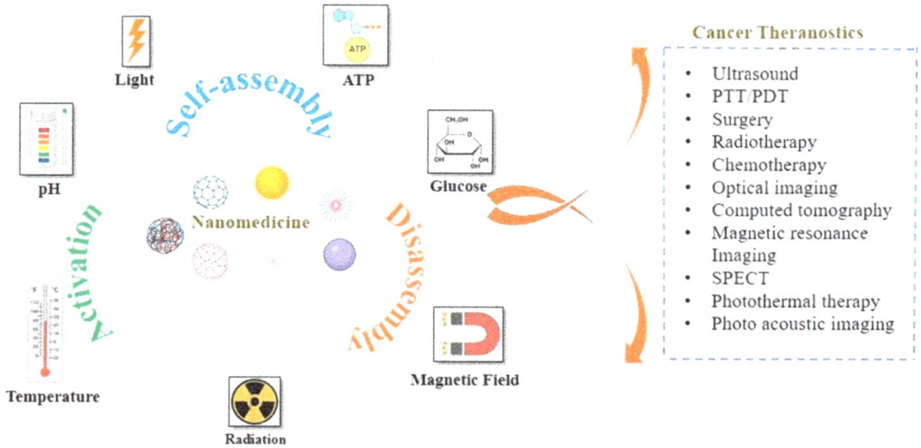

Figure 2.15. Stimuli-activation strategies of nanomedicine for cancer theranostics.

nanocarriers have the potential to address critical issues commonly faced in traditional drug treatments. These include problems such as drugs being distributed nonspecifically throughout the body, rapid elimination from circulation, uncontrolled release of the drug, and limited effectiveness due to low bioavailability. At the same time, the use of nanocarriers can also mitigate the toxicity and unwanted reactions associated with these drugs [124]. The intricate process of synthesizing these nanocarriers and concerns regarding drug toxicity resulting from chemical reactions have significantly limited their practical use in clinical settings [125]. Up to this point, the NP-based drug delivery systems that have gained approval for clinical use are primarily confined to DOX, which is basically liposomal doxorubicin and Abraxane, which is albumin-bound paclitaxel. These existing nanodrug delivery systems predominantly rely on passive targeting, which effectively diminishes toxicity and side effects. However, they do not bring about substantial enhancements in the therapeutic index [126]. Given these circumstances, there is an immediate need to create drug nanocarriers that exhibit strong biocompatibility and the capability to effectively target tumors [127]. NPs encompass polymeric NPs, liposomes, and micelles, each possessing distinct traits like encapsulating poorly soluble drugs, enabling targeted drug delivery, enhancing drug effectiveness by improving bioavailability, promoting better penetration through biological barriers, and facilitating controlled drug release. Many chemotherapy drugs primarily function by interacting with receptors on the cell surface, within the cell cytoplasm, or even within the cell nucleus. Tumors display a heterogeneous nature due to variations in the expression and mutation of oncogenes and tumor suppressor genes. These genetic alterations lead to changes in cellular processes such as programmed cell death (apoptosis), regulation of the cell cycle, development of resistance, and the ability to spread (metastasis). Drug actions occur during their circulation in the bloodstream, and the concentration of drugs at the tumor site directly influences their therapeutic effectiveness [128].

2.4.1.1 Nanocarriers in different types of cancer

2.4.1.1.1 Breast cancer

The advent of nanotechnology has sparked extensive exploration of diverse nanomaterials and their drug combinations as promising candidates for transporting drugs effectively to breast cancer locations. Both organic and inorganic nanostructures exhibit substantial promise for use in real-world medical scenarios, and they are at the forefront of groundbreaking advancements in cancer treatment discovery [129]. Nanomaterials hold significant appeal for drug delivery primarily due to their improved capacity to carry drugs efficiently and their capability to penetrate cells at the microscopic level, which is attributed to their nanoscale dimensions [130]. Numerous ongoing research endeavors have showcased the utilization of diverse nanomaterials combined with various drugs, highlighting their promising role in breast cancer treatment as efficient carriers for drug delivery. The specific therapeutic drugs employed for each breast cancer diagnosis varies based on the unique expression of protein biomarkers associated with the condition [131]. Typical chemotherapy drugs used to treat breast cancer belong to categories such as anthracyclines, taxanes, and cyclophosphamide. Anthracyclines constitute a class of anticancer medications that exert their effects by interacting with DNA, leading to therapeutic impacts against cancer. This interaction induces DNA damage, which, in turn, prompts cell apoptosis. While these drugs are successful in targeting cancerous cells, their toxicity does not differentiate between malignant and normal cells [132]. DOX is classified within the anthracycline family and is employed in breast cancer treatment. Nevertheless, its short duration of activity and the substantial harm it inflicts on healthy cells restrict its use in clinical settings. In light of this challenge, numerous investigations have been conducted over time to devise a strategy wherein DOX is linked to a carrier. This approach aims to enhance the drug's effectiveness while simultaneously diminishing its adverse effects [133]. To delve deeper into the impact of combining DOX with a nanocarrier, a particular study introduced a nanostructure comprising DOX and functionalized MWNTs. This nanostructure was examined thoroughly using MCF-7 human breast cancer cells and was observed to be successful in impeding cell proliferation by triggering apoptosis. Moreover, the study revealed that the nanostructure primarily directed its action toward cancer cells, largely leveraging the receptor-mediated endocytosis process [134]. The utilization of Doxorubicin-loaded lipid-polymer hybrid NPs (Dox-LPNs) against breast cancer cell lines that exhibit resistance to multiple drugs showed intriguing results. The Doxorubicin contained within these NPs managed to evade the Pgp (P-glycoprotein) found on the cell membrane. Notably, Doxorubicin encapsulated in the NPs exhibited better retention within cells overexpressing Pgp compared to using the drug on its own. This enhanced drug uptake in Pgp-overexpressing cells treated with Dox-LPNs was primarily facilitated through the process of phagocytosis [135]. Approximately 60–70% of breast cancer instances are managed through hormonal therapy, a medical approach that involves the use of medications to hinder hormones that fuel the proliferation of cancer cells, such as estrogen [136]. Deficiency of this type of treatment depends on the biological characteristics of patients with hormone receptor-positive (estrogen receptor-positive or ER+). Tamoxifen (TAM), aromatase inhibitors, and fulvestrant are frequently prescribed medications for this purpose [137]. TAM is designated as an 'anti-estrogen' compound and falls under the category of selective estrogen receptor modulators (SERMs). Its function revolves around attaching to estrogen receptors located in breast cancer cells, effectively impeding the hormone's functions. Currently, TAM finds widespread application in managing breast cancers characterized by estrogen receptor positivity (ER+). The efficacy of TAM has been examined across a variety of age groups among women, encompassing both the initial and advanced stages of the disease [138]. A comparative study was conducted in live mice, where some were treated with Doxil (Doxorubicin HCl liposome injection), while others received Doxil coupled with F5, which is scFV antibody F5, a type of ERBB2 recombinant antibody. It demonstrated that the mice receiving F5-modified Doxil exhibited a more rapid and substantial reduction in tumor volume compared to those treated with the unmodified Doxil [139]. NP systems have exhibited encouraging outcomes in terms of targeting HER2 (human epidermal growth factor 2). Administering toxin-loaded poly(lactic-co-glycolic acid) (PLGA) NPs, designed to target HER2, through intravenous injection to mice bearing HER-positive BT-474 cells, led to notable reductions in both tumor growth and overall systemic toxicity [140]. Promising outcomes in HER2 targeted therapy have also been witnessed with alternative NP systems. Noteworthy examples include the utilization of cross-linked human serum albumin NPs and chitosan NPs loaded with quantum dots and absorbed siRNA [141]. Beyond HER2, the luteinizing hormone-releasing hormone (LHRH) receptor has also garnered significant attention as a target for focused delivery of therapeutic agents and imaging tools aimed at treating both localized and metastatic breast cancer. This was demonstrated through *in vitro* as well as *in vivo* investigations employing LHRH-conjugated superparamagnetic iron oxide NPs (SPIONs). The SPIONs that were conjugated with LHRH exhibited distinct and specific accumulation (approximately nine times increase) within MDA-MB-435S.luc breast cancer cells in *in vitro* conditions, and they amassed at the main breast tumor areas having metastatic properties *in vivo*. In contrast, non-targeted SPIONs were found to be retained within the reticuloendothelial system (RES) during *in vivo* studies [142].

2.4.1.1.2 Prostate cancer

Numerous therapeutic NPs have emerged through nanotechnology, designed to precisely target and transport a range of agents, including chemotherapy drugs. This approach aims to selectively eliminate prostate cancer cells while minimizing harm to healthy cells [143]. The development of theranostic NPs has enabled targeted prostate cancer cell engagement using specialized ligands. These NPs facilitate the controlled and time-regulated release of anticancer agents, enhancing cancer treatment. Additionally, they incorporate assisted imaging to monitor therapy effectiveness in real time. Nanotechnology's role in prostate cancer extends to innovative stealth mechanisms that enhance the precision of therapeutic delivery [144]. The implementation of 'stealthing' techniques amplifies the nanoformulation's capacity to access tumor sites more effectively. This is achieved by employing hydrophilic polymers to coat the formulation, thereby extending its duration of circulation within the bloodstream. Consequently, this coating induces robust stealth effects [145]. Another strategic approach, in addition to stealthing, involves guiding NPs to bypass the trap set by the mononuclear phagocytic system. This strategy aims to prevent their premature elimination from the system [146]. Concerning prostate cancer, nanoparticles coated with poly(ethylene glycol) (PEG) for pegylation displayed significant NP accumulation at the tumor site, in stark contrast to non-stealth NPs that were not modified [147]. Furthermore, the stealth effect can also be achieved using various hydrophilic polymers like dextrans, heparins, and poly vinyl pyrrolidone [148]. Consequently, a diverse array of nanomedicines, spanning liposomes, polymeric nanospheres, and others, including niosomes, nanomicelles, lipid hybrid NPs, polymer–drug conjugates, and metallic NPs, along with immune-conjugates, have been skillfully developed. These advancements have notably improved the overall quality of life for individuals grappling with prostate cancer [149]. Up to the present moment, a considerable volume of research has been published delving into the utilization of nanomaterials for various applications within the realm of the environment [150]. Curcumin, a bioactive compound, exhibits anticancer properties against prostate cancer by impeding the proliferation, invasion, and angiogenesis of prostate cancer cell lines both *in vivo* and *in vitro* [151]. However, the precise pharmacokinetic effects and optimal dosages of curcumin remain largely undisclosed [152]. The potential of curcumin in cancer inhibition and therapy stems from its advantageous lack of dose-dependent toxicity. However, the biological impact of curcumin is hindered by its limited bioavailability [153]. Nanospheres loaded with curcumin exhibited a more pronounced effect on cancer cells in comparison to curcumin administered in its free form [154]. These nanospheres hold enhanced promise as adjunctive therapy for prostate cancer. Another approach involved crafting curcumin-loaded NPs using fibrinogen. These NPs demonstrated cytotoxicity against prostate cancer cells and displayed a favorable level of internalization, effectively retaining the NPs within the cells [155]. Noscapine, originally an antitussive agent, serves as an anticancer drug that binds to tubulin [156]. Derived from plants, this alkaloid can be taken orally and has exhibited the ability to restrain tumor growth in nude mice that were harboring prostate-derived human xenografts [157].

2.4.1.1.3 Colorectal cancer

Colorectal cancer (CRC) stands as one of the most debilitating diseases within the realm of prevalent malignancies. It holds the distressing status of being the second most significant contributor to cancer-related deaths in women and ranks as the third most prevalent ailment among men globally [158]. Current assessments project a disconcerting surge of 60% in the probability and mortality rates of CRC worldwide by the year 2030 [159]. Despite the existing diagnostic methods and treatment options, patients are subjected to prolonged invasive procedures accompanied by undesirable side effects in their battle against CRC. This pressing scenario underscores the necessity for further research to devise novel detection techniques that can enhance specificity and effectiveness [160]. Nanotechnology has ushered in a fresh avenue for creating innovative and highly structured nanomaterials that possess the potential to significantly enhance the efficacy of screening, detection, and treatment of CRC, as well as various other tumor types [161]. The involvement of nanotechnology in addressing CRC spans several aspects, encompassing nanomaterial-driven tumor screening, tailoring of targeted drug delivery platforms, and implementation of cutting-edge treatment methods [162]. Presently, nanotechnologies have garnered global attention owing to their capacity for enhancing established norms and approaches in CRC screening, diagnosis, and treatment. A specific example is iron oxide nanocrystals, which possess diameters ranging from 1 to 100 nm. These particles have attracted substantial interest across various domains due to their magnetic attributes and potential utility [163]. Gold nanotubes, specifically gold nanotubes with surface plasmon resonance (SPR) properties, feature a nanosilica core enveloped by an exceedingly thin gold outer layer. This category of plasmonic NPs serves diverse functions, spanning optical filters, sensing mechanisms, detection technologies, and even cancer treatment applications.

Hybrid magnetic gold nanoparticles (HNPs) are created by coupling magnetic properties with gold NPs. These HNPs are tethered to anti-MG1 antibodies and function as catalysts in the targeted elimination of liver metastases associated with colorectal cancer [164]. Gold nanoparticles (Au NPs) contribute to an enhanced delivery of chemotherapy drugs through their ability to compress vessels in colorectal cancer. Additionally, they have the potential to decrease the density of fibroblasts associated with colorectal cancer, along with diminishing collagen I production. By acting on the Akt signaling pathway, they also lower the expression of Transforming growth factor beta 1 (TGF-β1), connective tissue growth factor (CTGF), and vascular endothelial growth factor (VEGF) signals. This overall action reduces tumor pressure, subsequently boosting vascular permeability. As a result, the response to NP-based chemotherapy is improved. Au NPs exhibit a spherical morphology with consistent surface dispersion and display absorption peaks via surface plasmon resonance at approximately 517 nm wavelength [165]. The introduction of PEGylated gold NPs triggers oxidative stress and apoptosis in colon cancer cells. In the context of engineered nanomedicines, Au NP-PEG-RNase A prompts apoptosis in SW480 cells, consequently resulting in a noteworthy decline in cancer cell viability [166]. Gold NPs combined with RGD cyclic peptides serve the dual purpose of targeting and imaging intestinal cancer cells. The inclusion of small molecules on NP surfaces enhances their affinity for target cells. In a refined approach, plasmonic nanostructures coated with RGD (arginyl-glycyl-aspartic acid) cyclic peptides are designed as ligands attached to gold NPs, effectively directing them towards $\alpha v\beta 3$ integrin on colorectal cancer cells [167]. Carbon NPs, maintained in a consistently suspended form, encompass carbon particles with a diameter measuring 150 nm. Capitalizing on their permeability, these particles preferentially access lymph vessels as opposed to blood vessels. They amass within lymph nodes, especially those adjacent to cancer cells, consequently causing the affected lymph nodes to exhibit a distinct dark coloration. The utility of these carbon NPs lies in their capability to identify lymph node metastases in colorectal cases. Notably, no adverse toxic effects of these suspended NPs have been observed within the body.

Over a span of several months, carbon NPs undergo excretion via the pulmonary and intestinal routes [168].

Nano-sized probes loaded with near-infrared fluorescence (NIRF) offer enhanced diagnostic potential for colon cancer. Administering these NIRF nanoprobes via intracolonic means improves the accuracy of colon cancer diagnosis during colonoscopy. Conversely, intravenous infusion of NIRF nanoprobes heightens their EPR effect, facilitating accumulation within tumor and inflammatory regions. This, in turn, simplifies the imaging process for detecting colorectal cancer cells. In comparison, intracolonic administration of NIRF NPs holds a greater advantage over intravenous injection due to its prolonged and steady circulation, coupled with optimal color differentiation efficiency [169]. Chitosan NPs that harbor the dsNKG2D-IL-21 gene exhibit potential effects in activating lymphocytes and curbing tumor growth through gene delivery. This NP-mediated transmission of the gene holds the promise of facilitating these outcomes. The NP stands out due to its straightforward manufacturability, favorable biosafety profile, and effective biological distribution within the tumor environment [170]. Silica NPs with a dual-color composition (rhodamine B and cyanine 5) and an outer polyethylene glycol coating display a distinct propensity for specific accumulation within tumor tissue measuring less than 1 mm in dimension [171]. Functionalized fibrous nanosilica, known as KCC-1, has been utilized for precise electrochemical detection of HT-29 cancer cells, employing the interactions between folate (FA) and folate receptors (FRs). KCC-1 is synthesized via a hydrothermal approach and subsequently modified with FA molecules, yielding KCC-1-NH2-FA NPs. These NPs boast several advantages. Firstly, KCC-1-NH2-FA NPs exhibit an exceptional surface-to-volume ratio that facilitates adhesion to cancer cells, particularly those featuring elevated FR expression. Secondly, the positively charged FA and NH2 groups attached to the KCC-1 NP have an increased affinity for binding to the negatively charged cancer cell membrane. Thirdly, the association of HT-29 FR-positive cancer cells and KCC-1-NH2-FA NPs and can be verified with the help of techniques like fluorescent imaging and flow cytometry [172]. Mesoporous silica NPs encapsulating DM1 (designated as MSNPs-DM1@PDA-PEG-APT) constitute a strategic approach for treating colorectal cancer. These NPs are engineered with a surface comprising dopamine hydrochloride, polyethylene glycol, and an epithelial adhesion aptamer molecule (EPCAM), all aimed at targeted CRC therapy. The system incorporates a coating consisting of dopamine hydrochloride (PDA) which is pH-sensitive to govern active targeting as well as the controlled release of DM1 from MSNP, triggered by pH variations. This responsive feature enables enhanced DM1 delivery to colorectal cancer sites. The NP offers a host of benefits as a cancer treatment option, including substantial drug-loading capability, accelerated drug release at acidic pH, and the capacity to target SW480 tumors using both passive (EPR effect) and active (EpCAMaptamer-mediated) mechanisms [173].

2.4.1.1.4 Lung cancer

A variety of avenues have been explored to deliver anticancer drugs with the objective of targeting lung cancer cells. Among the numerous drug delivery approaches, systemic administration has garnered significant attention and investigation, primarily due to its effectiveness in transporting drug payloads to lung tumor cells. Nonetheless, even with high doses administered, only a restricted amount of the anticancer drug manages to reach the intended site. Furthermore, these anticancer agents also inadvertently impact noncancerous cells, leading to their detriment. In response to the complexities associated with oral drug delivery, the pulmonary route has also been investigated as an alternative means of administering drugs. The pulmonary drug delivery pathway involves targeting the respiratory tract, which serves either for addressing airway-related conditions or for the systemic absorption of drug components aimed at managing or treating different diseases. Garbuzenko and colleagues undertook an investigation encompassing diverse lipid- and non-lipid-based nano systems, which included liposomes, micelles, mesoporous silica NPs, dendrimers, poly (propyleneimine) (PPI), siRNA complexes, poly (ethylene glycol) polymers, and quantum dots. Their objective was to facilitate the delivery of the anticancer drug doxorubicin to the lungs via inhalation. Their findings indicated that, upon inhalation, lipid-based nanocarriers like micelles and liposomes exhibited superior lung accumulation and extended retention of the drug within lung cancer cells in comparison to non-lipid-based carriers. Dendrimers manifest as spherical structures, composed of numerous polymer branches emanating from a central atomic core. These branches consist of recurring polymeric units, forming inner shell cavities and an outer shell characterized by a multivalent functional group. These functional groups exhibit an affinity for charged polar molecules, while the inner shell adeptly encapsulates uncharged non-polar molecules. Notably, the functional groups play a pivotal role in orchestrating the controlled release of drugs under specific pH conditions or through the influence of particular enzymes. Noteworthy studies have revealed that copolymers of poly (glutamic acid)-b-poly (phenylalanine) dendrimers self-assemble into micelles, thereby enabling the controlled delivery of drugs at a regulated pace. Dendrimers function as a highly versatile delivery platform and can be tailored to attain desired pharmaceutical attributes. For instance, negatively charged and neutral dendrimers exhibit biocompatibility, while their positively charged counterparts can evoke toxicity. The steric properties of dendrimers intricately influence their pharmacokinetics and biodistribution patterns. By subjecting dendrimers to PEGylation, water solubility is enhanced, dendrimer size is increased, and both retention and biodistribution properties are improved. The surface modification of dendrimers with targeting moieties offers a strategic avenue for addressing cancer cells with heightened receptor expression. In recent years, dendrimers have increasingly found applications in the realm of cancer diagnosis and therapy. This encompasses their utilization in photothermal therapy, neutron capture therapy, and photodynamic therapy, demonstrating their growing significance in the treatment of cancer.

2.4.2 Combinatorial therapy

The landscape of cancer therapy has undergone a dynamic transformation, transitioning from the initial era of pre-genomic cytotoxic chemotherapy to the subsequent genomic and post-genomic phases. This evolution has led to a shift from the generalized approach to a personalized medicine paradigm and has culminated in the concurrent emergence of combination therapies. Progress in genetic sciences and biotechnology has unveiled novel molecular targets and therapeutic agents to address the challenges stemming from genetic diversity within various cancer subgroups. Nevertheless, while the concept of personalized medicine holds promise, its application remains largely experimental in the realm of oncology due to pragmatic limitations. To bridge the gap between the potential of personalized medicine and its practical implementation, a novel strategy is emerging—the concept of combination oncotherapy. Amid the pursuit of diminishing occurrences of tumor resistance, relapse, and treatment ineffectiveness encountered with single-agent therapies, a multitude of combination therapies have emerged as a potential solution. However, the feasibility of combination oncotherapy in clinical practice has been met with scrutiny due to challenges such as intricate dosage regimens, patient adherence concerns, suboptimal treatment responses, and the potential exacerbation of adverse effects. Upon reviewing literatures already existing on the same from a formulation perspective, it becomes evident that the achievement of successful combination therapy has often been impeded. This hindrance arises either from intricate dosing schedules, limitations in spatiotemporal delivery, or disparities in the pharmacokinetic and physicochemical attributes of the combined drugs.

2.4.2.1 NP platforms for combination cancer therapy

2.4.2.1.1 Liposomes

Over the past 20 years, the advent of nanotechnology has brought about substantial advancements in clinical therapeutics. Within this context, liposomes and polymeric NPs have emerged as pivotal agents at the nanoscale for enhancing the effectiveness and safety of drug delivery. Among the array of NP options, liposomes have established themselves as a well-recognized drug delivery platform, boasting numerous clinically available products. Comprising amphiphilic lipid molecules, liposomes self-assemble into bilayered spherical vesicles. The utilization of liposomes for drug delivery represents a notable enhancement attributed to their efficacy, biocompatibility, lack of immunogenicity, improved solubility of chemotherapeutic agents, and capacity to encapsulate a diverse spectrum of drugs. Moreover, liposomes have demonstrated remarkable therapeutic promise as carriers for cargo and targeted delivery to specific sites. The utilization of liposome-mediated drug delivery systems enhances the pharmacokinetic and pharmacodynamic characteristics of therapeutic payloads. This approach facilitates controlled and sustained drug release, resulting in reduced systemic toxicity as compared to free drug administration. For example, the incorporation of polyethylene glycol (PEG)-coated liposomes in drug delivery extends their *in vivo* circulation half-life from a mere few hours to approximately 45 h. Currently, a variety of liposomal products are employed for cancer treatment, encompassing Doxil, DaunoXome, DepoCyt, and ONCO-TCS. These formulations involve liposomal versions of doxorubicin (DOX), daunorubicin, cytarabine, and vincristine, respectively. Liposomes are cellular-mimicking constructs consisting of a lipid bilayer. The hydrophilic exterior layer facilitates smooth passage of the liposome within the human body, while drugs or markers can be encapsulated within the core or transmembrane region of these liposomes. Polymeric NPs exhibit notable drug loading efficiency and can readily undergo chemical conjugation with targeting or therapeutic agents, rendering them valuable for drug delivery applications. Another instance of combination therapy based on liposomes involves the simultaneous delivery of siRNA and chemodrugs. siRNA represents an emerging category of cancer therapeutics, functioning by targeting specific mRNA sequences to interfere with gene expression. A recent investigation by Saad *et al* showcased the creation of a liposomal system for co-delivering siRNA targeting BCL2 (a protein involved in anti-apoptotic cellular defense) and MRP1 (a protein associated with multidrug resistance) in conjunction with doxorubicin, aiming at human H69AR lung cancer cells. Utilizing a positively charged 1,2-dioleoyl-3-trimethylammonium-propane compound, a cationic liposome was constructed, followed by its loading with doxorubicin via an incubation approach, and subsequent interaction with siRNA. The assembly of the liposome–siRNA complex ensued through electrostatic interactions, as the negatively charged phosphate groups on siRNA molecules adhered to the positively charged surface of the liposome. A cytotoxicity evaluation conducted *in vitro* exhibited substantial reversal of cellular resistance in multidrug-resistant lung cancer cells. While the study is in its preliminary phases, it underscores the adaptability of liposomes as versatile nanocarriers for delivering multiple drugs.

2.4.2.1.2 Polymeric NPs

Progress in biomaterials exploration has given rise to the development of polymeric NPs that are both biocompatible and biodegradable, showcasing their potential in drug delivery roles. A range of synthetic polymers endorsed by the US FDA, including poly(lactic-co-glycolic acid) (PLGA) and polycaprolactone (PCL), alongside various natural polymers such as chitosan and polysaccharides, have undergone substantial investigation for the purpose of NP fabrication. In contrast to liposomes, polymeric NPs typically exhibit greater stability, more defined size distribution, enhanced adjustability of physicochemical attributes, and sustained and finely regulated drug release patterns, as well as heightened capacity for encapsulating poorly water-soluble drugs. The polymer-based platform additionally provides greater flexibility in synthesis, facilitating the customization of particles to meet specific requirements. Thanks to these distinctive traits, polymeric NPs have garnered considerable attention across academia, industry, and clinical realms, despite being in a relatively nascent stage of advancement. Polymeric NPs are commonly composed of amphiphilic diblock copolymers that spontaneously assemble into NPs when introduced to aqueous solutions. For *in vivo* drug delivery, hydrophobic and hydrophilic blocks are often formed using popular choices like PLGA and PEG, respectively. PLGA hydrolyzes into lactic acid, while PEG creates a stealth layer that significantly reduces non-specific cellular uptake. Polymer nanoparticles (PNPs) have sparked significant interest across various domains due to their capacity to modulate drug activity, regulate drug release kinetics, enhance drug adhesion, and prolong drug permanence on the skin. These PNPs have emerged as the preferred platform for NP-based drug delivery in cancer applications. Polymer nanoparticles (PNPs), with an average diameter below 1 μm, are classified as nanocapsules or nanospheres based on their composition. PNPs are generated using two primary approaches: dispersion of preformed polymers or polymerization of monomers. These PNPs find extensive utility in targeted delivery systems, functioning as effective carriers for cancer therapy. This preference stems from their inherent qualities, such as biodegradability, biocompatibility, non-toxicity, extended circulation, and versatile capacity to encapsulate a diverse range of therapeutic agents. Multidrug resistance (MDR) poses a significant challenge in cancer treatment. Gaining insight into the molecular mechanisms underpinning drug resistance is crucial, as this comprehension holds the potential to yield improved strategies for enhancing the efficacy of cancer therapy. Innovative formulations of polymer–lipid hybrid nanoparticles (PLNs) were harnessed for the administration of DOX, a cytotoxic drug, GG918, a chemosensitizer, and a combination of DOX and GG918. These PLNs effectively enhance the encapsulation and therapeutic efficacy of DOX and GG918 within a human multidrug-resistant breast cancer cell line known as MDA435/LCC6/MDR1. It is noteworthy that the advancement of polymeric NP platforms has witnessed rapid progress, driven by the continuous exploration of novel techniques in synthesizing polymer–drug conjugates by polymer chemists. Polymeric NPs can be employed as a delivery platform in conjunction with a combination of small interfering (si) RNA and chemotherapy. In this context, the utilization of poly(ethylene oxide)-modified poly(beta-amino ester) (PEO-PbAE) and PEO-modified poly(epsilon-caprolactone) (PEO–PCL) NPs, loaded with MDR1 silencing siRNA and paclitaxel, led to a substantial enhancement in the cytotoxic effectiveness of paclitaxel against resistant SKOV3 cells, similar to the results observed in drug-sensitive SKOV3 cells. Several nanoparticulate formulations loaded with dual drugs have been developed, including: (i) polymeric NPs targeted to the epidermal growth factor receptor (EGFR) and carrying ionidamine and paclitaxel, which demonstrated targeted antitumor effects by reducing MDR in human breast and ovarian tumor cells and (ii) PLGA NPs encapsulating vincristine and verapamil, exhibiting moderate MDR reversal activity on MCF-7/ADR cells that are resistant to vincristine. Some polymers used in the preparation of NPs are PLGA and polylactide acid (PLA), polymers approved by the US FDA, which are utilized in a range of therapeutic devices due to their biodegradability and biocompatibility. PLA is a lactic acid-based polymer, while PLGA is created through the copolymerization of glycolic and lactic acids' cyclic dimers (1,4-dioxane-2,5 dione). The specific form of PLGA obtained depends on the ratio of lactide to glycolide used in the polymerization process. PLGA/PLA experiences ester linkage hydrolysis in the presence of water, and the degradation timeline is linked to the monomer ratio in the formulation. A higher glycolide unit content leads to faster degradation. As a result, PLGA/PLA breaks down in the body, yielding lactic acid and glycolic acid monomers. These byproducts are part of different metabolic pathways, ensuring minimal systemic toxicity [174].

1. *Poly 1-caprolactone*

This represents another category of FDA-approved polymers known for their biocompatibility and biodegradability, offering potential for NP formulation. Poly(1-caprolactone) (PCL), functioning as a homopolymer of 1-caprolactone, demonstrates an advantage for prolonged delivery systems due to its slower degradation compared to polyglycolic acid and polyglycolic acid-co-lactic acid. Moreover, PCL boasts compatibility with a wide array of other polymers [175]. In recent times, there has been progress in the development of biodegradable poly(ethylene oxide)-modified poly(1-caprolactone) (PEO–PCL) NPs aimed at delivering TX and ceramide (CER) to address drug resistance issues in ovarian cancer. TX and the apoptotic signaling molecule C(6)-CER were introduced intravenously, either individually or in combination, using both aqueous solution and PEO–PCL NPs, in mice bearing tumors. A noteworthy reduction in tumor growth was observed ($P<0.05$) in both wildtype SKOV3 and multidrug-resistant SKOV3 (TR) models following a single dose co-administration of TX (20 $mg\,kg^{-1}$) and CER (100 $mg\,kg^{-1}$) within NP formulations, in comparison to individual agent administration and aqueous solution administration. The outcomes of their investigation demonstrated the potential of combining TX and CER within biodegradable polymeric NPs as a highly effective therapeutic approach to counter drug resistance in ovarian cancer. Biodegradable poly(ε-caprolactone)/poly(ethylene glycol) (PCL/PEG) copolymer NPs have shown promise in drug delivery applications. Through a solvent extraction approach utilizing acetone as the organic solvent, monodisperse poly(ε-caprolactone)/poly(ethylene glycol)/poly(ε-caprolactone) (PCL/PEG/PCL, PCEC) NPs with a size of approximately 40 nm were generated. These PCL/PEG/PCL NPs exhibited no hemolysis *in vitro* and demonstrated no toxicity both *in vitro* and *in vivo*. These engineered PCL/PEG/PCL NPs were utilized for loading doxorubicin using a pH-induced self-assembly technique. The *in vitro* release study indicated that the release of doxorubicin from NPs was faster at pH 5.5 compared to pH 7.0. Encapsulation of doxorubicin within PCL/PEG/PCL NPs increased its cytotoxicity against the C-26 cell line *in vitro*. Furthermore, in comparison to free doxorubicin, doxorubicin within the NPs exhibited more effective treatment of mice with subcutaneous C-26 tumors. These doxorubicin-loaded PCL/PEG/PCL NPs offer a potential novel formulation for cancer therapy. The biodegradable poly(ε-caprolactone)/poly(ethylene glycol) (PCL/PEG) copolymer NPs demonstrated promising applicability in drug delivery systems. In this study, monodisperse poly(ε-caprolactone)/poly(ethylene glycol)/poly(ε-caprolactone) (PCL/PEG/PCL, PCEC) NPs with a size of approximately 40 nm were synthesized through a solvent extraction method using acetone as the organic solvent. These PCL/PEG/PCL NPs exhibited no hemolysis *in vitro* and demonstrated no toxicity both *in vitro* and *in vivo*. The prepared PCL/PEG/PCL NPs were utilized to encapsulate doxorubicin using a pH-triggered self-assembly technique. *In vitro* release experiments indicated that the release of doxorubicin from the NPs was more rapid at pH 5.5 than at pH 7.0. The incorporation of doxorubicin within PCL/PEG/PCL NPs enhanced its cytotoxicity against the C-26 cell line *in vitro*. Moreover, compared to free doxorubicin, doxorubicin delivered via NPs exhibited more effective treatment of mice carrying subcutaneous C-26 tumors. These doxorubicin-loaded PCL/PEG/PCL NPs hold potential as an innovative doxorubicin formulation for cancer therapy [176].

2. *Chitosan*

Chitosan, a polysaccharide derived from the partial N-deacetylation of chitin [177], is chosen as a material for NP formulation due to its favorable characteristics as a polymeric carrier. These properties include biocompatibility, biodegradability, and non-toxicity. Furthermore, chitosan exhibits remarkable mucoadhesive properties and the capacity to facilitate the penetration of larger molecules through mucosal surfaces. Chitosan NPs have demonstrated robust cytotoxic effects on diverse tumor cell lines in both *in vitro* and *in vivo* settings [178]. Furthermore, chitosan serves as a defense elicitor and exhibits antimicrobial activity. Chitosan possesses intriguing attributes, including biodegradability, biocompatibility, bioactivity, non-toxicity, and a polycationic nature. This section provides an exploration of the structural features and physicochemical attributes of chitosan. Elaborated insights into the techniques for fabricating chitosan NPs are presented. The applications of chitosan NPs are thoroughly examined, encompassing drug delivery, encapsulation, antimicrobial roles, utilization as a plant growth enhancer, and its efficacy as a plant protective agent [179]. Chitosan NPs have demonstrated significant applications in diverse fields, including parenteral drug delivery, oral administration of drugs, non-viral gene delivery, vaccine administration, ocular drug delivery, electrodeposition, brain-targeted drug delivery, stability enhancement, mucosal drug delivery, controlled drug release, tissue engineering, and efficient insulin delivery. This comprehensive description delves into the characteristics of chitosan and its NPs, elucidating their innovative drug delivery applications across diverse domains [180]. Due to their favorable attributes such as biocompatibility, degradability, and lack of toxicity, chitosan NPs have garnered growing interest as a drug delivery system. These NPs have the potential to enhance the absorption and bioavailability of encapsulated drugs, including proteins and genes, safeguarding them against enzymatic degradation *in vivo*. Presently, chitosan NPs are undergoing modifications to enable sustained and controlled release, as well as targeted delivery. With ongoing discoveries and advancements in the active antitumor constituents of plant-based drugs, there is a future prospect for developing targeted chitosan carriers that ensure sustained and controlled release of such plant-derived therapeutics. Despite significant advances in utilizing chitosan NPs as drug carriers, several challenges still require prompt resolution. A notable issue is the limited solubility of chitosan, which restricts unmodified chitosan NPs to effectively encapsulate only certain hydrophilic drugs. While chitosan can be readily adapted to encapsulate hydrophobic drugs, additional research is necessary to thoroughly assess the biocompatibility of modified chitosan and its derivatives. In summary, chitosan and its derivatives exhibit promising potential as versatile drug carriers with broader applicability [181].

3. *Human serum albumin*

   Recent research has explored the potential of human serum albumin (HSA) NPs as viable drug carrier systems. A study focused on the preparation, characterization, and preservation of drug efficacy in DOX-loaded HSA NPs, with the resulting NPs having a size range of 150–500 nm and a loading efficiency of 70–90%. The impact on cell viability was evaluated in two distinct neuroblastoma cell lines, revealing that the NP-loaded drug exhibited enhanced anticancer effects compared to a DOX solution [182]. With a molecular weight of 66.5 kDa, HSA stands as the most abundant protein in the human body. Synthesized by the liver, it exhibits a half-life of approximately 19 days [183]. X-ray structural analysis has unveiled HSA's composition, characterized by three domains—denoted as I, II, and III. Within each of these domains, two subdomains (Ia, Ib, IIa, IIb, IIIa, and IIIb) assemble to create binding sites on the HSA molecules [184]. HSA exhibits the capability to bind with both metabolic substrates and therapeutic drugs, encompassing hydrophobic and hydrophilic compounds alike. The assembly of HSA NPs arises through the aggregation of HSA molecules in solution, giving rise to intermolecular disulfide bonds [185]. HSA NPs possess attributes such as biocompatibility, biodegradability, and non-immunogenicity [186]. The selectivity of HSA towards the glycoprotein 60 (gp60) receptor found on cancer cell surfaces facilitates the transportation of diverse anticancer drugs, including docetaxel, paclitaxel, and noscapine, all while avoiding an immune reaction [187]. Paclitaxel, marketed as Taxol, is a prominent anticancer medication extensively employed as a chemotherapy agent to address various cancer forms like breast, ovarian, and lung cancer. To counteract the detrimental impact of this formulation on healthy cells, Paclitaxel was combined with HSA NPs (known as Abraxane) for precise, targeted delivery [188]. As a result, this approach has resulted in enhanced tumor targeting, achieved by augmenting the EPR effect, in contrast to the administration of unbound drugs [189].

4. *Other polymers*

   Numerous other polymers have also been employed in the formulation of NPs for cancer therapy. In a study, NPs were developed utilizing a degradable poly(beta-amino ester) polymer named poly(butane dioldiacrylate-co-amino pentanol) (C32) [190]. These NPs were designed to deliver a diphtheria toxin suicide gene (DT-A) under the control of a prostate-specific promoter to target cells. The C32/DT-A NPs were administered via direct injection into both normal prostate tissue and prostate tumors in mice. The outcomes demonstrated that approximately 50% of normal prostates exhibited a notable reduction in size due to cellular apoptosis, while injection of naked DT-A-encoding DNA had minimal impact. Furthermore, notable apoptosis was also detected in prostate tumors that were injected with C32/DT-A NPs, and there was no observed harm to the neighboring tissue. The *in vivo* effectiveness and potential toxicity of a polymer–lipid hybrid NP formulation loaded with DOX (DOX-PLN) were investigated in a murine solid tumor model following intratumoral injection [191]. Unwanted drug-associated effects were carefully assessed, including the examination of histological and structural changes in tumor and heart tissues, along with the intratumoral (IT) distribution of DOX-PLN after IT treatment. The introduction of DOX-PLN through IT delivery resulted in remarkable tumor growth delays (TGDs) of 70% and 100% ($P<0.01$) for DOX doses of 0.1 and 0.2 mg, respectively. The study demonstrates the substantial *in vivo* cytotoxic efficacy of DOX-PLN against solid tumors, with minimal systemic repercussions. Tumors treated with DOX-PLN displayed significantly larger central necrotic regions compared to untreated tumors, and the remains of DOX-PLN were extensively distributed among the disintegrated cell debris. This suggests that the anticancer influence of DOX-PLN primarily arises from the combined outcomes of NP distribution via IT administration and the sustained drug release over a concise range.

2.4.2.1.3 Polymeric micelles

Polymeric micelles (PMs) are nanoscale core–shell structures that result from the self-assembly of amphiphilic block copolymers or graft copolymers. They exhibit an average diameter ranging from 10 to 100 nm and display a spherical morphology. PMs possess notable thermodynamic and kinetic properties and have found application in the targeted delivery of anticancer drugs to tumor sites [192]. Composite micelles, which include both a cisplatin (CP) (IV) prodrug and PTX, offer a mechanism for the release of effective anticancer compound CP (II) within cancer cells through intracellular reduction, and PTX is released via acid hydrolysis. The combined micelles exhibited a synergistic impact, resulting in decreased systemic toxicity and heightened effectiveness against tumors [193]. PMs possess the capability to function as intelligent drug carriers, enabling them to selectively target particular cancerous locations through a range of stimuli (both internal and external). This characteristic enhances the precision and effectiveness of targeted drug delivery based on micelles. This section also encompasses a comprehensive exploration of diverse types of triggers, along with the interactions between PM–anticancer drug complexes and these triggers, and their corresponding pharmacodynamics. To sum up, the potential strategy of commercializing engineered micelle nanoparticles (MNPs) for therapeutic and imaging purposes holds promise as a means to enhance the therapeutic index of anticancer medications [194]. The effectiveness of micelles as nanocarriers stems from their capacity to encapsulate hydrophobic drugs with low water solubility. These hydrophobic drug molecules are housed within the core, promoting improved solubility and stability of the micelles within the biological milieu. The hydrophilic segment shields the cargo by preventing its interaction with blood components. The nanoscale size of PMs allows them to evade the mononuclear phagocytic system (MPS), resulting in prolonged circulation times within the *in vivo* environment. This phenomenon is a result of the transition from blood circulation to the target tissue, facilitated by the EPR effect commonly observed in various tumors. The EPR effect is influenced by two pivotal factors: the nanoscale size of PMs and the distinct tumor pathophysiology. Tumor pathophysiology is characterized by compromised vascular integrity, atypical architecture, and the absence of a functional lymphatic drainage system. As a consequence, the nanoscale dimensions of PMs allow them to extravasate into the tumor interstitium, exploiting the leakiness of tumor vasculature and thereby augmenting their permeability within the tumor environment. Furthermore, the absence of functional lymphatic drainage within tumors contributes to the prolonged retention of PMs within the tumor microenvironment, thereby facilitating enhanced retention. This combined enhancement in permeability and retention effectively results in the passive localization of PMs at the intended target site [195]. Additionally, PMs can be surface-engineered through the incorporation of diverse ligands, enabling active targeting and consequently enabling the precise delivery of anticancer medications to specific sites.

2.4.2.1.4 Multifunctional polymeric micelles targeted for multidrug resistance in tumors

By combining various attributes, including active targeting ligands, the micelles can achieve site-specific drug release and on-demand release upon reaching the tumor, facilitated by trigger mechanisms. The incorporation of imaging agents further enables the *in vivo* tracking and localization of the micelles [196]. By incorporating both siRNA and drug resistance modulators alongside the chemotherapeutic agent, it becomes possible to concurrently suppress anti-apoptotic proteins and drug resistance genes. The potential of polymeric micelles as nanocarriers is comparable to that of NPs, liposomes, and other similar carriers in terms of commercial viability and availability. In fact, polymeric micelles stand out as one of the extensively researched delivery systems for effectively addressing diverse cancer types and non-cancer ailments [197]. Diverse targeting ligands can be affixed to facilitate cellular or intracellular accumulation at desired sites. Furthermore, integrating imaging agents or chelating moieties into the micelle architecture permits *in vivo* biodistribution investigations. Additionally, the incorporation of pH-responsive, temperature-sensitive, ultrasound-sensitive, enzyme-responsive, and light-responsive block copolymers enables controlled micelle breakdown and triggered drug release, responding to specific stimuli inherent to pathological environments or external signals. By combining these strategies, the potential to enhance both specificity and efficacy of drug delivery via micelles is heightened, promoting the advancement of intelligent multifunctional micelle platforms [198].

2.4.2.1.5 Dendrimers

Dendrimers are precisely engineered synthetic macromolecules characterized by their nanoscale size, radial symmetry, and uniform, well-defined structure featuring tree-like arms or branches. Within their compact molecular arrangement, dendrimers possess an array of functional groups, offering a diverse combination of properties [199]. A carrier composed of H(2)N-PEG-dendrimer-(COOH)(4), a PEG-dendrimer, was employed to deliver a combination of PTX and alendronate (ALN).

The PTX–PEG–ALN conjugate demonstrated an enhanced pharmacokinetic profile compared to free drugs, providing a solution for cancer bone metastases without requiring additional solubilizing agents. Dendritic polymers, akin to proteins, enzymes, and viruses, are easily functionalized and offer multiple advantages, including prolonged drug efficacy, high stability, water solubility, reduced immunogenicity, and diminished antigenicity. With these attributes, dendrimers have garnered significant interest for diverse biomedical applications such as drug and gene delivery, magnetic resonance imaging contrast agents, and sensor development [200]. The nanotheranostics platform is meticulously engineered to surpass diverse biological obstacles, precisely direct the payload to the intended site, and concurrently facilitate treatment planning, monitoring, and validation. This approach showcases improved therapeutic effectiveness by amalgamating targeted delivery with the ability to track and confirm treatment administration [201]. Therefore, a nanotheranostic platform holds the promise to facilitate targeted drug delivery, image-guided focal therapy, tracking drug release and distribution, foreseeing treatment response, and stratifying patients. Among these, dendrimers, a class of highly branched nanocarriers, stand out as an advanced nanotheranostic solution with the potential to revolutionize the field of oncology due to their distinctive and intriguing attributes. Dendrimers exhibit a well-defined three-dimensional globular chemical structure, exceptional uniformity in size, precise size regulation, and customizable surface functionalities. The consistent characteristics of dendrimers result in a predictable pharmacokinetic pattern, which in turn guarantees the intended biodistribution and effectiveness. This has led to the utilization of dendrimers as a nanotheranostic framework encompassing a wide array of therapeutic, imaging, and targeting components for the purpose of cancer diagnosis and treatment [202]. Dendrimers find significant utility as carriers for diverse anticancer drugs, constituting one of their primary applications. The modifiable structure and surface properties of dendrimers facilitate the encapsulation or coupling of numerous components, either within their core or on their surface, making them well-suited carriers for a variety of anticancer drugs. Developing drug delivery systems based on dendrimers involves incorporating drugs through either physical adsorption or chemical conjugation. In conventional dendrimer-mediated drug delivery systems for cancer treatment, the primary objectives include enhancing the solubility of anticancer agents, bolstering the stability of sensitive drugs, augmenting drug bioavailability, and mitigating adverse effects. Given that numerous anticancer drug compounds lack reactive functional groups, the physical adsorption approach holds greater appeal and is extensively employed for loading hydrophobic anticancer drugs, as opposed to chemical conjugation [203]. The interaction between dendrimers and drug molecules is influenced by factors such as drug polarity, size, and chemical structure, leading to varied approaches for physically incorporating anticancer drugs within dendrimers—either within the central cavity or on the outer surface. For instance, utilizing polyester dendrimers to encapsulate the hydrophobic antitumor drug camptothecin enhances its water solubility from 20 to 240 $\mu mol\ l^{-1}$ [204]. Immunodendrimers were developed for ovarian cancer therapy by attaching mAbK1 to half-generation poly(propyleneimine) (PPI) dendrimers. Paclitaxel

(PTX) was encapsulated within the hydrophobic nanodomains of PPI dendrimers, with approximately 30% of the drug being captured within the dendrimers at a ratio of 4:1 (drug to dendrimer). The resulting formulation, mAbK1–PPI–PTX, underwent testing in an ovarian cancer model, demonstrating notable reduction in tumor volume and extended survival in animals. These outcomes were attributed to the improved drug uptake within the tumor site [205]. Dendrimers are intricate three-dimensional molecules characterized by extensive branching, ranging from 1 to 10 nm in size. They exhibit distinctive physicochemical attributes, including: (1) minimal cytotoxicity, (2) exceptional cellular penetration efficiency, and (3) an inherent 'autofluorescence capability' that permits tracking of their behavior within cells and living organisms [206]. Dendrimers can be synthesized through various approaches, among which are the divergent growth method, convergent method, hypercore and branched method, and double and mixed exponential growth method. However, the widely employed techniques are the divergent and convergent methods [207]. The divergent method initiates dendrimer synthesis from the core, gradually adding individual monomers under precise physicochemical conditions until the desired generation of dendrimer is attained. As each subsequent dendrimer generation is created, the number of branches is doubled. This approach offers the advantage of potentially achieving greater reaction efficiency, although it comes at the cost of synthesized compound purity and the possibility of structural defects arising from the inherent nature of the reaction [208].

2.5 Conclusion

In conclusion, nanoplatform-based imaging for cancer diagnosis is a rapidly evolving and promising field that utilizes nanoscale materials to revolutionize cancer detection and monitoring. The integration of nanomaterials with various imaging modalities offers numerous advantages, such as enhanced sensitivity and accuracy, improved targeting capabilities, and multimodal imaging options. This innovative approach holds great potential for advancing early cancer detection and facilitating personalized medicine for improved patient outcomes.

One of the fundamental aspects of nanoplatform-based imaging is the selection of appropriate nanomaterials. These materials should possess specific properties, such as biocompatibility, stability, and the ability to carry imaging agents or therapeutic payloads. NPs, quantum dots, and nanotubes are examples of nanomaterials that have shown promise in cancer imaging applications.

Imaging modalities are another critical factor in nanoplatform-based cancer diagnosis. Techniques like fluorescence imaging, computed tomography (CT), magnetic resonance imaging (MRI), and photoacoustic imaging (PAI) can be integrated with nanoplatforms to provide complementary information and improve overall diagnostic accuracy. Each imaging modality has its strengths and weaknesses, and the selection of the appropriate imaging method depends on the specific requirements of the cancer diagnosis. Targeting strategies play a pivotal role in nanoplatform-based imaging for cancer diagnosis. By incorporating targeting ligands or antibodies onto the nanoplatforms' surface, specific cancer cells or tissues can be selectively labeled, enhancing the imaging contrast and minimizing off-target effects. This targeted approach improves the accuracy of cancer diagnosis and allows for early detection of tumors. Contrast enhancement is a crucial aspect of nanoplatform-based imaging. Nanomaterials can act as contrast agents, significantly improving the visibility of cancerous tissues during imaging procedures. The use of contrast agents helps distinguish between healthy and cancerous tissues, enabling precise tumor localization and facilitating early intervention.

The concept of multimodal imaging, which combines two or more imaging modalities, further enhances the diagnostic capabilities of nanoplatforms. Multimodal imaging provides comprehensive information about the tumor microenvironment, improving the accuracy of cancer staging and treatment planning. Nanoplatforms' theranostic approach, which integrates both diagnosis and therapy, is particularly promising for cancer management. Nanoplatforms can simultaneously carry imaging agents for diagnosis and therapeutic agents for targeted treatment. This approach allows for real-time monitoring of treatment efficacy and enhances the potential for personalized therapy. Ensuring the biocompatibility and safety of nanoplatforms is of utmost importance for clinical translation. Thorough preclinical evaluations are necessary to assess potential toxicities and immune responses. Biocompatible nanoplatforms are essential for their safe use in cancer diagnosis and therapy.

In conclusion, nanoplatform-based imaging for cancer diagnosis holds immense promise for improving cancer detection, staging, and treatment monitoring. By harnessing the unique properties of nanomaterials and integrating various imaging modalities, nanoplatforms offer a multifunctional and precise approach to cancer diagnosis, opening new frontiers in personalized medicine and advancing patient care. However, further research and clinical trials are needed to fully realize the potential of nanoplatform-based imaging and ensure its safe and effective implementation in cancer diagnostics.

Acknowledgments

Ranjan G and Dasgupta S contributed equally to this work. Pattanayak S P revised the whole manuscript. We are grateful for financial support from the Department of Science and Technology under the DST-INSPIRE Fellowship (DST/INSPIRE FELLOWSHIP/2020/IF200148).

Conflict of interest

The authors declare that there are no conflicts of interest.

References

[1] Mansoori G A and Soelaiman T A F 2005 *Nanotechnology—An Introduction for the Standards Community* (West Conshohocken, PA: ASTM International)

[2] Gnach A, Lipinski T, Bednarkiewicz A, Rybka J and Capobianco J A 2015 Upconverting nanoparticles: assessing the toxicity *Chem. Soc. Rev.* **44** 1561–84

[3] Liu Z, Tabakman S, Welsher K and Dai H 2009 Carbon nanotubes in biology and medicine: *in vitro* and *in vivo* detection, imaging and drug delivery *Nano Res.* **2** 85–120
[4] Orive G, Gascon A R, Hernández R M, Domínguez-Gil A and Pedraz J L 2004 Techniques: new approaches to the delivery of biopharmaceuticals *Trends Pharmacol. Sci.* **25** 382–7
[5] Patra J K and Baek K-H 2015 Green nanobiotechnology: factors affecting synthesis and characterization techniques *J. Nanomater.* **2014** 219
[6] Mirza A Z and Siddiqui F A 2014 Nanomedicine and drug delivery: a mini review *Int. Nano Lett.* **4** 1–7
[7] Jahangirian H, Lemraski E G, Webster T J, Rafiee-Moghaddam R and Abdollahi Y 2017 A review of drug delivery systems based on nanotechnology and green chemistry: green nanomedicine *Int. J. Nanomed.* 2957–78
[8] Lam P-L, Wong W-Y, Bian Z, Chui C-H and Gambari R 2017 Recent advances in green nanoparticulate systems for drug delivery: efficient delivery and safety concern *Nanomedicine* **12** 357–85
[9] Astefanei A, Núñez O and Galceran M T 2015 Characterisation and determination of fullerenes: a critical review *Anal. Chim. Acta* **882** 1–21
[10] Ibrahim K S 2013 Carbon nanotubes? Properties and applications: a review *Carbon Lett.* **14** 131–44
[11] Aqel A, Abou El-Nour K M M, Ammar R A A and Al-Warthan A 2012 Carbon nanotubes, science and technology, part I: structure, synthesis and characterisation *Arab. J. Chem.* **5** 1–23
[12] Elliott J A, Shibuta Y, Amara H, Bichara C and Neyts E C 2013 Atomistic modelling of CVD synthesis of carbon nanotubes and graphene *Nanoscale* **5** 6662–76
[13] Saeed K and Khan I 2016 Preparation and characterization of single-walled carbon nanotube/nylon 6, 6 nanocomposites *Instrum Sci. Technol.* **44** 435–44
[14] Saeed K and Khan I 2014 Preparation and properties of single-walled carbon nanotubes/ poly (butylene terephthalate) nanocomposites *Iran. Polym. J.* **23** 53–8
[15] Mabena L F, Sinha Ray S, Mhlanga S D and Coville N J 2011 Nitrogen-doped carbon nanotubes as a metal catalyst support *Appl. Nanosci.* **1** 67–77
[16] Thomas S C, Mishra P K and Talegaonkar S 2015 Ceramic nanoparticles: fabrication methods and applications in drug delivery *Curr. Pharm. Des* **21** 6165–88
[17] Ali S, Khan I, Khan S A, Sohail M, Ahmed R, ur Rehman A *et al* 2017 Electrocatalytic performance of Ni@ Pt core–shell nanoparticles supported on carbon nanotubes for methanol oxidation reaction *J. Electroanal. Chem.* **795** 17–25
[18] Sun S, Murray C B, Weller D, Folks L and Moser A 2000 Monodisperse FePt nanoparticles and ferromagnetic FePt nanocrystal superlattices *Science* **287** 1989–92
[19] Hisatomi T, Kubota J and Domen K 2014 Recent advances in semiconductors for photocatalytic and photoelectrochemical water splitting *Chem. Soc. Rev.* **43** 7520–35
[20] Mansha M, Khan I, Ullah N and Qurashi A 2017 Synthesis, characterization and visible-light-driven photoelectrochemical hydrogen evolution reaction of carbazole-containing conjugated polymers *Int. J. Hydrogen Energy* **42** 10952–61
[21] Rao J P and Geckeler K E 2011 Polymer nanoparticles: preparation techniques and size-control parameters *Prog. Polym. Sci.* **36** 887–913
[22] Abd Ellah N H and Abouelmagd S A 2017 Surface functionalization of polymeric nanoparticles for tumor drug delivery: approaches and challenges *Expert Opin. Drug Deliv* **14** 201–14

[23] Silva A M, Alvarado H L, Abrego G, Martins-Gomes C, Garduño-Ramirez M L, García M L *et al* 2019 *In vitro* cytotoxicity of oleanolic/ursolic acids-loaded in PLGA nanoparticles in different cell lines *Pharmaceutics* **11** 362

[24] Carbone C, Martins-Gomes C, Pepe V, Silva A M, Musumeci T, Puglisi G *et al* 2018 Repurposing itraconazole to the benefit of skin cancer treatment: a combined azole-DDAB nanoencapsulation strategy *Colloids Surf. B Biointerfaces* **167** 337–44

[25] Doktorovova S, Souto E B and Silva A M 2014 Nanotoxicology applied to solid lipid nanoparticles and nanostructured lipid carriers—a systematic review of *in vitro* data *Eur. J. Pharm. Biopharm.* **87** 1–18

[26] Rawat M K, Jain A and Singh S 2011 Studies on binary lipid matrix based solid lipid nanoparticles of repaglinide: *in vitro* and *in vivo* evaluation *J. Pharm. Sci.* **100** 2366–78

[27] Puri A, Loomis K, Smith B, Lee J-H, Yavlovich A, Heldman E *et al* 2009 Lipid-based nanoparticles as pharmaceutical drug carriers: from concepts to clinic *Crit. Rev. Ther. Drug Carr. Syst.* **26** 523–580

[28] Gujrati M, Malamas A, Shin T, Jin E, Sun Y and Lu Z-R 2014 Multifunctional cationic lipid-based nanoparticles facilitate endosomal escape and reduction-triggered cytosolic siRNA release *Mol. Pharm* **11** 2734–44

[29] Wang Y and Xia Y 2004 Bottom-up and top-down approaches to the synthesis of monodispersed spherical colloids of low melting-point metals *Nano Lett.* **4** 2047–50

[30] Siafaka P I, Üstündağ Okur N, Karavas E and Bikiaris D N 2016 Surface modified multifunctional and stimuli responsive nanoparticles for drug targeting: current status and uses *Int. J. Mol. Sci.* **17** 1440

[31] Chen X, Wang T, Le W, Huang X, Gao M, Chen Q *et al* 2020 Smart sorting of tumor phenotype with versatile fluorescent Ag nanoclusters by sensing specific reactive oxygen species *Theranostics* **10** 3430

[32] Qi B, Crawford A J, Wojtynek N E, Talmon G A, Hollingsworth M A, Ly Q P *et al* 2020 Tuned near infrared fluorescent hyaluronic acid conjugates for delivery to pancreatic cancer for intraoperative imaging *Theranostics* **10** 3413

[33] Muthu M S, Leong D T, Mei L and Feng S-S 2014 Nanotheranostics-application and further development of nanomedicine strategies for advanced theranostics *Theranostics* **4** 660

[34] Shao L, Li Q, Zhao C, Lu J, Li X, Chen L *et al* 2019 Auto-fluorescent polymer nanotheranostics for self-monitoring of cancer therapy via triple-collaborative strategy *Biomaterials* **194** 105–16

[35] Fu F, Wu Y, Zhu J, Wen S, Shen M and Shi X 2014 Multifunctional lactobionic acid-modified dendrimers for targeted drug delivery to liver cancer cells: investigating the role played by PEG spacer *ACS Appl. Mater. Interfaces* **6** 16416–25

[36] Wang J T W, Hodgins N O, Maher J, Sosabowski J K and Al-Jamal K T 2020 Organ biodistribution of radiolabelled $\gamma\delta$ T cells following liposomal alendronate administration in different mouse tumour models *Nanotheranostics* **4** 71

[37] Costa P M, Wang J T-W, Morfin J-F, Khanum T, To W, Sosabowski J *et al* 2018 Functionalised carbon nanotubes enhance brain delivery of amyloid-targeting Pittsburgh compound B (PiB)-derived ligands *Nanotheranostics* **2** 168

[38] Li G, Pei M and Liu P 2020 pH/Reduction dual-responsive comet-shaped PEGylated CQD–DOX conjugate prodrug: synthesis and self-assembly as tumor nanotheranostics *Mater. Sci. Eng.* C **110** 110653

[39] Govindasamy M, Manavalan S, Chen S-M, Rajaji U, Chen T-W, Al-Hemaid F M A *et al* 2018 Determination of neurotransmitter in biological and drug samples using gold nanorods decorated f-MWCNTs modified electrode *J. Electrochem. Soc.* **165** B370

[40] Karthik R, Govindasamy M, Chen S-M, Chen T-W, Elangovan A, Muthuraj V *et al* 2017 A facile graphene oxide based sensor for electrochemical detection of prostate anti-cancer (anti-testosterone) drug flutamide in biological samples *RSC Adv.* **7** 25702–9

[41] Sung S-Y, Su Y-L, Cheng W, Hu P-F, Chiang C-S, Chen W-T *et al* 2018 Graphene quantum dots-mediated theranostic penetrative delivery of drug and photolytics in deep tumors by targeted biomimetic nanosponges *Nano Lett.* **19** 69–81

[42] Filippousi M, Papadimitriou S A, Bikiaris D N, Pavlidou E, Angelakeris M, Zamboulis D *et al* 2013 Novel core–shell magnetic nanoparticles for Taxol encapsulation in biodegradable and biocompatible block copolymers: preparation, characterization and release properties *Int. J. Pharm.* **448** 221–30

[43] Filippousi M, Altantzis T, Stefanou G, Betsiou M, Bikiaris D N, Angelakeris M *et al* 2013 Polyhedral iron oxide core–shell nanoparticles in a biodegradable polymeric matrix: preparation, characterization and application in magnetic particle hyperthermia and drug delivery *RSC Adv.* **3** 24367–77

[44] Pelaz B, Alexiou C, Alvarez-Puebla R A, Alves F, Andrews A M, Ashraf S *et al* 2017 Diverse applications of nanomedicine *ACS Nano* **11** 2313–81

[45] Zhao Y, Fletcher N L, Liu T, Gemmell A C, Houston Z H, Blakey I *et al* 2018 *In vivo* therapeutic evaluation of polymeric nanomedicines: effect of different targeting peptides on therapeutic efficacy against breast cancer *Nanotheranostics* **2** 360

[46] Sharma M, Dube T, Chibh S, Kour A, Mishra J and Panda J J 2019 Nanotheranostics, a future remedy of neurological disorders *Expert Opin. Drug Deliv.* **16** 113–28

[47] Paul A, Hasan A, Kindi H, Al Gaharwar A K, Rao V T S, Nikkhah M *et al* 2014 Injectable graphene oxide/hydrogel-based angiogenic gene delivery system for vasculogenesis and cardiac repair *ACS Nano* **8** 8050–62

[48] Ge J, Zhang Q, Zeng J, Gu Z and Gao M 2020 Radiolabeling nanomaterials for multimodality imaging: new insights into nuclear medicine and cancer diagnosis *Biomaterials* **228** 119553

[49] Han N, Yang Y Y, Wang S, Zheng S and Fan W 2013 . Polymer-based cancer nanotheranostics: retrospectives of multi-functionalities and pharmacokinetics *Curr. Drug Metab.* **14** 661–74

[50] Ferlay J, Colombet M, Soerjomataram I, Mathers C, Parkin D M, Piñeros M *et al* 2019 Estimating the global cancer incidence and mortality in 2018: GLOBOCAN sources and methods *Int. J. Cancer* **144** 1941–53

[51] Siegel R L, Miller K D and Jemal A 2018 Cancer statistics *CA Cancer J. Clin.* **68** 7–30

[52] Cheng L, Wang C, Feng L, Yang K and Liu Z 2014 Functional nanomaterials for phototherapies of cancer *Chem. Rev.* **114** 10869–939

[53] Yun S H and Kwok S J J 2017 Light in diagnosis, therapy and surgery *Nat. Biomed. Eng.* **1** 8

[54] Allhoff F 2007 On the autonomy and justification of nanoethics *Nanoethics* **1** 185–210

[55] American Cancer Society 2008 *Cancer Facts & Figures* (Atlanta, GA: American Cancer Society)

[56] Chen H, Zhang W, Zhu G, Xie J and Chen X 2017 Rethinking cancer nanotheranostics *Nat. Rev. Mater* **2** 1–18

[57] Shi J, Kantoff P W, Wooster R and Farokhzad O C 2017 Cancer nanomedicine: progress, challenges and opportunities *Nat. Rev. Cancer* **17** 20–37

[58] Thu M S, Bryant L H, Coppola T, Jordan E K, Budde M D, Lewis B K *et al* 2012 Self-assembling nanocomplexes by combining ferumoxytol, heparin and protamine for cell tracking by magnetic resonance imaging *Nat. Med.* **18** 463–7

[59] Khurana A, Nejadnik H, Gawande R, Lin G, Lee S, Messing S *et al* 2012 Intravenous ferumoxytol allows noninvasive MR imaging monitoring of macrophage migration into stem cell transplants *Radiology* **264** 803–11

[60] Bobo D, Robinson K J, Islam J, Thurecht K J and Corrie S 2016 Nanoparticle-based medicines: a review of FDA-approved materials and clinical trials to date *Pharm. Res.* **33** 2373–87

[61] Kim D-H, Nikles D E, Johnson D T and Brazel C S 2008 Heat generation of aqueously dispersed $CoFe_2O_4$ nanoparticles as heating agents for magnetically activated drug delivery and hyperthermia *J. Magn. Magn. Mater.* **320** 2390–6

[62] Kim D-H, Nikles D E and Brazel C S 2010 Synthesis and characterization of multifunctional chitosan-$MnFe_2O_4$ nanoparticles for magnetic hyperthermia and drug delivery *Materials (Basel)* **3** 4051–65

[63] Park W, Cho S, Huang X, Larson A C and Kim D 2017 Branched gold nanoparticle coating of *Clostridium novyi*-NT spores for CT-guided intratumoral injection *Small* **13** 1602722

[64] Kim D-H, Rozhkova E A, Ulasov I V, Bader S D, Rajh T, Lesniak M S *et al* 2010 Biofunctionalized magnetic-vortex microdiscs for targeted cancer-cell destruction *Nat. Mater.* **9** 165–71

[65] Kim D-H, Vitol E A, Liu J, Balasubramanian S, Gosztola D J, Cohen E E *et al* 2013 Stimuli-responsive magnetic nanomicelles as multifunctional heat and cargo delivery vehicles *Langmuir* **29** 7425–32

[66] Kim D, Guo Y, Zhang Z, Procissi D, Nicolai J, Omary R A *et al* 2014 Temperature-sensitive magnetic drug carriers for concurrent gemcitabine chemohyperthermia *Adv. Healthc. Mater* **3** 714–24

[67] Sun J, Kim D-H, Guo Y, Teng Z, Li Y, Zheng L *et al* 2015 A C (RGDfE) conjugated multi-functional nanomedicine delivery system for targeted pancreatic cancer therapy *J. Mater. Chem.* B **3** 1049–58

[68] Egusquiaguirre S P, Igartua M, Hernández R M and Pedraz J L 2012 Nanoparticle delivery systems for cancer therapy: advances in clinical and preclinical research *Clin. Transl. Oncol.* **14** 83–93

[69] Silverman S G, Deuson T E, Kane N, Adams D F, Seltzer S E, Phillips M D *et al* 1998 Percutaneous abdominal biopsy: cost-identification analysis *Radiology* **206** 429–35

[70] Link R E, Permpongkosol S, Gupta A, Jarrett T W, Solomon S B and Kavoussi L R 2006 Cost analysis of open, laparoscopic, and percutaneous treatment options for nephron-sparing surgery *J. Endourol.* **20** 782–9

[71] Lee J, Gordon A C, Kim H, Park W, Cho S, Lee B *et al* 2016 Targeted multimodal nano-reporters for pre-procedural MRI and intra-operative image-guidance *Biomaterials* **109** 69–77

[72] Hu Z, Chi C, Liu M, Guo H, Zhang Z, Zeng C *et al* 2017 Nanoparticle-mediated radiopharmaceutical-excited fluorescence molecular imaging allows precise image-guided tumor-removal surgery *Nanomed. Nanotechnol. Biol. Med.* **13** 1323–31

[73] Park W, Gordon A C, Cho S, Huang X, Harris K R, Larson A C *et al* 2017 Immunomodulatory magnetic microspheres for augmenting tumor-specific infiltration of natural killer (NK) cells *ACS Appl. Mater. Interfaces* **9** 13819–24
[74] Tomitaka A, Arami H, Raymond A, Yndart A, Kaushik A, Jayant R D *et al* 2017 Development of magneto-plasmonic nanoparticles for multimodal image-guided therapy to the brain *Nanoscale* **9** 764–73
[75] Cho S, Park W and Kim D-H 2017 Silica-coated metal chelating-melanin nanoparticles as a dual-modal contrast enhancement imaging and therapeutic agent *ACS Appl. Mater. Interfaces* **9** 101–11
[76] Li Y, Lin T, Luo Y, Liu Q, Xiao W, Guo W *et al* 2014 A smart and versatile theranostic nanomedicine platform based on nanoporphyrin *Nat. Commun.* **5** 4712
[77] Kim D-H and Larson A C 2015 Deoxycholate bile acid directed synthesis of branched Au nanostructures for near infrared photothermal ablation *Biomaterials* **56** 154–64
[78] Zhao K, Cho S, Procissi D, Larson A C and Kim D 2017 Non-invasive monitoring of branched Au nanoparticle-mediated photothermal ablation *J. Biomed. Mater. Res. Part B Appl. Biomater.* **105** 2352–9
[79] White S B, Kim D-H, Guo Y, Li W, Yang Y, Chen J *et al* 2017 Biofunctionalized hybrid magnetic gold nanoparticles as catalysts for photothermal ablation of colorectal liver metastases *Radiology* **285** 809–19
[80] Detappe A, Thomas E, Tibbitt M W, Kunjachan S, Zavidij O, Parnandi N *et al* 2017 Ultrasmall silica-based bismuth gadolinium nanoparticles for dual magnetic resonance–computed tomography image guided radiation therapy *Nano Lett.* **17** 1733–40
[81] Zhou H, Qian W, Uckun F M, Wang L, Wang Y A, Chen H *et al* 2015 IGF1 receptor targeted theranostic nanoparticles for targeted and image-guided therapy of pancreatic cancer *ACS Nano* **9** 7976–91
[82] Gao N, Bozeman E N, Qian W, Wang L, Chen H, Lipowska M *et al* 2017 Tumor penetrating theranostic nanoparticles for enhancement of targeted and image-guided drug delivery into peritoneal tumors following intraperitoneal delivery *Theranostics* **7** 1689
[83] Kim D-H, Li W, Chen J, Zhang Z, Green R M, Huang S *et al* 2016 Multimodal imaging of nanocomposite microspheres for transcatheter intra-arterial drug delivery to liver tumors *Sci. Rep.* **6** 29653
[84] Kim D-H, Chen J, Omary R A and Larson A C 2015 MRI visible drug eluting magnetic microspheres for transcatheter intra-arterial delivery to liver tumors *Theranostics* **5** 477
[85] Jeon M J, Gordon A C, Larson A C, Chung J W, Kim Y and Kim D-H 2016 Transcatheter intra-arterial infusion of doxorubicin loaded porous magnetic nano-clusters with iodinated oil for the treatment of liver cancer *Biomaterials* **88** 25–33
[86] Chen X S 2011 Introducing theranostics journal—from the editor-in-chief *Theranostics* **1** 1
[87] Zhang F, Zhu L, Liu G, Hida N, Lu G, Eden H S *et al* 2011 Multimodality imaging of tumor response to doxil *Theranostics* **1** 302
[88] Ferrari M 2005 Cancer nanotechnology: opportunities and challenges *Nat. Rev. Cancer* **5** 161–71
[89] Yang J, Lee C, Ko H, Suh J, Yoon H, Lee K *et al* 2007 Multifunctional magneto-polymeric nanohybrids for targeted detection and synergistic therapeutic effects on breast cancer *Angew Chem. Int. Ed.* **46** 8836–9
[90] Namiki Y, Namiki T, Yoshida H, Ishii Y, Tsubota A, Koido S *et al* 2009 A novel magnetic crystal–lipid nanostructure for magnetically guided *in vivo* gene delivery *Nat. Nanotechnol.* **4** 598–606

[91] Day E S, Bickford L R, Slater J H, Riggall N S, Drezek R A and West J L 2010 Antibody-conjugated gold–gold sulfide nanoparticles as multifunctional agents for imaging and therapy of breast cancer *Int. J. Nanomed.* **2010:5** 445–54

[92] Kim S, Ohulchanskyy T Y, Pudavar H E, Pandey R K and Prasad P N 2007 Organically modified silica nanoparticles co-encapsulating photosensitizing drug and aggregation-enhanced two-photon absorbing fluorescent dye aggregates for two-photon photodynamic therapy *J. Am. Chem. Soc.* **129** 2669–75

[93] Loo C, Lowery A, Halas N, West J and Drezek R 2005 Immunotargeted nanoshells for integrated cancer imaging and therapy *Nano Lett.* **5** 709–11

[94] Huang X, El-Sayed I H, Qian W and El-Sayed M A 2006 Cancer cell imaging and photothermal therapy in the near-infrared region by using gold nanorods *J. Am. Chem. Soc.* **128** 2115–20

[95] Kenny G D, Kamaly N, Kalber T L, Brody L P, Sahuri M, Shamsaei E *et al* 2011 Novel multifunctional nanoparticle mediates siRNA tumour delivery, visualisation and therapeutic tumour reduction *in vivo J. Control. Release* **149** 111–6

[96] McCarthy J R, Perez J M, Brückner C and Weissleder R 2005 Polymeric nanoparticle preparation that eradicates tumors *Nano Lett.* **5** 2552–6

[97] Robinson J T, Welsher K, Tabakman S M, Sherlock S P, Wang H, Luong R *et al* 2010 High performance *in vivo* near-IR (>1 μm) imaging and photothermal cancer therapy with carbon nanotubes *Nano Res.* **3** 201779–93

[98] Kim J-H, Kim Y-S, Park K, Lee S, Nam H Y, Min K H *et al* 2008 Antitumor efficacy of cisplatin-loaded glycol chitosan nanoparticles in tumor-bearing mice *J. Control. Release* **127** 41–9

[99] Huh M S, Lee S-Y, Park S, Lee S, Chung H, Lee S *et al* 2010 Tumor-homing glycol chitosan/polyethylenimine nanoparticles for the systemic delivery of siRNA in tumor-bearing mice *J. Control. Release* **144** 134–43

[100] Gianella A, Jarzyna P A, Mani V, Ramachandran S, Calcagno C, Tang J *et al* 2011 Multifunctional nanoemulsion platform for imaging guided therapy evaluated in experimental cancer *ACS Nano* **5** 4422–33

[101] Sanson C, Diou O, Thevenot J, Ibarboure E, Soum A, Brûlet A *et al* 2011 Doxorubicin loaded magnetic polymersomes: theranostic nanocarriers for MR imaging and magneto-chemotherapy *ACS Nano* **5** 1122–40

[102] Hwu J R, Lin Y S, Josephrajan T, Hsu M-H, Cheng F-Y, Yeh C-S *et al* 2009 Targeted paclitaxel by conjugation to iron oxide and gold nanoparticles *J. Am. Chem. Soc.* **131** 66–8

[103] Lee J-H, Huh Y-M, Jun Y, Seo J, Jang J, Song H-T *et al* 2007 Artificially engineered magnetic nanoparticles for ultra-sensitive molecular imaging *Nat. Med.* **13** 95–9

[104] Piao Y, Kim J, Na H B, Kim D, Baek J S, Ko M K *et al* 2008 Wrap–bake–peel process for nanostructural transformation from β-FeOOH nanorods to biocompatible iron oxide nanocapsules *Nat. Mater.* **7** 242–7

[105] Canese R, Vurro F and Marzola P 2021 Iron oxide nanoparticles as theranostic agents in cancer immunotherapy *Nanomaterials* **11** 1950

[106] Zhang L, Xiao S, Kang X, Sun T, Zhou C, Xu Z *et al* 2021 Metabolic conversion and removal of manganese ferrite nanoparticles in RAW264. 7 cells and induced alteration of metal transporter gene expression *Int. J. Nanomed.* 1709–24

[107] Roy I, Ohulchanskyy T Y, Pudavar H E, Bergey E J, Oseroff A R, Morgan J *et al* 2003 Ceramic-based nanoparticles entrapping water-insoluble photosensitizing anticancer drugs: a novel drug-carrier system for photodynamic therapy *J. Am. Chem. Soc.* **125** 7860–5
[108] Park J-H, Gu L, Von Maltzahn G, Ruoslahti E, Bhatia S N and Sailor M J 2009 Biodegradable luminescent porous silicon nanoparticles for *in vivo* applications *Nat. Mater.* **8** 331–6
[109] Schipper M L, Nakayama-Ratchford N, Davis C R, Kam N W S, Chu P, Liu Z *et al* 2008 A pilot toxicology study of single-walled carbon nanotubes in a small sample of mice *Nat. Nanotechnol.* **3** 216–21
[110] Guo W, Chen Z, Tan L, Gu D, Ren X, Fu C *et al* 2022 Emerging biocompatible nanoplatforms for the potential application in diagnosis and therapy of deep tumors *View* **3** 20200174
[111] Rieffel J, Chitgupi U and Lovell J F 2015 Recent advances in higher-order, multimodal, biomedical imaging agents *Small* **11** 4445–61
[112] Yin S, Song G, Yang Y, Zhao Y, Wang P, Zhu L *et al* 2019 Persistent regulation of tumor microenvironment via circulating catalysis of $MnFe_2O_4$@ metal–organic frameworks for enhanced photodynamic therapy *Adv. Funct. Mater.* **29** 1901417
[113] Sun P, Wu Q, Sun X, Miao H, Deng W, Zhang W *et al* 2018 J-Aggregate squaraine nanoparticles with bright NIR-II fluorescence for imaging guided photothermal therapy *Chem. Commun.* **54** 13395–8
[114] Wang H-S, Li J, Li J-Y, Wang K, Ding Y and Xia X-H 2017 Lanthanide-based metal–organic framework nanosheets with unique fluorescence quenching properties for two-color intracellular adenosine imaging in living cells *NPG Asia Mater.* **9** e354–4
[115] Li Y-A, Zhao C-W, Zhu N-X, Liu Q-K, Chen G-J, Liu J-B *et al* 2015 Nanoscale UiO–MOF-based luminescent sensors for highly selective detection of cysteine and glutathione and their application in bioimaging *Chem. Commun.* **51** 17672–5
[116] Ai T, Shang W, Yan H, Zeng C, Wang K, Gao Y *et al* 2018 Near infrared-emitting persistent luminescent nanoparticles for hepatocellular carcinoma imaging and luminescence-guided surgery *Biomaterials* **167** 216–25
[117] Shen Z, Song J, Zhou Z, Yung B C, Aronova M A, Li Y *et al* 2018 Dotted core–shell nanoparticles for T1-weighted MRI of tumors *Adv. Mater.* **30** 1803163
[118] Liu Y, Bhattarai P, Dai Z and Chen X 2019 Photothermal therapy and photoacoustic imaging via nanotheranostics in fighting cancer *Chem. Soc. Rev.* **48** 2053–108
[119] Yang M, Fan Q, Zhang R, Cheng K, Yan J, Pan D *et al* 2015 Dragon fruit-like biocage as an iron trapping nanoplatform for high efficiency targeted cancer multimodality imaging *Biomaterials* **69** 30–7
[120] Wang W, Hao C, Sun M, Xu L, Xu C and Kuang H 2018 Spiky Fe_3O_4@ Au supraparticles for multimodal *in vivo* imaging *Adv. Funct. Mater.* **28** 1800310
[121] Sun X, Hong Y, Gong Y, Zheng S and Xie D 2021 Bioengineered ferritin nanocarriers for cancer therapy *Int. J. Mol. Sci.* **22** 7023
[122] Villavicencio T C R and Paredes G C 2019 Initial prehospital management of pain in patients over 12 years old with trauma *Rev. Inv. Acad. Educ. ISTCRE* **3** 84–5 https://www.revistaacademica-istcre.edu.ec/articulo/35
[123] Webster D M, Sundaram P and Byrne M E 2013 Injectable nanomaterials for drug delivery: carriers, targeting moieties, and therapeutics *Eur. J. Pharm. Biopharm.* **84** 1–20

[124] Yong K-T, Wang Y, Roy I, Rui H, Swihart M T, Law W-C *et al* 2012 Preparation of quantum dot/drug nanoparticle formulations for traceable targeted delivery and therapy *Theranostics* **2** 681

[125] Yezhelyev M V, Gao X, Xing Y, Al-Hajj A, Nie S and O'Regan R M 2006 Emerging use of nanoparticles in diagnosis and treatment of breast cancer *Lancet Oncol.* **7** 657–67

[126] Ligresti G, Libra M, Militello L, Clementi S, Donia M, Imbesi R *et al* 2008 Breast cancer: molecular basis and therapeutic strategies *Mol. Med. Rep.* **1** 451–8

[127] Tan J M, Arulselvan P, Fakurazi S, Ithnin H and Hussein M Z 2014 A review on characterizations and biocompatibility of functionalized carbon nanotubes in drug delivery design *J. Nanomater.* **2014** 111

[128] Perk J, De Backer G, Gohlke H, Graham I, Reiner Ž, Verschuren M *et al* 2012 European guidelines on cardiovascular disease prevention in clinical practice (version 2012) *Eur. Heart J.* **33** 1635–701

[129] Wong H L, Bendayan R, Rauth A M and Wu X Y 2006 Simultaneous delivery of doxorubicin and GG918 (Elacridar) by new polymer–lipid hybrid nanoparticles (PLN) for enhanced treatment of multidrug-resistant breast cancer *J. Control. Release* **116** 275–84

[130] Vanitha M K, Sakthisekaran D and Anandakumar P 2014 Breast cancer: types, epidemiology and aeitiology, a review *Adv. J. Pharm. Life Sci. Res.* **2** 29–38

[131] Casals-Molina M L, Cab C, Canto G, Medina J and Tapia A 2018 Carbon nanomaterials for breast cancer treatment *J. Nanomater.* **2018** 1–9

[132] Ronchi A, Pagliuca F, Marino F Z, Accardo M, Cozzolino I and Franco R 2021 Current and potential immunohistochemical biomarkers for prognosis and therapeutic stratification of breast carcinoma *Seminars in Cancer Biology* (Amsterdam: Elsevier) pp 114–22

[133] Nielsen U B, Kirpotin D B, Pickering E M, Hong K, Park J W, Shalaby M R *et al* 2002 Therapeutic efficacy of anti-ErbB2 immunoliposomes targeted by a phage antibody selected for cellular endocytosis *Biochim. Biophys. Acta (BBA)—Mol. Cell Res.* **1591** 109–18

[134] Chen H, Gao J, Lu Y, Kou G, Zhang H, Fan L *et al* 2008 Preparation and characterization of PE38KDEL-loaded anti-HER2 nanoparticles for targeted cancer therapy *J. Control. Release* **128** 209–16

[135] Steinhauser I, Spänkuch B, Strebhardt K and Langer K 2006 Trastuzumab-modified nanoparticles: optimisation of preparation and uptake in cancer cells *Biomaterials* **27** 4975–83

[136] Leuschner C, Kumar C S S R, Hansel W, Soboyejo W, Zhou J and Hormes J 2006 LHRH-conjugated magnetic iron oxide nanoparticles for detection of breast cancer metastases *Breast Cancer Res. Treat.* **99** 163–76

[137] Cui J, Björnmalm M, Ju Y and Caruso F 2018 Nanoengineering of poly (ethylene glycol) particles for stealth and targeting *Langmuir* **34** 10817–27

[138] Rosenblum D, Joshi N, Tao W, Karp J M and Peer D 2018 Progress and challenges towards targeted delivery of cancer therapeutics *Nat. Commun.* **9** 1410

[139] Peng L, Liu D, Cheng H, Zhou S and Zu M 2018 A multilayer film based selective thermal emitter for infrared stealth technology *Adv. Opt. Mater.* **6** 1801006

[140] Huckaby J T and Lai S K 2018 PEGylation for enhancing nanoparticle diffusion in mucus *Adv. Drug Deliv. Rev.* **124** 125–39

[141] Ghimici L and Nichifor M 2018 Dextran derivatives application as flocculants *Carbohydr. Polym.* **190** 162–74

[142] Adjei I M, Temples M N, Brown S B and Sharma B 2018 Targeted nanomedicine to treat bone metastasis *Pharmaceutics* **10** 205

[143] Kyzas G Z and Matis K A 2016 Electroflotation process: a review *J. Mol. Liq.* **220** 657–64

[144] Caruthers S D, Wickline S A and Lanza G M 2007 Nanotechnological applications in medicine *Curr. Opin. Biotechnol.* **18** 26–30

[145] Viswanath B, Kim S and Lee K 2016 Recent insights into nanotechnology development for detection and treatment of colorectal cancer *Int. J. Nanomed.* **2016:11** 2491–504

[146] Zhao X, Pan J, Li W, Yang W, Qin L and Pan Y 2018 Gold nanoparticles enhance cisplatin delivery and potentiate chemotherapy by decompressing colorectal cancer vessels *Int. J. Nanomed.* **2018:13** 6207–21

[147] Biscaglia F, Ripani G, Rajendran S, Benna C, Mocellin S, Bocchinfuso G *et al* 2019 Gold nanoparticle aggregates functionalized with cyclic RGD peptides for targeting and imaging of colorectal cancer cells *ACS Appl. Nano Mater.* **2** 6436–44

[148] Osumi H, Shinozaki E, Yamaguchi K and Zembutsu H 2019 Early change in circulating tumor DNA as a potential predictor of response to chemotherapy in patients with metastatic colorectal cancer *Sci. Rep.* **9** 17358

[149] Chen J, Wang D, Xi J, Au L, Siekkinen A, Warsen A *et al* 2007 Immuno gold nanocages with tailored optical properties for targeted photothermal destruction of cancer cells *Nano Lett.* **7** 1318–22

[150] Tan L, Han S, Ding S, Xiao W, Ding Y, Qian L *et al* 2017 Chitosan nanoparticle-based delivery of fused NKG2D–IL-21 gene suppresses colon cancer growth in mice *Int. J. Nanomed.* 3095–107

[151] Soster M, Juris R, Bonacchi S, Genovese D, Montalti M, Rampazzo E *et al* 2012 Targeted dual-color silica nanoparticles provide univocal identification of micrometastases in preclinical models of colorectal cancer *Int. J. Nanomed.* **2012:7** 4797–807

[152] Soleymani J, Hasanzadeh M, Somi M H, Shadjou N and Jouyban A 2019 Highly sensitive and specific cytosensing of HT 29 colorectal cancer cells using folic acid functionalized-KCC-1 nanoparticles *Biosens. Bioelectron.* **132** 122–31

[153] Li Y, Duo Y, Bao S, He L, Ling K, Luo J *et al* 2017 EpCAM aptamer-functionalized polydopamine-coated mesoporous silica nanoparticles loaded with DM1 for targeted therapy in colorectal cancer *Int. J. Nanomed.* **2017:12** 6239–57

[154] Tseng C-L, Wu S Y-H, Wang W-H, Peng C-L, Lin F-H, Lin C-C *et al* 2008 Targeting efficiency and biodistribution of biotinylated-EGF-conjugated gelatin nanoparticles administered via aerosol delivery in nude mice with lung cancer *Biomaterials* **29** 3014–22

[155] Shoyele S A and Slowey A 2006 Prospects of formulating proteins/peptides as aerosols for pulmonary drug delivery *Int. J. Pharm.* **314** 1–8

[156] Garbuzenko O B, Mainelis G, Taratula O and Minko T 2014 Inhalation treatment of lung cancer: the influence of composition, size and shape of nanocarriers on their lung accumulation and retention *Cancer Biol. Med.* **11** 44

[157] Markman J L, Rekechenetskiy A, Holler E and Ljubimova J Y 2013 Nanomedicine therapeutic approaches to overcome cancer drug resistance *Adv. Drug Deliv. Rev.* **65** 1866–79

[158] Wolinsky J B and Grinstaff M W 2008 Therapeutic and diagnostic applications of dendrimers for cancer treatment *Adv. Drug Deliv. Rev.* **60** 1037–55

[159] Al-Lazikani B, Banerji U and Workman P 2012 Combinatorial drug therapy for cancer in the post-genomic era *Nat. Biotechnol.* **30** 679–92

[160] Davis J L, Paris H L, Beals J W, Binns S E, Giordano G R, Scalzo R L *et al* 2016 Liposomal-encapsulated ascorbic acid: influence on vitamin C bioavailability and capacity to protect against ischemia–reperfusion injury *Nutr. Metab. Insights* **9** NMI-S39764

[161] Deshpande P P, Biswas S and Torchilin V P 2013 Current trends in the use of liposomes for tumor targeting *Nanomedicine* **8** 1509–28

[162] Voinea M and Simionescu M 2002 Designing of 'intelligent' liposomes for efficient delivery of drugs *J. Cell. Mol. Med.* **6** 465–74

[163] Couvreur P and Vauthier C 2006 Nanotechnology: intelligent design to treat complex disease *Pharm. Res.* **23** 1417–50

[164] Hubert A, Lyass O, Pode D and Gabizon A 2000 Doxil (Caelyx): an exploratory study with pharmacokinetics in patients with hormone-refractory prostate cancer *Anticancer Drugs* **11** 123–7

[165] Hwang T, Park T-J, Koh W-G, Cheong I W, Choi S-W and Kim J H 2011 Fabrication of nano-scale liposomes containing doxorubicin using Shirasu porous glass membrane *Colloids Surf. A: Physicochem. Eng. Asp.* **392** 250–5

[166] Saad M, Garbuzenko O B and Minko T 2008 Co-delivery of siRNA and an anticancer drug for treatment of multidrug-resistant cancer *Nanomedicine* **3** 761–776

[167] Adel A L, Dorr R T and Liddil J D 1993 The effect of anticancer drug sequence in experimental combination chemotherapy *Cancer Invest* **11** 15–24

[168] Guterres S S, Alves M P and Pohlmann A R 2007 Polymeric nanoparticles, nanospheres and nanocapsules, for cutaneous applications *Drug Target Insights* **2** 117739280700200000

[169] Masood F 2016 Polymeric nanoparticles for targeted drug delivery system for cancer therapy *Mater. Sci. Eng.* C **60** 569–78

[170] Baguley B C 2010 Multiple drug resistance mechanisms in cancer *Mol. Biotechnol.* **46** 308–16

[171] Tong R and Cheng J 2008 Paclitaxel-initiated, controlled polymerization of lactide for the formulation of polymeric nanoparticulate delivery vehicles *Angew Chem. Int. Ed.* **47** 4830–4

[172] Yadav S, van Vlerken L E, Little S R and Amiji M M 2009 Evaluations of combination MDR-1 gene silencing and paclitaxel administration in biodegradable polymeric nanoparticle formulations to overcome multidrug resistance in cancer cells *Cancer Chemother. Pharmacol.* **63** 711–22

[173] Song X R, Cai Z, Zheng Y, He G, Cui F Y, Gong D Q *et al* 2009 Reversion of multidrug resistance by co-encapsulation of vincristine and verapamil in PLGA nanoparticles *Eur. J. Pharm. Sci.* **37** 300–5

[174] Park T G 1995 Degradation of poly (lactic-co-glycolic acid) microspheres: effect of copolymer composition *Biomaterials* **16** 1123–30

[175] Devalapally H, Duan Z, Seiden M V and Amiji M M 2007 Paclitaxel and ceramide co-administration in biodegradable polymeric nanoparticulate delivery system to overcome drug resistance in ovarian cancer *Int. J. Cancer* **121** 830(8)

[176] Gou M 2009 Poly (ε-caprolactone)/poly (ethylene glycol)/poly (ε-caprolactone) nanoparticles: preparation, characterization, and application in doxorubicin delivery *J. Phys. Chem. B* **113** 12928–33

[177] Agnihotri S A, Mallikarjuna N N and Aminabhavi T M 2004 Recent advances on chitosan-based micro-and nanoparticles in drug delivery *J. Controll. Rel.* **100** 5–28

[178] Dodane V and Vilivalam V D 1998 Pharmaceutical applications of chitosan *Pharmaceut. Sci. Technol. Today* **1** 246–53

[179] Divya K and Jisha M S 2018 Chitosan nanoparticles preparation and applications *Environ. Chem. Lett.* **16** 101–12
[180] Nagpal K, Singh S K and Mishra D N 2010 Chitosan nanoparticles: a promising system in novel drug delivery *Chem. Pharmaceut. Bull.* **58** 1423–30
[181] Xu Y and Du Y 2003 Effect of molecular structure of chitosan on protein delivery properties of chitosan nanoparticles *Int. J. Pharmaceut.* **250** 215–26
[182] Dreis S, Rothweiler F, Michaelis M, Cinatl Jr J, Kreuter J and Langer K 2007 Preparation, characterisation and maintenance of drug efficacy of doxorubicin-loaded human serum albumin (HSA) nanoparticles *Int. J. Pharmaceut.* **341** 207–14
[183] Kratz F 2008 Albumin as a drug carrier: design of prodrugs, drug conjugates and nanoparticles *J. Controll. Rel.* **132** 171–83
[184] Dockal M, Carter D C and Ruker F 1999 The three recombinant domains of human serum albumin: structural characterization and ligand binding properties *J. Biol. Chem.* **274** 29303–10
[185] Elzoghby A O, Samy W M and Elgindy N A 2012 Albumin-based nanoparticles as potential controlled release drug delivery system *J. Controll. Rel.* **157** 168–82
[186] Haley B and Frenkel E 2008 Nanoparticles for drug delivery in cancer treatment *Urologic Oncology: Seminars and Original Investigations* **vol 26** (Elsevier) pp 57–64
[187] Abbasi S, Paul A, Shao W and Prakash S 2012 Cationic albumin nanoparticles for enhanced drug delivery to treat breast cancer: preparation and in vitro assessment *J. Drug Del.* **2012** 686108
[188] Desai N P, Tao C, Yang A, Louie L, Zheng T, Yao Z, Soon-Shiong P and Magdassi S 1999 Vivorx Pharmaceuticals Inc, assignee. Protein stabilized pharmacologically active agents, methods for the preparation thereof and methods for the use thereof *US patent US 5* **916** 596
[189] Maeda H, Wu J, Sawa T, Matsumura Y and Hori K 2000 Tumor vascular permeability and the EPR effect in macromolecular therapeutics: a review *J. Controll. Rel.* **65** 271–84
[190] Peng W, Anderson D G, Bao Y, Padera R F, Jr, Langer R and Sawicki J A 2007 Nanoparticulate delivery of suicide DNA to murine prostate and prostate tumors *Prostate* **67** 855–62
[191] Wong H L, Bendayan R, Rauth A M, Li Y and Wu X Y 2007 Chemotherapy with anticancer drugs encapsulated in solid lipidnanoparticles *Adv. Drug Deliv. Rev.* **59** 491–504
[192] Kwon G S and Okano T 1996 Polymeric micelles as new drug carriers *Adv. Drug Deliv. Rev.* **21** 107–16
[193] Xiao H *et al* 2012 A prodrug strategy to deliver cisplatin (IV) and paclitaxel in nanomicelles to improve efficacy and tolerance *Biomaterials* **33** 6507–19
[194] Hari S K, Gauba A, Shrivastava N, Tripathi R M, Jain S K and Pandey A K 2023 Polymeric micelles and cancer therapy: An ingenious multimodal tumor-targeted drug delivery system *Drug Deliv. Translat. Res.* **13** 135–63
[195] Li X, Li P, Zhang Y, Zhou Y, Chen X, Huang Y and Liu Y 2010 Novel mixed polymeric micelles for enhancing delivery of anticancer drug and overcoming multidrug resistance in tumor cell lines simultaneously *Pharmaceut. Res.* **27** 1498–511
[196] Thipparaboina R, Chavan R B, Kumar D, Modugula S and Shastri N R 2010 Micellar carriers for the delivery of multiple therapeutic agents *Coll. Surf.* B **1** 291–308
[197] Gothwal A, Khan I and Gupta U 2016 Polymeric micelles: recent advancements in the delivery of anticancer drugs *Pharmaceut. Res.* **33** 18 39

[198] Movassaghian S, Merkel O M and Torchilin V P 2015 Applications of polymer micelles for imaging and drug delivery *Wiley Interdiscip. Rev. Nanomed. Nanobiotechnol.* **7** 691–707
[199] Tomalia D A and Fréchet J M 2002 Discovery of dendrimers and dendritic polymers: A brief historical perspective *J. Polymer Sci.* A **40** 2719–28
[200] Clementi C, Miller K, Mero A, Satchi-Fainaro R and Pasut G 2011 Dendritic poly (ethylene glycol) bearing paclitaxel and alendronate for targeting bone neoplasms *Mol. Pharmaceut.* **8** 1063–72
[201] Abbasi E *et al* 2014 Dendrimers: synthesis, applications, and properties *Nanoscale Res. Lett.* **9** 1–10
[202] Saluja V, Mishra Y, Mishra V, Giri N and Nayak P 2021 Dendrimers based cancer nanotheranostics: An overview *Int. J. Pharmaceut.* **600** 120485
[203] Na K, Lee K H, Lee D H and Bae Y H 2006 Biodegradable thermo-sensitive nanoparticles from poly (L-lactic acid)/poly (ethylene glycol) alternating multi-block copolymer for potential anti-cancer drug carrier *Eur. J. Pharmaceut. Sci.* **27** 115–22
[204] Morgan M T *et al* Dendrimer-encapsulated camptothecins: increased solubility, cellular uptake, and cellular retention affords enhanced anticancer activity in vitro *Cancer Res* **66** 11913–21
[205] Jain N K, Tare M S, Mishra V and Tripathi P K 2015 The development, characterization and in vivo anti-ovarian cancer activity of poly (propylene imine)(PPI)-antibody conjugates containing encapsulated paclitaxel *Nanomed. Nanotechnol. Biol. Med.* **11** 207–18
[206] Kalomiraki M, Thermos K and Chaniotakis N A 2016 Dendrimers as tunable vectors of drug delivery systems and biomedical and ocular applications *Int. J. Nanomed.* **22** 1–2
[207] Ranjan G, Ranjan S, Sunita P and Pattanayak S P 2024 Thiazolidinedione derivatives in cancer therapy: exploring novel mechanisms, therapeutic potentials, and future horizons in oncology *Naunyn-Schmiedeberg's Arch. Pharmacol.* **2** 1–21
[208] Gupta V and Nayak S K 2015 Dendrimers: A review on synthetic approaches *J. Appl. Pharmaceut. Sci.* **5** 117–22

IOP Publishing

Nanoplatforms for Cancer Imaging

Nanasaheb D Thorat and Sandeep B Somvanshi

Chapter 3

Nanoplatforms for precision imaging and targeted therapy in oncology

Kovuri Umadevi, Dola Sundeep, Mulukala Swetha, Eravalli Sudhakar Rao, Eswaramoorthy K Varadharaj, C Chandrasekhara Sastry, Umesh Kumar and Alluru Gopala Krishna

The fusion of nanotechnology and imaging has opened new avenues for precision diagnostics in cancer care. Nanoplatform-based imaging enhances the capabilities of traditional diagnostic methods by offering molecular-level accuracy and improving contrast and resolution. This chapter explores recent innovations in nanotechnology applications for cancer diagnosis, including the use of nanoparticles, quantum dots, and hybrid nanomaterials to improve the sensitivity of imaging techniques such as magnetic resonance imaging (MRI), positron emission tomography (PET), and optical imaging. We examine how targeted imaging, made possible by ligand-functionalized nanomaterials, enables the early detection of tumors and improves the monitoring of therapeutic outcomes. Furthermore, the chapter addresses challenges such as the biocompatibility and toxicity of nanomaterials, while also discussing regulatory and clinical considerations. The integration of nanoplatforms into cancer diagnosis marks a significant step toward personalized medicine and theranostics, where diagnosis and treatment are closely linked. Future trends, including artificial intelligence-driven imaging analysis and the development of novel nanomaterials, are also highlighted.

3.1 Introduction

3.1.1 The convergence of nanotechnology and cancer imaging

Biomedical imaging stands as a cornerstone in comprehensive cancer management due to its numerous advantages. One of the most significant benefits of imaging is its ability to monitor biological processes in real time, allowing clinicians to track changes and progression with minimal or no invasiveness [1, 2]. This capability not only reduces the need for destructive tissue biopsies but also provides a clear window

doi:10.1088/978-0-7503-5864-4ch3

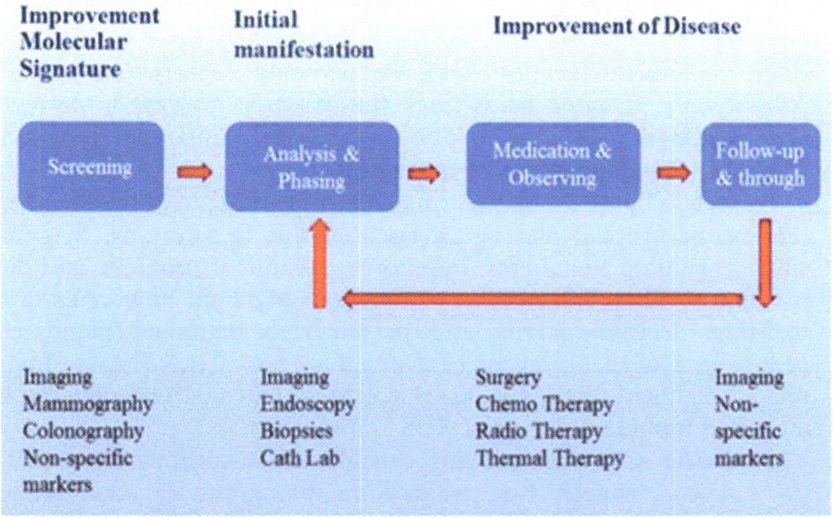

Figure 3.1. An overview of the disease management process, illustrating the progression from initial screening and diagnosis through treatment and follow-up, utilizing imaging and molecular markers at each stage for enhanced precision in care.

into the body's internal workings without disrupting normal functions [2]. A remarkable feature of biomedical imaging is its ability to function across a vast spectrum of time and size scales. In terms of time, imaging technologies can capture rapid biological events such as protein binding and chemical reactions that occur within milliseconds [3]. At the other end of the spectrum, they can also track the progression of diseases like cancer, which may unfold over several years [2]. When it comes to size, imaging techniques are versatile enough to explore processes occurring at the molecular and cellular levels, as well as providing detailed images of entire organs or even the whole body. This range makes imaging an indispensable tool in both diagnosing and managing cancer at various stages [4].

As illustrated in figure 3.1, the present-day role of imaging in cancer care spans both the screening of asymptomatic individuals and the management of those with symptomatic disease. Imaging is key to early detection, allowing for timely interventions that can significantly improve outcomes. Moreover, its role extends into disease management, helping to determine the stage of cancer, guide treatment decisions, and monitor response to therapy. Through this dual role of screening and management, biomedical imaging has become an integral component in the continuum of cancer care [2, 5].

3.1.2 Historical perspective on cancer imaging

(a) **Cancer imaging: an overview**

Detecting cancer early is crucial for increasing the chances of effective treatment, especially for certain cancer types [2]. Imaging techniques, which involve creating detailed pictures of the body's internal structures, play a vital role not only in early detection but also in determining the cancer stage, its precise location, and the planning of surgeries or therapies. Additionally, imaging helps track the cancer's progression or recurrence after treatment [6].

(b) **The role of imaging in cancer management**

As seen in figure 3.2, cancer imaging forms the core of the diagnostic and therapeutic process, playing an essential role in screening, diagnosis and staging, guiding treatments, monitoring treatment progress, and detecting recurrence. These interconnected functions highlight how imaging enables real-time decision-making and personalized treatment plans, ensuring precise and efficient cancer care at all stages of the disease. Imaging is not a treatment itself, but a critical tool that aids clinicians in making informed treatment decisions [7].

1. **Cancer screening**: imaging can identify suspicious areas that might indicate cancer. For instance, mammograms, a common imaging method, are widely used for breast cancer screening. People at higher risk, due to factors like genetics or lifestyle, often undergo regular screenings to detect potential cancers early [8].
2. **Diagnosis and staging**: imaging allows clinicians to pinpoint where cancer is located, whether it has spread, and the extent of the disease. It can help in staging cancer, which is essential for planning treatment

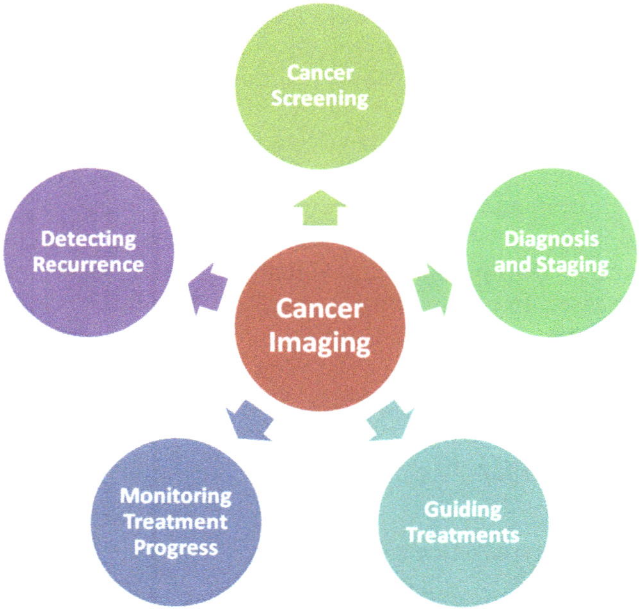

Figure 3.2. The central role of cancer imaging in comprehensive cancer care.

[5]. Additionally, imaging assists in guiding biopsies by helping doctors locate the tumor and extract tissue samples for laboratory analysis [9].

3. **Guiding treatments**: imaging techniques are valuable for accurately targeting cancer treatments. By identifying the tumor's exact location, methods such as ultrasound, magnetic resonance imaging (MRI), or computed tomography (CT) scans can focus treatments like radiation therapy on the tumor while sparing surrounding healthy tissue [10].
4. **Monitoring treatment progress**: after starting treatment, imaging helps assess whether the tumor is shrinking or responding as expected. Periodic imaging tests such as x-rays, MRI, or CT scans are often performed during cancer therapy to monitor changes in the tumor. Techniques like positron emission tomography (PET) and magnetic resonance spectroscopy track how the tumor is using the body's resources, providing deeper insights into its behavior post-treatment [11].
5. **Detecting recurrence**: post-treatment, imaging is used to check whether cancer has returned or if it has metastasized to other parts of the body.

(c) **X-ray imaging: a common tool**

X-rays are perhaps the most familiar imaging method, widely used for diagnosing various health conditions. X-ray images are produced based on the different absorption rates of tissues [12]. For example, bones, rich in calcium, absorb more x-rays and appear white, while soft tissues absorb less and appear gray. Air, on the other hand, absorbs the least, rendering the lungs black in x-ray images. Beyond broken bones, x-rays also help in cancer detection. Chest x-rays and mammograms, for instance, are regularly used to screen for lung and breast cancers, respectively [13].

(d) **CT scans: a step beyond x-rays**

CT scans offer a more detailed three-dimensional view compared to standard x-rays. While x-rays provide two-dimensional images, CT scans allow doctors to examine the body in cross-sectional slices [14]. These scans are particularly useful in determining the size, depth, and exact location of a tumor. During a CT scan, contrast agents may be used to enhance the clarity of the images, allowing better visualization of the tumor's boundaries and its relationship to surrounding tissues, as shown in figure 3.3 [15].

(e) **Molecular and nuclear imaging: PET and SPECT scans**

Molecular and nuclear imaging techniques, such as PET and single-photon emission computed tomography (SPECT), provide unique insights by using radioactive substances [17]. These substances are either linked to compounds that cancer cells absorb or compounds that are preferentially taken up by tumors. This imaging approach reveals metabolic activities or chemical changes within tumors, offering a more detailed perspective than traditional imaging methods [18].

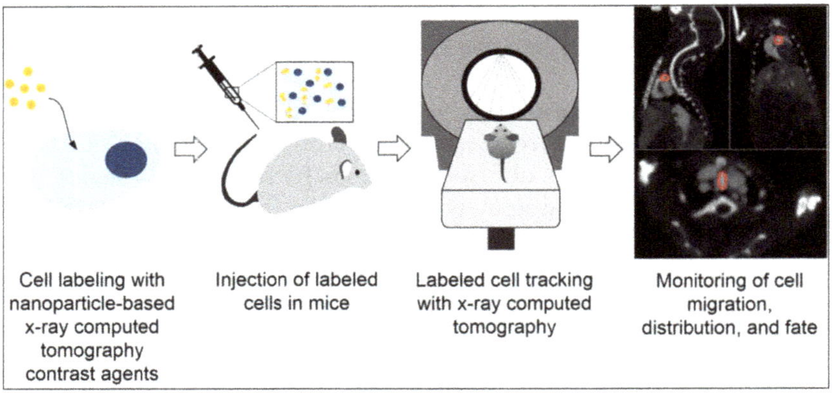

Figure 3.3. Illustration of cell labeling with nanoparticle-based x-ray computed tomography (CT) contrast agents, followed by the injection of labeled cells into mice for tracking. The process allows real-time monitoring of cell migration, distribution, and fate using CT imaging. Reproduced with permission from [16]. © 2017 American Chemical Society.

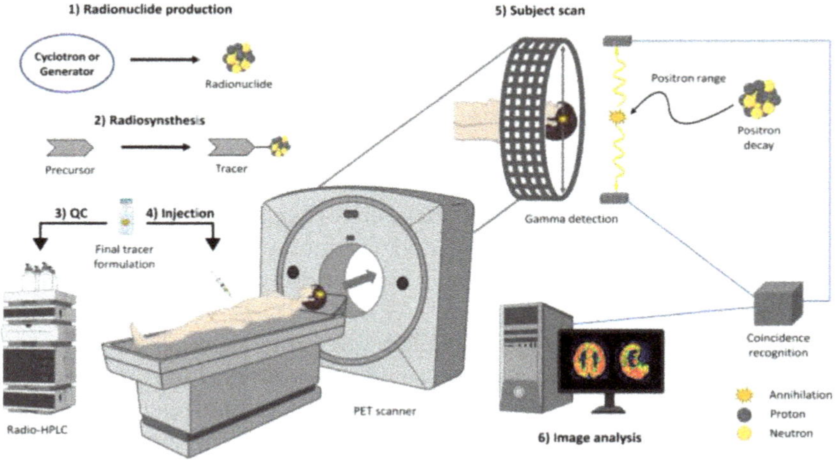

Figure 3.4. Illustration of the PET imaging workflow, including radionuclide production, radiosynthesis of tracers, quality control, and injection of the tracer into the subject. The process is followed by a subject scan in a PET scanner, detecting gamma rays from positron decay, and concluding with image analysis to visualize the tracer distribution in the body. Reproduced from [19]. CC BY 4.0.

Figure 3.4 provides a detailed illustration of the workflow involved in PET, a crucial technique in molecular and nuclear imaging, which is often paired with SPECT. The process begins with the production of radionuclides in a cyclotron or generator. These radionuclides, which emit positrons or gamma rays, are then used to create radioactive tracers through a process called radiosynthesis, where a precursor is combined with the radionuclide. These tracers are designed to target specific biological markers or processes within the body, making them indispensable in diagnosing diseases such as cancer, cardiovascular conditions, and neurological disorders. After the tracer is synthesized, it undergoes stringent quality control using methods like high-performance liquid chromatography (HPLC) to ensure its purity, safety, and efficacy before it can be injected into the patient. Once the tracer is cleared, it is administered to the patient, typically via intravenous injection. The tracer circulates through the bloodstream, accumulating in areas with high biological activity, such as tumors or areas of inflammation, allowing for targeted imaging.

The subject is then placed into a PET or SPECT scanner, where gamma rays emitted from the decay of the radionuclide are detected. In PET imaging, the emitted positrons interact with electrons in the body, producing gamma rays through a process called annihilation. These gamma rays are detected by the PET scanner, and the data are processed to create high-resolution images. For SPECT imaging, gamma rays emitted directly from the tracer are detected, providing valuable functional information about organ systems and tissues. Finally, advanced image analysis is conducted, using software to reconstruct the tracer's distribution throughout the body. These images provide clinicians with precise visual information on metabolic and biochemical activities, enabling early detection of diseases, assessment of treatment efficacy, and even monitoring of disease progression. The integration of molecular and nuclear imaging techniques such as PET and SPECT offers unparalleled insights into the functional processes of the body, making these tools essential in modern diagnostics and personalized treatment planning.

(f) **PET scans**

PET scans are used to visualize metabolic processes in the body. For cancer detection, patients are typically injected with a small amount of radioactive sugar. Cancer cells, due to their higher rate of glucose uptake, absorb more of this sugar, making tumors visible in PET scans. PET scans are particularly effective at identifying aggressive or larger tumors and can be used to evaluate whether cancer treatment is working by observing the tumor's metabolic activity over time [20] (figure 3.5).

The figure illustrates the process of PET imaging using 124I-labeled cRGDY-PEG-C-dots as targeted nanoparticles designed for tumor imaging. In panel (a), a syringe containing the nanoparticle formulation is injected into the patient, where the particles are specifically directed towards integrin-bearing tumor cells. The nanoparticles are functionalized with cyclic RGD peptides (cRGDY), which target integrin receptors commonly overexpressed in tumor cells. The nanoparticles also contain Cy5, a fluorescent dye within a silica core, and are stabilized with PEG chains to enhance circulation time and biocompatibility.

a)

b)

c)

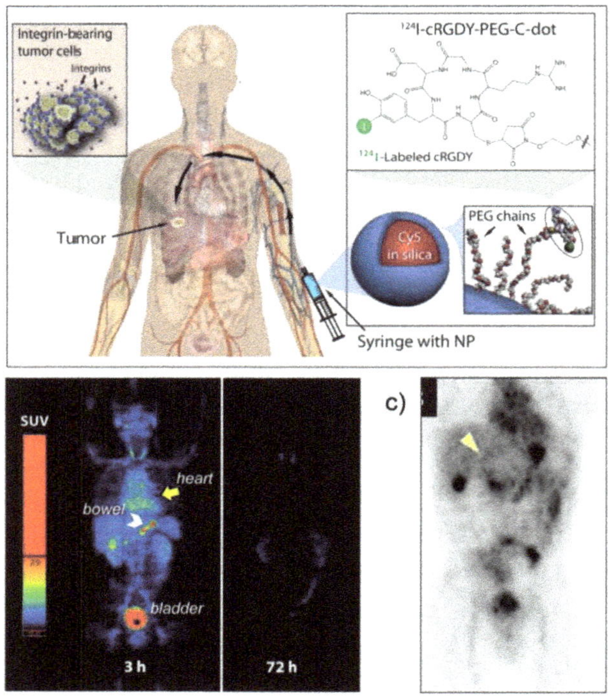

Figure 3.5. Illustrating the use of 124I-labeled cRGDY-PEG-C-dots for targeted tumor imaging. (a) Nanoparticle injection and accumulation in integrin-bearing tumor cells, highlighted by Cy5 fluorescence and PEG chains for stability. (b) PET imaging at 3 and 72 h post-injection showing biodistribution in the heart, bowel, and bladder. (c) PET scan of the tumor site demonstrating the localized uptake of nanoparticles for precise imaging. Reproduced from [21].

Panel (b) shows PET imaging of the patient at two different time points —3 and 72 h post-injection. The scan at 3 h reveals the biodistribution of the nanoparticles, with accumulation in the heart, bowel, and bladder, indicating the nanoparticle's initial circulation and clearance pathways. By 72 h, the imaging shows minimal background signal, highlighting the prolonged retention of the nanoparticles at the tumor site and efficient clearance from non-targeted tissues. Panel (c) further emphasizes the precise targeting of the nanoparticles to the tumor, as shown by the distinct localization of the PET signal at the tumor site. This demonstrates the efficacy of the cRGDY-PEG-C-dots in specifically binding to tumor cells, providing high-resolution imaging for accurate tumor diagnosis and treatment monitoring. The use of PET scans in this context allows for detailed visualization of nanoparticle distribution and tumor uptake over time, supporting its potential as a powerful tool in cancer theranostics [21].

(g) **SPECT scans**

SPECT scans, similar to PET scans, utilize radioactive tracers, but they differ in how the data are captured. These scans provide information about blood flow and chemical activity in tissues. In cancer detection, antibodies linked to radioactive substances can be used to specifically target cancer cells. The radioactive substance attached to the antibodies allows the tumor to be detected in SPECT images, providing critical information about tumor location and spread.

Imaging technologies are indispensable tools in cancer detection, diagnosis, and treatment planning. From early screening with mammograms to the precise targeting of tumors with MRI or CT scans, these techniques offer clinicians the ability to not only detect cancer early but also tailor treatment strategies. Advances in molecular imaging like PET and SPECT add an additional layer of insight, enabling a deeper understanding of cancer biology and the effectiveness of therapies. As technology continues to evolve, imaging will remain a cornerstone of personalized cancer care, helping clinicians improve outcomes through earlier detection and more targeted interventions.

Figure 3.6 illustrates transaxial brain perfusion images obtained using [99mTc]Tc-HMPAO SPECT under resting conditions. Following an intravenous dose of 740 MBq of [99mTc]Tc-HMPAO, dynamic images were captured using the AnyScan S Flex SPECT system (Mediso Ltd, Budapest, Hungary). The images reveal no detectable perfusion abnormalities, with symmetrical and uniform radiotracer distribution observed in both the right and left hemispheres. Notably, the cortical grey matter, basal ganglia, and visual cortex exhibit high radiotracer uptake, whereas the white matter and ventricular regions display minimal radioactivity [22].

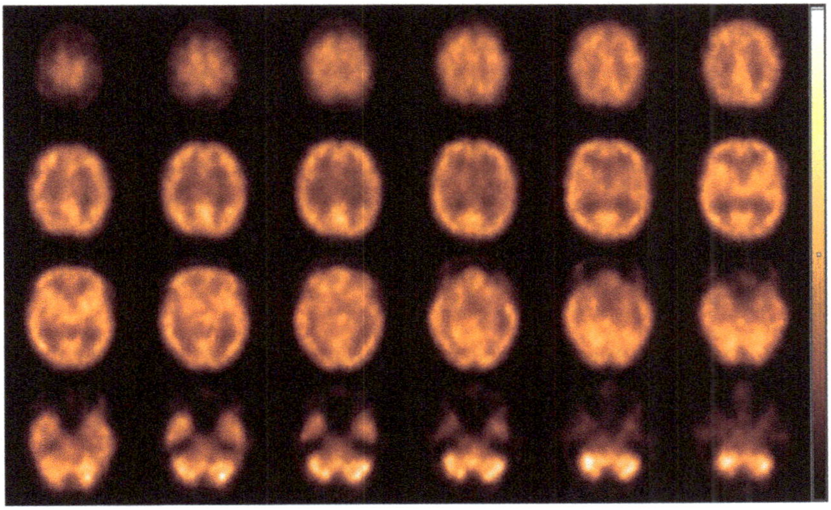

Figure 3.6. SPECT imaging of a normal brain, illustrating typical radiotracer distribution in different regions of the brain. Reproduced from [22]. CC BY 4.0.

3.2 The role of nanotechnology in disease diagnosis and treatment

Nanotechnology is already making significant strides in the medical field, particularly in the areas of disease detection, diagnosis, and treatment. This technology allows for early diagnosis of diseases and more precise therapies, which are crucial for successful outcomes [1]. Applications of nanotechnology extend across various medical disciplines, including surgery, cancer treatment, bio-detection of disease markers, molecular imaging, implant technology, tissue engineering, and the development of advanced drug delivery systems [22]. The use of nanomaterials in organic, inorganic, and biological sciences has become indispensable due to their unique properties, which vary depending on their size. These materials offer unprecedented capabilities in detecting disease markers, pre-cancerous cells, viruses, proteins, and antibodies, all of which are vital for early diagnosis. Over the next few years, the impact of nanotechnology on medical diagnostics is expected to grow even more substantially [23].

Nanotechnology offers a broad range of applications in biomedicine and biotechnology, including regenerative medicine, which promises new solutions for patients suffering from organ failure or serious injuries. Innovations like nanoparticle-reinforced polymers, orally administered insulin, and nano-engineered artificial joints are already transforming medical treatments [24–27]. Moreover, commercially available nanotechnology products, such as surgical tools, bone replacement materials, wound dressings, antimicrobial textiles, and contrast agents for imaging, have already demonstrated the versatility and power of nanotechnology. Additionally, nano-based diagnostic devices like micro-cantilevers and chips for *in vitro* diagnostics are revolutionizing the way diseases are detected and managed [28–31].

Nanotechnology has the potential to address some of the most challenging issues in health and medicine by offering solutions such as imaging, sensing, targeted drug delivery, and gene delivery systems [1]. In the context of cancer, nanoparticles are being used in new therapies, allowing for the precise targeting of cancer cells while sparing healthy tissues [2]. Moreover, bioengineered nanoparticles serve as transport vehicles for diagnostic or therapeutic agents, offering a new approach to treatment and management of diseases. These advancements represent only the beginning of nanotechnology's impact on healthcare [32].

3.2.1 Emerging nanodiagnostics for early detection

Accurate disease diagnosis is essential for effective treatment and management. The diagnostic process typically involves gathering information about the patient's medical history, conducting physical examinations, and using various diagnostic tools to identify signs and symptoms [33]. Ideally, these tools should be sensitive, specific, accurate, easy to use, and cost-effective. Traditional diagnostic methods, while useful, often fall short in terms of speed, accuracy, cost, and the need for specialized professionals, which can be especially challenging in developing nations [29–31].

Nanodiagnostics, an emerging field that leverages the unique properties of nanomaterials, offers a solution to these limitations. With their distinct physio-chemical and optical characteristics, nanomaterials have the ability to provide highly accurate and timely disease detection [32]. This technology is particularly vital in developing countries, where socioeconomic factors, geographic conditions, and limited access to healthcare contribute to increased vulnerability to diseases. Nanotechnology-based diagnostics are poised to meet the growing demand for fast, sensitive, and cost-effective diagnostic solutions, particularly for point-of-care testing in community settings [33, 34].

As many diseases in developing nations lead to widespread epidemics, it is critical to have diagnostic tools that are not only effective but also accessible and affordable. Nanotechnology-based diagnostics can provide rapid results, require fewer resources, and are more robust and user-friendly than traditional methods [33]. These features are especially important in countries with limited healthcare infrastructure, where early diagnosis and intervention can significantly reduce the burden of disease on the population.

3.2.2 Nanoplatforms and cancer treatment: a new frontier

Cancer remains one of the most formidable challenges in healthcare, posing significant threats to human life. The lack of efficient early detection and screening methods often leads to a delayed diagnosis, with many cancers only being discovered at advanced stages [2]. Consequently, patients frequently miss the optimal window for treatment, which severely compromises their chances of recovery. Traditional cancer treatment modalities such as surgery, chemotherapy, and radiation therapy (RT) have shown success in treating tumors but come with a myriad of side effects [35]. These include drug resistance, toxicity to healthy tissues, and high rates of metastasis and recurrence. The limitations of these conventional treatments are particularly evident when treating deep-seated tumors, where outcomes can be less favorable [36]. In response, recent advances in cancer research have shifted toward combining diagnostics and therapy, referred to as theranostics. This approach, particularly when combined with imaging guidance, offers the promise of targeted treatment for deep tumors with minimal side effects, potentially revolutionizing cancer therapy [37, 38].

Figure 3.7 provides an overview of the various nanoplatforms currently being explored for cancer therapy. These include micelles, DNA origami, dendrimers, polymeric nanoparticles, lipid nanoparticles, gold nanoparticles, and responsive nanoparticles, each with unique properties that enhance their ability to target cancer cells effectively. Micelles are small, spherical nanocarriers composed of amphiphilic molecules that can encapsulate hydrophobic drugs, improving their solubility and delivery to tumor sites. DNA origami, a novel nanoplatform, uses precisely folded DNA structures to deliver drugs or therapeutic agents to specific cells, offering high targeting accuracy. Dendrimers, tree-like branched molecules, can carry multiple drug molecules or imaging agents simultaneously, enhancing their therapeutic efficiency. Polymeric nanoparticles, made from biodegradable polymers, allow for

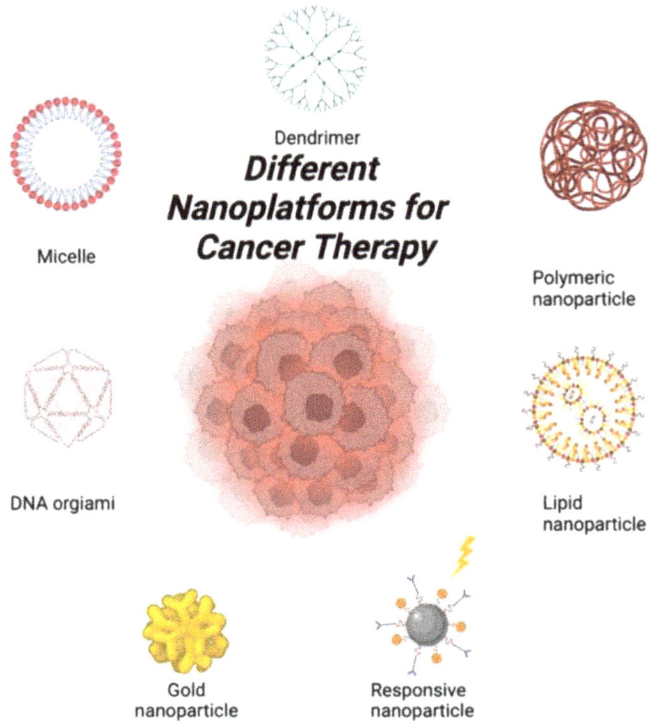

Figure 3.7. Overview of different nanoplatforms used in cancer therapy. Reprinted by permission from Springer Nature, [39], Copyright (2024).

controlled drug release and enhanced stability. Lipid nanoparticles are composed of lipid bilayers and have been used extensively in delivering RNA-based therapies and chemotherapeutics due to their biocompatibility. Gold nanoparticles possess unique optical properties that make them useful in both imaging and photothermal therapy, providing a dual-function theranostic approach.

Responsive nanoparticles are designed to react to specific stimuli, such as pH, temperature, or light, allowing for controlled drug release in the tumor microenvironment. Together, these nanoplatforms offer versatile options for improving the targeting and efficacy of cancer treatments while minimizing off-target effects and systemic toxicity. Nanoplatforms, which merge materials science and nanotechnology, have gained significant attention in oncology due to their remarkable biocompatibility and versatile applications. By exploiting the unique physical and chemical properties of nanomaterials, nanoplatforms can act as carriers to deliver contrast agents and anticancer drugs directly to tumor sites. This capability allows for precise treatment under imaging guidance, ensuring a more targeted and effective approach. The diversity of nanomaterials available, including nanogels, dendrimers, carbon nanotubes, graphene, SiO_2 nanoparticles, and nanoscale metal–organic frameworks (NMOFs), allows researchers to select the most suitable nanoplatforms for diagnostic and therapeutic purposes [40]. These platforms exhibit excellent physicochemical and biological properties, making them particularly effective in reducing toxicity and side effects, further enhancing their potential for cancer diagnosis and treatment.

3.2.3 Advances in tumor diagnosis using nanoplatforms

In vivo imaging is indispensable in biomedicine, especially for cancer diagnosis and treatment. By providing real-time monitoring and precise localization of lesions, imaging technologies are crucial for formulating effective treatment strategies and improving prognosis. Early detection, enabled by advanced imaging, allows for personalized treatment plans tailored to the individual characteristics of the tumor [41]. Common imaging techniques such as fluorescence imaging (FI), CT, MRI, and photoacoustic imaging (PAI) are widely employed for real-time monitoring during cancer therapy, enhancing treatment accuracy [2].

Nanomaterials have become central to biomedicine due to their structural versatility, biocompatibility, and ability to accumulate in tumors. They serve as platforms for both imaging and therapeutic delivery, enhancing the precision of cancer treatments. However, relying solely on a single imaging method often falls short in terms of accuracy and resolution [42]. As a result, researchers are increasingly exploring the combination of multiple imaging modalities, known as multimodal imaging, to guide cancer therapy. This multimodal approach integrates different imaging techniques, improving treatment outcomes by leveraging the strengths of each method [43].

3.2.4 Theranostics: combining diagnosis and therapy

In recent years, the integration of diagnosis and therapy into a single, unified approach—theranostics—has emerged as a promising solution for treating cancer. This imaging-guided method allows for the precise targeting of tumors, particularly those located deep within the body [38]. By using nanoplatforms, which combine both diagnostic and therapeutic functions, scientists can minimize side effects while enhancing treatment efficacy. The development of biocompatible nanomaterials has played a pivotal role in advancing theranostics, allowing for the safe and effective delivery of drugs and contrast agents directly to tumor sites [18].

The use of nanoplatforms in cancer treatment is not limited to specific types of nanomaterials; rather, a wide range of materials are being explored to improve the precision and effectiveness of cancer therapies. These include advanced nanomaterials such as microbubbles, dendrimers, nanogels, and carbon-based structures, which are designed to carry both imaging elements and therapeutic agents [36]. This approach ensures that cancer treatments are guided by imaging, leading to more accurate targeting of tumors and reduced damage to surrounding tissues [44].

Figure 3.8 illustrates the key advantages of using responsive therapeutic nanoparticles in medical applications, particularly in cancer therapy. These nanoparticles are designed to react to specific stimuli, such as pH changes, temperature, or external signals, to deliver drugs more precisely and effectively. The diagram highlights several benefits of this technology, including enhanced therapeutic efficacy, which

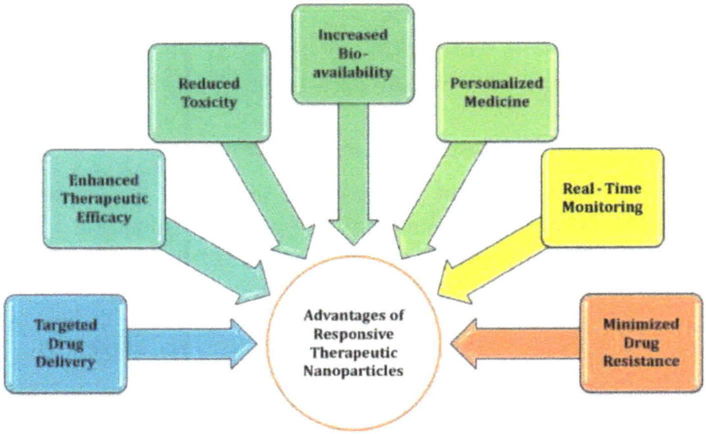

Figure 3.8. Showcasing the various advantages of responsive therapeutic nanoparticles, including enhanced therapeutic efficacy, targeted drug delivery, reduced toxicity, increased bioavailability, personalized medicine, real-time monitoring, and minimized drug resistance. Reprinted by permission from Springer Nature, [45], Copyright (2023).

ensures better treatment outcomes, and targeted drug delivery, which allows the nanoparticles to focus on the disease site, reducing systemic exposure. Additionally, reduced toxicity and increased bioavailability improve patient safety and drug absorption.

Responsive nanoparticles also support personalized medicine, tailoring treatments based on the individual characteristics of a patient's disease, and facilitate real-time monitoring, allowing for continuous observation of the treatment's effectiveness. Lastly, these nanoparticles help minimize drug resistance, a common challenge in long-term cancer therapy, by delivering drugs more precisely and in response to changing tumor conditions. This combination of features makes responsive therapeutic nanoparticles a powerful tool in modern medicine [45].

3.2.5 Multimodal imaging for precision cancer treatment

While monomodal imaging techniques have been the standard in cancer diagnosis, their limitations have prompted the exploration of multimodal imaging. Multimodal imaging combines two or more imaging modalities to provide a more comprehensive view of the tumor, enhancing diagnostic accuracy and treatment precision [46]. For example, combining MRI with CT or PAI can offer both high-resolution images and detailed information about the tumor's metabolic state, allowing clinicians to tailor treatment strategies more effectively. This combination of imaging techniques is particularly valuable for guiding therapy in real time, ensuring that treatments are administered with optimal precision [47].

The integration of nanotechnology with advanced imaging techniques is transforming the landscape of cancer diagnosis and treatment. Nanoplatforms, with their unique properties and biocompatibility, offer a promising avenue for theranostics,

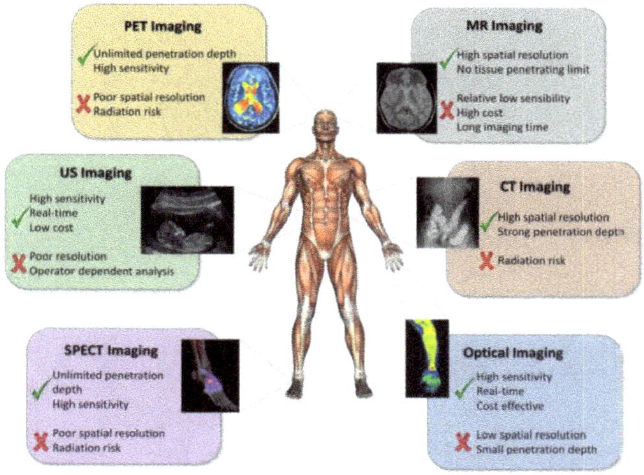

Figure 3.9. Comparison of different imaging modalities, including positron emission tomography (PET), single-photon emission computed tomography (SPECT), computed tomography (CT), magnetic resonance (MR), ultrasound (US), and optical imaging, highlighting their advantages and limitations in terms of sensitivity, resolution, cost, and potential risks [1].

enabling precise, targeted treatment with fewer side effects. As the field of nanomedicine continues to evolve, it is poised to play an increasingly important role in combating cancer, improving both patient outcomes and the overall efficacy of cancer therapies [36, 43].

Figure 3.9 provides a comparative overview of several imaging modalities used in medical diagnostics, including PET, SPECT, CT, MR, ultrasound (US), and optical imaging. Each modality is assessed based on key factors such as spatial resolution, sensitivity, cost, and associated risks. PET and SPECT imaging offer high sensitivity and unlimited penetration depth but suffer from poor spatial resolution and radiation risk. CT and MR imaging provide excellent spatial resolution, with CT offering strong penetration depth but with radiation exposure, while MR is limited by high cost and long imaging times. US and optical imaging are noted for their real-time capabilities and cost-effectiveness, though both face challenges with resolution and, in the case of optical imaging, limited tissue penetration depth. This figure helps illustrate the strengths and weaknesses of each modality for use in specific clinical scenarios [1].

3.3 Key nanomaterials in imaging applications

3.3.1 Overview of nanoparticles used in cancer imaging

Nanoparticles have emerged as a powerful tool in cancer diagnosis, especially for cancers like breast, colon, and cervical cancers. A wide variety of nanoparticles, including metallic, magnetic, polymeric, metal oxide, quantum dots (QDs), graphene, fullerene, liposomes, carbon nanotubes, and dendrimers, have been developed and applied for improved diagnostic capabilities [1]. These nanoparticles play

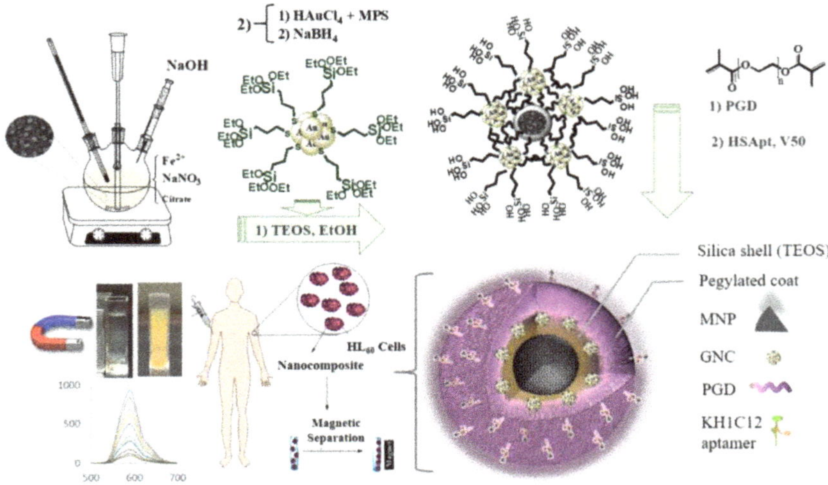

Figure 3.10. Illustrates the synthesis and functionalization of a nanocomposite, integrating magnetic nanoparticles (MNPs), gold nanoclusters (GNCs), and silica shells with a PEGylated coating. The process involves magnetic separation, with the nanocomposite targeting HL-60 cells using the KH1C12 aptamer for selective delivery. Reproduced from [56]. © IOP Publishing Ltd. All rights reserved.

an essential role in imaging functions due to their unique properties. One of their most significant advantages is their ability to remain in the bloodstream for extended periods before reaching their target cells, allowing them to pass through biological barriers such as cell membranes and interact effectively with biological systems [48]. Additionally, when conjugated with cancer-specific antibodies, nanoparticles enhance cancer cell targeting and detection, leading to better diagnostic outcomes.

Recent research has highlighted the ability of nanoparticles and nanosensors to improve the sensitivity of cancer detection. For example, certain nanoparticles can be used to detect specific methylation patterns and mutations, which serve as markers for cancer diagnosis [49]. However, further studies are needed before newer diagnostic methods, such as using extracellular vesicles, circulating tumor cells, and cell-free RNA, can be incorporated into clinical practices. Studies also show that fluorescent gold nanoclusters (GNCs) or superparamagnetic Fe_3O_4/GNCs have been developed using (γ-mercaptopropyl) trimethoxysilane (MPS) as a stabilizing agent [50]. These GNCs were further conjugated onto the surface of $Fe_3O_4@SiO_2$ nanoparticles, followed by the addition of poly ethylene glycol dimethacrylate (PGD) to form nanoprobes [51]. These nanoprobes, known as Fe_3O_4/GNCs/aptamer, as shown in figure 3.10, have demonstrated successful uptake in HL60 cancer cells, indicating their potential in cancer diagnostics [52].

3.3.2 Quantum dots and their applications

Figure 3.11 illustrates the diverse applications of QDs, highlighting their roles in areas such as light-emitting diodes (LEDs), photoconductors and photodetectors, photovoltaics, biomedicine, environmental applications, and catalysis. These versatile

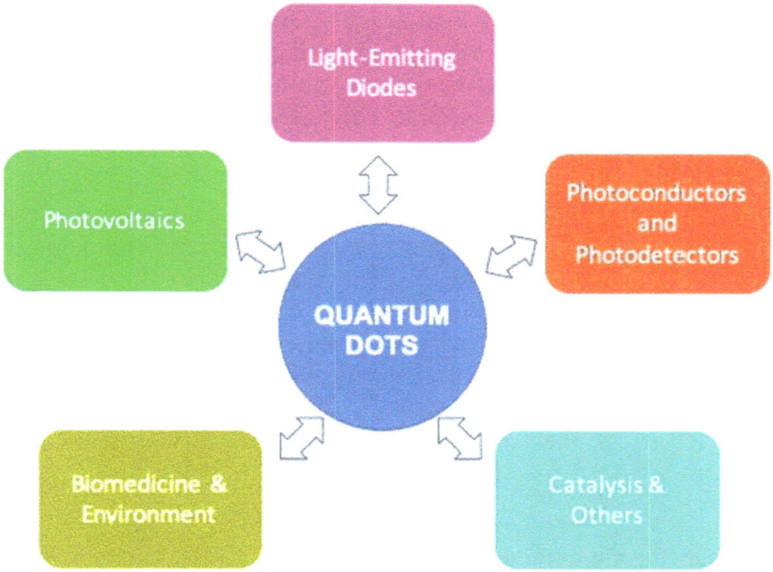

Figure 3.11. Overview of the various applications of quantum dots, including their use in light-emitting diodes, photoconductors and photodetectors, photovoltaics, biomedicine and environmental applications, and catalysis. Reprinted with permission from [54]. Copyright (2020) American Chemical Society.

nanomaterials are utilized across multiple fields due to their unique optical and electronic properties. Clinical cancer imaging techniques such as x-ray, CT, MRI, and PET have been instrumental in providing detailed morphological data about cancer cells and tissues [53]. However, when cancerous tissues closely resemble healthy tissues, these imaging methods face limitations in terms of resolution and contrast. This presents a significant challenge in clinical diagnostics. To overcome these issues, the development of advanced imaging probes that enhance signal intensity, stability, and tissue penetration is crucial for broader clinical applications [5, 43].

QDs, often referred to as 'artificial atoms,' represent one of the most promising solutions in this regard. These semiconductor nanocrystals, typically less than 10 nm in size, are categorized as zero-dimensional nanostructures. QDs exhibit several attractive optical characteristics that make them ideal for fluorescent imaging probes. These properties include tunable emission in the near-infrared (NIR) region, broad excitation range, narrow emission spectrum, high photoluminescence quantum yield, long photoluminescence lifetimes, and compatibility with biomolecular functionalization through the enhanced permeability and retention (EPR) effect. Furthermore, QDs can enhance signal intensity through mechanisms such as participating in reactions as catalysts, acting as energy acceptors, or direct oxidation with simultaneous energy transfer.

The ability of QDs to emit light at longer wavelengths following broad-spectrum excitation further enhances their utility in tissue penetration, a critical factor for deep-tissue imaging. Additionally, the large surface area of QDs enables them to bind covalently to various biorecognition molecules, including peptides, antibodies, nucleic acids, and small-molecule ligands [55]. This property significantly expands their application as fluorescent probes in cancer diagnostics. The synthesis of QDs is typically achieved through methods such as molecular beam epitaxy (MBE), ion implantation, electron-beam lithography, x-ray lithography, wet-chemical methods, and vapor-phase processes, which can be generally categorized into top-down and bottom-up approaches [56].

In recent years, QDs have been studied extensively and applied across various fields such as biosensing, *in vitro* diagnostics, cancer therapy, bioimaging, and drug delivery. Of particular importance is their role in optical imaging of cancer cells, which holds great potential for improving clinical diagnosis. Several types of QDs, including semiconductor-based, carbon-based, chalcogenide, and black phosphorus QDs, have been developed for this purpose [57]. Each type of QD has its own set of synthesis methods and modifications to improve performance, while researchers continue to assess their cytotoxicity to ensure their safe use in medical applications [58].

3.3.3 Semiconductor quantum dots: synthesis, modifications, cytotoxicity, and applications in cancer imaging

Semiconductor quantum dots (SQDs) are widely used in biomedical applications, particularly in cancer cell imaging, due to their unique properties, as shown in figure 3.12. These nanocrystals typically consist of a core–shell structure. The biocompatible fluorescent core, often made from elements in groups II–IV (like CdSe) or III–V (like InP), is coated with a semiconductor shell such as ZnS or ZnSe

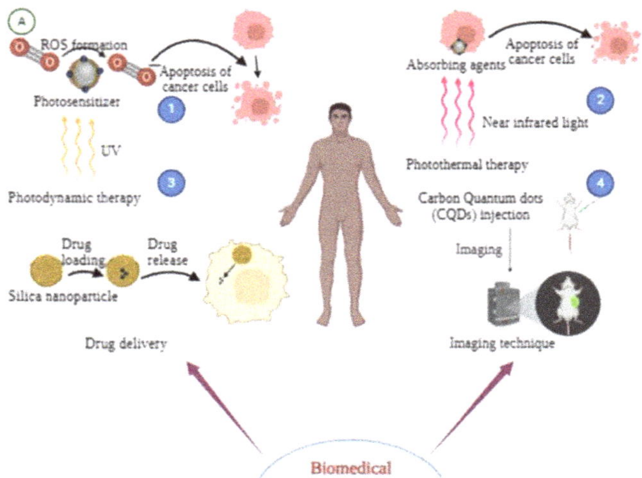

Figure 3.12. Overview of the biomedical applications of carbon quantum dots (CQDs). Reprinted from [60], Copyright (2024), with permission from Elsevier.

[59–61]. This shell enhances both the photostability and efficiency of the core. Additionally, an outer layer, usually silica, provides a large surface area for functionalization, allowing these SQDs to be dispersed in water and conjugated with biomolecules such as peptides, antibodies, and nucleic acids. This functionalization enables the targeting of specific proteins on the surface of cancer cells, making SQDs highly useful for imaging applications [61].

The synthesis of SQDs varies depending on the desired size, material composition, and quantum yield, as well as their intended application. Common methods include high-temperature synthesis, γ-irradiation, microwave-assisted synthesis, the sol–gel technique, and the core–shell technique. In the high-temperature method, a NaHTe solution is injected into an N_2-saturated Cd^{2+} precursor, which is then heated under atmospheric conditions, with the resulting QDs being precipitated and collected [61]. The gamma irradiation method, on the other hand, uses gamma rays to synthesize QDs from an aerated solution of $CdCl_2$ and SeO_2 [62]. Meanwhile, the microwave-assisted method involves exposing a pre-prepared NaHTe solution to microwave irradiation at varying temperatures and durations to obtain monodispersed QDs. Other techniques, such as the sol–gel and core–shell methods, are also widely employed in synthesizing Au, Cu, and Zn-based QDs [63, 64].

Modifications to the surface of SQDs can significantly enhance their luminous efficiency and stability. These modifications can be organic, involving ligands, polymers, and proteins, or inorganic, with elements such as Co^{2+}, Ni^{2+}, Mn^{2+}, and Cu^{2+} being doped into the structure. However, while SQDs offer benefits such as high sensitivity and stability, those containing cadmium (Cd) present significant cytotoxicity risks [65, 66]. The release of toxic Cd ions from these QDs has been shown to cause cellular damage, especially in normal cells. Studies have indicated that smaller CdTe-QDs (2.2 nm) are more toxic than larger particles (5.2 nm), and research has shown that CdTe-QDs can generate reactive oxygen species (ROS), which damage the DNA of cells like human umbilical vein endothelial cells (HUVECs). Therefore, due to the inherent cytotoxicity of heavy metals like cadmium, alternative materials are being explored for safer applications in clinical treatments [67, 68].

One promising alternative to cadmium-based SQDs is copper indium sulfide ($CuInS_2$ or CIS) QDs, which have been found to exhibit lower toxicity. When coated with a ZnS shell, CIS/ZnS QDs demonstrate high photoluminescence quantum yield and can be easily dispersed in aqueous solutions, making them suitable for biological imaging [69]. In one study, researchers synthesized $CuInS_2$/ZnS QDs coated with bovine serum albumin (BSA) and poly(ε-caprolactone) and labeled them with Arg–Gly–Asp (RGD) [70, 71]. These QDs were then used to evaluate cytotoxicity and tumor targeting in U87 and HeLa cells [72]. The presence of cRGD significantly increased the internalization of the QDs in both cancer cell lines, while BSA reduced non-specific binding and improved biocompatibility.

Another study explored the application of Cd-free CuInS2/ZnS core–shell QDs for *in vivo* tumor targeting in cancer cell xenograft mice, as presented in figure 3.13 [73]. The results showed increased NIR fluorescence emission over time following intravenous injection, indicating high tumor uptake. Similarly, Zhao *et al*

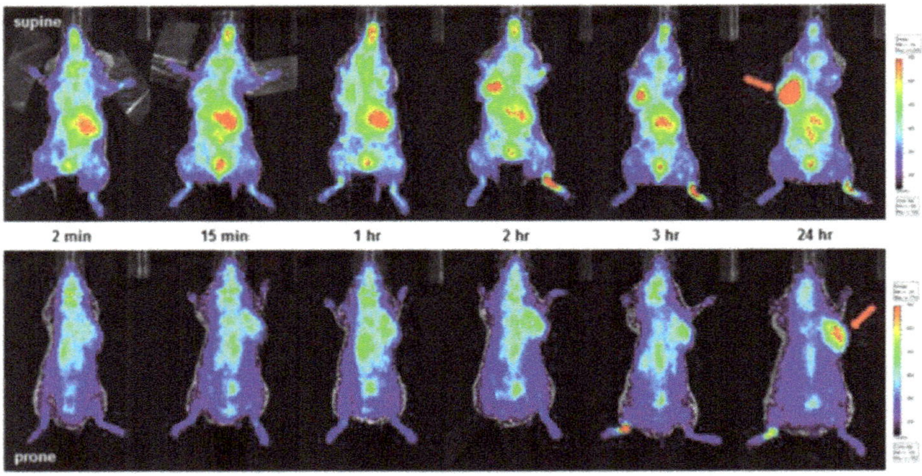

Figure 3.13. NIR fluorescence images of an RR1022 tumor-bearing mouse after intravenous injection of cRGDyk-GCM-QDs. Reprinted by permission from Springer Nature, [77], Copyright (2017).

investigated the ability of GSH-capped CuInS2/ZnS QDs for cancer cell imaging, finding that the QDs were primarily localized in the cytoplasm of the cells [74]. However, it is important to note that CIS QDs without ZnS shells tend to degrade rapidly, leading to increased toxicity in blood chemistry, organ weight, and histology. This highlights the need for caution when considering their clinical use.

3.3.4 Carbon quantum dots: properties and applications in cancer detection

Carbon quantum dots (CQDs), also known as carbon dots (CDs), were initially discovered accidentally during the separation and purification of single-walled carbon nanotubes (SWCNTs) [1, 3]. Since their discovery, their properties—such as low toxicity, biocompatibility, fluorescence, and chemical stability—have made them highly valuable in the field of theranostics. Fluorescent CQDs, in particular, have become preferred over traditional organic dyes for imaging applications due to their hydrophilicity, ease of preparation, biocompatibility, and reduced toxicity. These characteristics make CQDs promising candidates for cancer detection and imaging [74, 75].

One of the key applications of CQDs is their use as imaging probes for cancer cells. For instance, researchers have explored combining CQDs with metals like gadolinium, which not only enhances the imaging properties of CQDs but also reduces their toxicity and prevents leakage into surrounding tissues. This combination proves useful in ensuring safer and more effective imaging in clinical settings. Furthermore, CQDs have shown potential in the development of fluorescent sensors for detecting Fe^{3+} ions [76, 77]. Abnormal levels of Fe^{3+} are associated with cancer development and other diseases, and CQD-based sensors are being developed to detect these abnormal levels. For example, a solution containing CQDs doped with

Fe^{3+} has been used to differentiate cancer cells from normal cells, primarily due to variations in glutathione (GSH) levels between the two types of cells [78].

In addition to their diagnostic applications, CQDs have demonstrated anticancer properties *in vitro*, where they have been found to suppress cancer cell growth. Green fluorescent CDs have been designed as probes for visual cancer detection, utilizing their fluorescence properties to image cancer cells [79]. In one such study, CQDs were engineered to interact with folic acid, a well-known cancer cell marker. This interaction enabled the detection of folate receptor (FR)-positive cancer cells through turn-on fluorescence, providing a clear visual distinction between healthy and cancerous cells. Additionally, fluorescent CDs conjugated with folic acid have shown excellent biocompatibility, allowing them to bind specifically to cancer cells expressing FR, further distinguishing them from normal cells [80, 81]. The ability of CQDs to target cancer cells selectively, combined with their fluorescence and biocompatibility, makes them a promising tool for cancer detection and imaging. Ongoing research continues to explore their potential, not only for diagnostic purposes but also for therapeutic applications. As CQDs become more refined, their role in cancer treatment may expand, offering new avenues for early detection and precise treatment.

3.3.5 Graphene quantum dots in cancer therapy and diagnosis

Graphene quantum dots (GQDs), derived from graphene, are recognized for their excellent biocompatibility, luminescence, and ease of dispersion in various solvents. These properties make them highly suitable for applications in anti-cancer therapy, especially due to their intrinsic fluorescence, which allows for effective cell tracking *in vitro* [82, 83]. Studies have demonstrated the potential of GQDs in enhancing the efficiency of anticancer drugs, while their low cytotoxicity and strong optical absorption further solidify their role in bioimaging applications. This makes GQDs highly favorable for imaging cancer cells and supporting therapeutic interventions [84, 85].

One of the most promising uses of GQDs is in photodynamic therapy and tumor diagnosis. *In vivo* experiments have shown that GQDs can significantly inhibit the growth of breast cancer in mice, providing hope for their application in human cancer treatment. Nitrogen-doped GQDs have also been developed as nanocarriers for delivering the anticancer drug methotrexate, showing promising results. Additionally, sulfur-doped GQDs conjugated with folic acid have been synthesized for targeting FR-positive cancer cells [86, 87]. These GQDs enter the cancer cells via endocytosis, making them highly effective for early cancer detection and diagnosis. Their large surface area-to-volume ratio allows them to carry substantial amounts of anticancer drugs, improving drug delivery efficiency [88]. Furthermore, functionalizing GQDs with targeted ligands enables them to selectively target cancer cells that overexpress specific receptors. This targeted approach enhances the effectiveness of cancer therapies, reducing off-target effects and improving patient outcomes. Recently, biosensors utilizing GQDs in combination with gold nanoparticles were

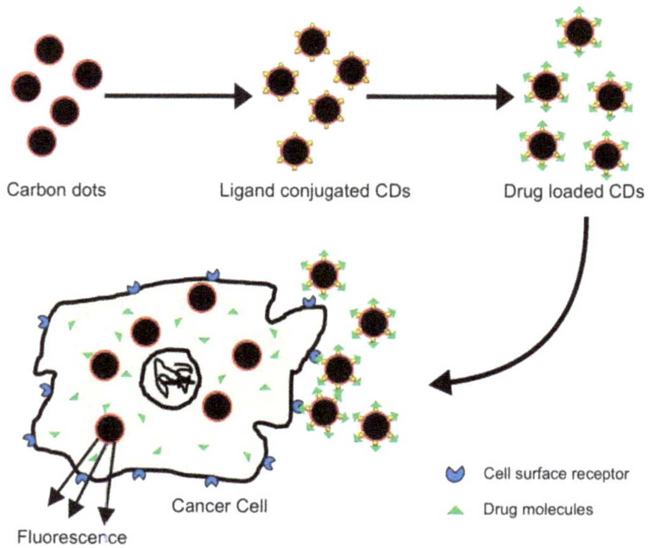

Figure 3.14. Illustration of carbon dot (CD) drug delivery to cancer cells. Reproduced from [89]. CC BY 4.0.

designed for 'turn on fluorescence' detection of lung cancer biomarkers, demonstrating the versatility and diagnostic potential of GQD-based nanomaterials [89].

Figure 3.14 illustrates the process of utilizing CDs for targeted drug delivery in cancer therapy. Initially, bare CDs are functionalized by conjugating them with ligands, allowing for specific targeting of cancer cells. These ligand-conjugated CDs are subsequently loaded with therapeutic drug molecules. Upon administration, the drug-loaded CDs target cancer cells by binding to specific cell surface receptors. Once inside the cancer cells, the CDs release the therapeutic agents, facilitating localized treatment. Additionally, the fluorescent properties of the CDs enable real-time imaging, allowing for the tracking of the CDs' distribution and interaction with the cancer cells. This approach enhances the precision of drug delivery while providing an integrated method for treatment and diagnosis [89].

3.3.6 Fullerenes in cancer therapy and drug delivery

Fullerenes (C_{60}) have emerged as promising candidates for cancer treatment, particularly as drug carriers. By conjugating drugs like paclitaxel and doxorubicin (DOX) with fullerenes, researchers have enhanced the therapeutic efficacy of these drugs. For example, fullerene-based paclitaxel formulations have demonstrated improved performance in drug delivery, while conjugating doxorubicin with fullerenes has made the drug more hydrophilic and less cytotoxic [90, 91]. Additionally, fullerenes facilitate the efficient delivery of DNA into cells, which opens up new possibilities for gene therapy applications in cancer treatment. Beyond drug delivery, fullerenes also hold promise in photodynamic therapy, a cancer treatment that uses light-activated compounds to generate ROS to kill cancer cells [92, 93].

When conjugated with polyethylene glycol (PEG), fullerenes exhibit enhanced photosensitivity, making them more effective in photodynamic applications. In some studies, endohedral fullerenes have been shown to inhibit angiogenesis, thereby reducing blood vessel density within tumors, which can help suppress tumor growth [94].

Fullerenes have also demonstrated potential as immunomodulators. By generating ROS, fullerenes activate immune cells and enhance their ability to target and destroy cancer cells. This ability to modulate the immune response, combined with their capacity to overcome tumor resistance to chemotherapeutic drugs, makes fullerenes valuable in combination therapies [95]. Furthermore, derivatives of fullerenes have been studied for their antioxidant properties, offering potential benefits in reducing the harmful side effects of traditional chemotherapy. One notable study found that fullerene conjugation with anticancer drugs significantly increased phagocyte activity. This process not only promotes the immune system's ability to clear cancer cells but also enhances ROS production by phagocytes, further amplifying the cancer-fighting effects. This dual mechanism of promoting phagocytosis and generating ROS makes fullerenes a promising strategy in the development of new cancer treatments [93–95].

3.3.7 Carbon nanotubes in cancer therapy and imaging

Carbon nanotubes (CNTs) have garnered significant attention as contrast agents in medical imaging due to their unique properties. They offer numerous advantages over other nanoscale detection agents, primarily because of their exceptionally high surface area and their ability to incorporate additional therapeutic and diagnostic components, either on their surface or within their inner cavity [96, 97]. Functionalized CNTs show promise as ultrasound contrast agents, laying the foundation for their future applications as theranostic tools. Their application in PAI further enhances accurate tumor targeting, while conjugation with MRI contrast agents enables efficient tumor localization in magnetic fields. CNTs also improve drug delivery, facilitating targeted delivery to cancer cells and prolonging circulation time in the bloodstream after successful uptake by malignant cells [98, 99].

CNTs are particularly useful in cancer photothermal therapy, where they help in efficiently targeting and killing cancer cells using heat. Based on their structure and diameter, CNTs are categorized into two main types: SWCNTs, consisting of a single graphene sheet in a tubular form with diameters ranging from 0.4 to 3 nm, and multi-walled carbon nanotubes (MWCNTs), which are composed of multiple layers of graphite with inner diameters of 1–3 nm and outer diameters of 2–100 nm [100, 101]. Like other nanoparticles, CNTs are not easily soluble in aqueous media, which necessitates functionalization or modification to improve their biocompatibility.

SWCNTs have shown great promise in delivering drugs, proteins, and siRNA into target cells. For instance, SWCNTs conjugated with the anticancer drug DOX demonstrated significantly improved clinical outcomes compared to DOX alone. SWCNTs have also been effectively employed *in vivo* for cancer therapy, where they aid in administering therapeutic agents with high precision and reduced toxicity

[102, 103]. Another anticancer drug, Paclitaxel (PTX), when conjugated with SWCNTs, effectively suppressed tumors without causing damage to other organs, providing evidence that CNT-based drug delivery systems offer high treatment efficacy with minimal toxicity [104]. MWCNTs, on the other hand, have been used to develop magnetic nanocarriers by incorporating iron oxide nanoparticles. These MWCNT-based nanocarriers demonstrated dual-targeted delivery capabilities, making them useful for cancer therapy. Additionally, a novel method using MWCNTs for delivering DNA and siRNA into microglial cells for brain cancer therapy has been developed, opening new avenues for treating challenging cancers, such as those affecting the brain [105].

Figure 3.15 demonstrates the internalization of MWCNTs by BV2 microglia cells. Panel (a) shows confocal microscopy images of BV2 cells incubated with pMWCNTs-PKH for 48 h, revealing increasing internalization of the nanoparticles over time. Panel (b) presents transmission electron microscopy (TEM) images of the cells after 2, 6, and 24 h of incubation, where single MWCNTs can be observed penetrating the cell membrane. Panel (c) provides a highly magnified TEM image, illustrating the detailed process of MWCNTs penetrating the cell surface. This figure highlights the ability of MWCNTs to effectively enter microglia cells, which is crucial for understanding their potential applications in drug delivery and therapeutic interventions [106].

Their ability to penetrate cell membranes, as shown in figure 3.15, makes them an effective vehicle for intracellular drug delivery. The image demonstrates how MWCNTs can enter BV2 microglia cells over time, providing a visual representation of their capacity to penetrate cell surfaces. This property is crucial in cancer

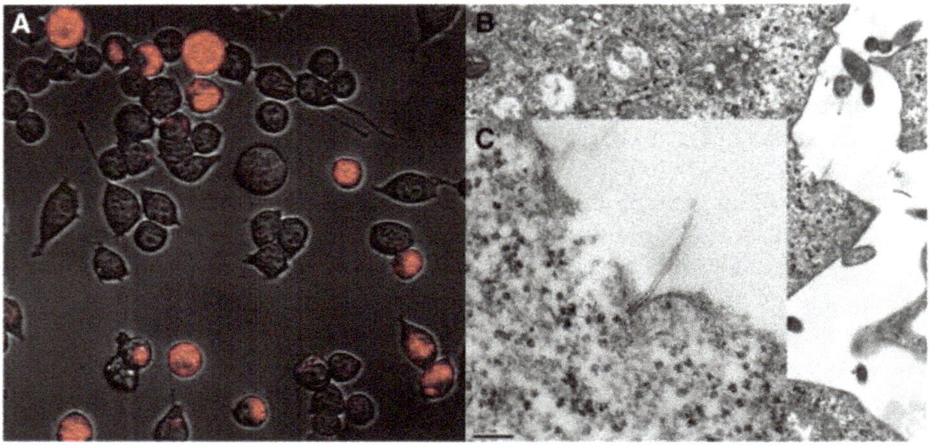

Figure 3.15. MWCNT internalization by BV2 microglia cells. (a) Confocal microscopy images of BV2 cells incubated with pMWCNTs-PKH for 48 h, revealing increasing internalization of the nanoparticles over time. (b) Transmission electron microscopy (TEM) images of the cells after 2, 6, and 24 h of incubation. Single MWCNTs can be observed penetrating the cell membrane. (c) A highly magnified TEM image, illustrating the detailed process of MWCNTs penetrating the cell surface. Reprinted from [106], copyright (2007), with permission from Elsevier.

therapy, where effective drug delivery directly into tumor cells can significantly improve treatment outcomes. Additionally, CNTs can be used for photothermal therapy, where they absorb NIR light and convert it into heat, effectively killing cancer cells without harming surrounding healthy tissue.

3.3.8 Magnetic nanoparticles in cancer diagnosis and treatment

Magnetic nanoparticles (MNPs) have become a significant breakthrough in oncology, offering various applications in cancer diagnosis, screening, targeted drug delivery, and treatment. One of their most prominent uses is in tumor targeting, made possible by advanced imaging technologies that enable early detection of cancer. MNPs, particularly superparamagnetic iron oxide nanoparticles (SPIONs), are commonly used as contrast agents in imaging techniques such as MRI, magneto-acoustic tomography (MAT), CT, and NIR imaging [107, 108]. In addition to their role in imaging, MNPs are increasingly employed in drug delivery systems, where they act as carriers, delivering therapeutic agents to specific target sites in the body through the use of an external magnetic field (EMF). Functionalizing MNPs with antibodies and chemotherapeutic drugs enhances their specificity, allowing them to target cancer cells with greater precision [109].

Figure 3.16 illustrates two key strategies for fabricating multifunctional MNPs and their potential applications in biomedical fields. The first strategy involves conjugating biomolecules, such as antibodies, ligands, receptors, or dyes, to the MNP surface, enabling applications like specific binding for targeted drug delivery, bacteria detection, protein separation, and multimodal imaging. The second approach integrates nanocomponents such as QDs or metal nanoparticles, creating hybrid structures that enhance functionality for multimodal imaging and drug delivery. These versatile nanoparticles offer a range of applications, including MRI and targeted cancer therapy, making them valuable tools in both diagnostics and treatment.

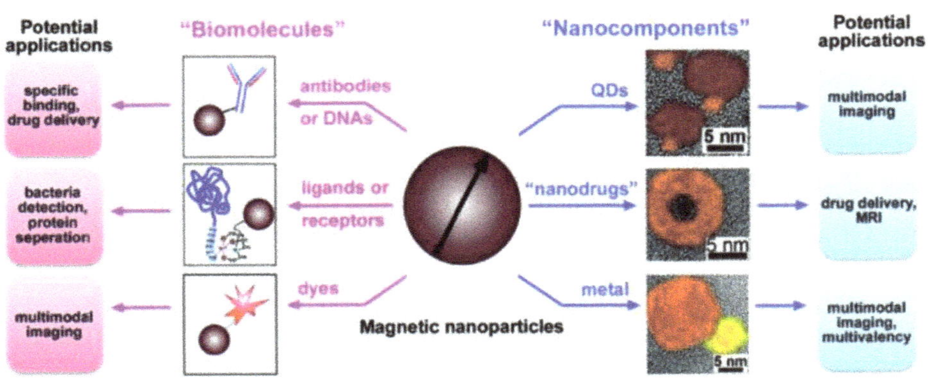

Figure 3.16. Two commonly used strategies for fabricating multifunctional magnetic nanoparticles. Reproduced with permission from [109]. © 2021 The Author(s). Published by Elsevier B.V.

MNPs also hold promise in cancer treatment through methods such as magnetically induced hyperthermia (MHT), photodynamic therapy (PDT), and photothermal therapy (PTT). These strategies can be combined with other treatments, such as chemotherapy and imaging, to achieve more effective outcomes [110]. The unique design of MNPs allows them to perform multiple functions simultaneously, enhancing their therapeutic impact [111]. For example, MRI can be used for early cancer diagnosis, while chemotherapy can be administered alongside it, optimizing treatment speed and efficacy. The synthesis of MNPs significantly influences their properties, such as superparamagnetism, high magnetic moment, and magnetocaloric effect, which make them ideal for medical applications [112]. These nanoparticles, typically smaller than 100 nm, are magnetized in the presence of an EMF and lose magnetization when the field is removed, preventing clustering [113]. The magnetocaloric effect of MNPs, which allows them to change temperature based on the EMF, is particularly useful in cancer therapy, especially for hyperthermia treatments, where localized heating is used to kill cancer cells [114].

In targeted drug delivery systems, MNPs are transported *in vivo* to specific sites within the body using an external magnetic field. Their small size—comparable to biological entities such as proteins, viruses, and cells—allows for efficient diffusion and distribution in tissues near the targeted area [107]. Parameters such as particle size, composition, and surface functionalization can be adjusted to improve their magnetic properties and optimize their behavior *in vivo*. Among the most commonly used MNPs are iron oxide nanoparticles, particularly magnetite (Fe_3O_4) and maghemite (γ-Fe_2O_3), which are favored for their biocompatibility, low toxicity, and ease of preparation [115]. MNPs are also being applied in cancer thermotherapy, or hyperthermia, where they serve as mediators for localized heating to treat tumors. Additionally, MNPs are now being developed as platforms for biosensors and immunoassays, with ligands such as aptamers and antibodies immobilized on their surfaces to target tumor cells more effectively. These ligands enable MNPs to accumulate in specific locations within cancerous tissues, improving the accuracy of diagnostics and therapy [116, 117].

Figure 3.17 presents an overview of the molecular subtypes in cancer and their corresponding therapeutic strategies. The figure classifies cancers into four primary subtypes: luminal androgen receptor, immune-enriched, PI3K/AKT/mTOR activated, and DNA repair deficiency. For each subtype, specific treatment approaches are highlighted. For example, the luminal androgen receptor subtype is targeted with anti-androgen therapy and combinations with CDK 4/6 inhibitors. The immune-enriched subtype benefits from immune checkpoint inhibitors due to increased immune response genes and PD-L1 expression. The PI3K/AKT/mTOR activated subtype can be treated with selective inhibitors for PI3KCA and AKT mutations, while DNA repair-deficient cancers, particularly those with BRCA1 and BRCA2 mutations, are treated using PARP inhibitors and platinum-based therapies. This figure emphasizes the importance of molecular profiling for selecting personalized treatment strategies in oncology [117].

Furthermore, MNPs have shown significant potential in gene delivery and therapy. For instance, viral vectors carrying therapeutic genes can be attached to

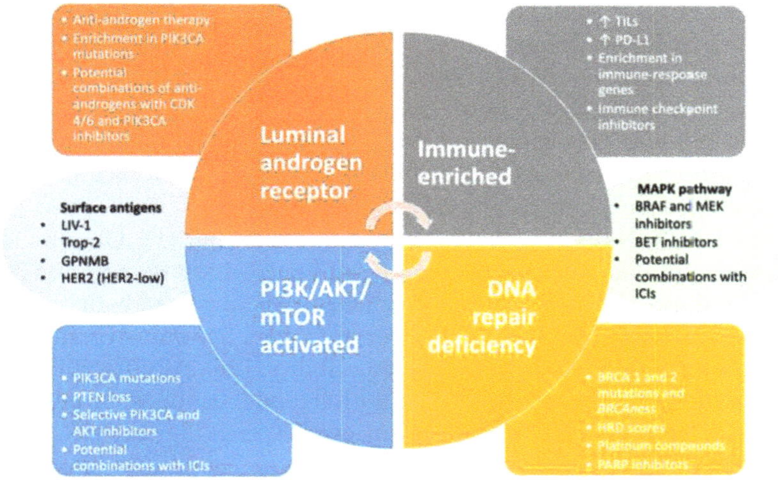

Figure 3.17. Overview of molecular subtypes in cancer and corresponding therapeutic strategies. Reproduced with permission from [117]. © 2021 The Author(s). © The Royal Society of Chemistry 2022.

MNPs, facilitating gene transfection and expression in target cells. This approach, known as magnetic transfection or magnetofection, has been explored for the treatment of lung, gastrointestinal, and blood cancers [118, 119]. The potential for using MNPs in non-viral transfection methods, including for DNA and siRNA delivery, is also under investigation. MNPs offer a versatile and multifaceted approach to cancer detection, diagnosis, and treatment. Their multifunctional properties make them ideal for use in MRI, hyperthermia, drug delivery, tissue repair, immunoassays, and biosensors [120, 121]. As research progresses, MNPs are expected to continue revolutionizing the field of cancer biomedicine, enabling more effective and targeted treatments that could improve patient outcomes.

3.4 Nanotechnology-enhanced imaging techniques

3.4.1 Magnetic resonance imaging with nanoparticle contrast agents

MRI is a widely used diagnostic tool in modern medicine, known for its ability to create detailed images of soft tissues without the use of ionizing radiation. In recent years, the incorporation of nanomaterials as contrast agents has significantly enhanced MRI's efficacy, particularly for the early detection and monitoring of cancers [122, 123]. Nanomaterial-based contrast agents, particularly MNPs like SPIONs, have transformed the field of MRI by improving image contrast, increasing diagnostic accuracy, and enabling multifunctional applications such as drug delivery and hyperthermia therapy [124].

3.4.1.1 Properties of magnetic nanoparticles for MRI

Nanoparticles used as contrast agents in MRI have several intrinsic properties that make them ideal for enhancing imaging contrast. These include superparamagnetism, high surface area, and the ability to be functionalized with targeting molecules. SPIONs, which typically range between 10–100 nm in size, are among the most commonly used MNPs for MRI [124]. They exhibit a phenomenon called superparamagnetism, meaning they become magnetized only in the presence of an external magnetic field but lose their magnetization once the field is removed. This property ensures that SPIONs do not aggregate in the body after the MRI scan, which makes them safe and effective for medical use [125].

The core of SPIONs is usually composed of magnetite (Fe_3O_4) or maghemite (γ-Fe_2O_3), which provide the magnetic properties needed to affect proton relaxation times in tissues during MRI. These nanoparticles are then coated with biocompatible materials such as dextran, PEG, or other polymers to improve their stability, dispersibility in biological fluids, and biocompatibility [126]. Additionally, the surface of the nanoparticles can be functionalized with ligands, peptides, or antibodies that enable them to target specific tissues or cancer cells, making the MRI scan highly specific to areas of interest such as tumors [127].

3.4.1.2 Mechanism of action in magnetic resonance imaging

MNPs enhance MRI images by affecting the relaxation times of hydrogen protons in water molecules within tissues. When these nanoparticles are injected into the body, they accumulate in the target tissue (such as a tumor) due to their magnetic properties and surface modifications [128, 129]. Once in the presence of an external magnetic field, such as during an MRI scan, the nanoparticles alter the local magnetic environment, shortening the transverse (T2) and longitudinal (T1) relaxation times. This results in enhanced contrast in the images, allowing for more precise visualization of tissues and abnormalities [127–129].

For T1-weighted MRI imaging, the use of nanoparticles increases the brightness of the tissue by enhancing proton relaxation. For T2-weighted images, which are particularly useful for identifying tumors, the nanoparticles cause a darkening effect due to proton dephasing, helping to differentiate between normal and diseased tissues [130]. The ability to manipulate the imaging properties based on the type of nanoparticle and the intended application gives healthcare providers the flexibility to adapt MRI scans to various diagnostic needs [131].

3.4.1.3 Advantages of nanomaterial-based contrast agents

Nanoparticle-based MRI contrast agents offer several advantages over traditional contrast agents. Their small size, typically on the scale of a few nanometers, allows for better penetration into tissues and more accurate targeting of disease sites [129, 131]. In cancer imaging, where precise detection of tumor margins is crucial, the ability of nanoparticles to be functionalized with ligands for tumor-specific markers (such as folic acid or antibodies targeting cancer cell receptors) enhances diagnostic accuracy. This targeting ability also reduces off-target effects and minimizes damage to surrounding healthy tissues [132].

The versatility of nanoparticles also extends to theranostic applications, where diagnostic and therapeutic functionalities are combined. For example, MNPs can be loaded with chemotherapeutic drugs, enabling them to not only serve as contrast agents for MRI but also deliver drugs directly to the tumor site [133]. This dual functionality can be monitored in real time during MRI, allowing clinicians to track the effectiveness of treatment and make adjustments as necessary. SPIONs and other MNPs are biocompatible and have relatively low toxicity, especially compared to traditional gadolinium-based contrast agents, which have been linked to nephrogenic systemic fibrosis in patients with kidney disease. Once the nanoparticles have fulfilled their role, they can be metabolized and excreted from the body without causing long-term adverse effects [130–132].

3.4.1.4 Applications in cancer diagnosis and treatment

Nanoparticle contrast agents are particularly beneficial in the field of oncology. For early detection of tumors, MNPs can be engineered to specifically target cancerous cells, enabling the detection of small, early-stage tumors that may not be visible with conventional MRI. This capability is critical for improving patient outcomes, as early diagnosis is often linked to higher survival rates [130]. Furthermore, MNPs are being used in magnetic hyperthermia therapy, a treatment modality where localized heating of cancer cells is achieved by applying an alternating magnetic field to the nanoparticles. The heat generated by the MNPs helps destroy cancer cells while sparing the surrounding healthy tissues [134]. This treatment can be combined with MRI for precise monitoring, ensuring that the heat is delivered exactly where it is needed. In addition to their role in hyperthermia, MNPs can also be used in gene delivery for cancer therapy. By attaching DNA or RNA to the surface of these nanoparticles, genetic material can be delivered to target cells, offering potential treatments for genetic disorders or cancers with known genetic mutations [135].

3.4.1.5 Challenges and future directions

While nanomaterial-based MRI contrast agents offer many advantages, there are still challenges to overcome. One of the primary concerns is the potential toxicity and long-term effects of nanoparticles, particularly if they accumulate in organs such as the liver or spleen. Ongoing research is focused on developing biodegradable nanoparticles that can break down safely in the body after fulfilling their role [129–131]. Another challenge is the complexity of manufacturing nanoparticles with precise size, shape, and surface properties. Variability in these parameters can affect their behavior in the body and their performance as contrast agents. Researchers are working to develop more controlled synthesis methods to ensure uniformity in nanoparticle production [136].

The integration of nanomaterials in MRI as contrast agents represents a significant advancement in medical imaging, particularly in cancer diagnosis and treatment. Their ability to enhance image contrast, target specific tissues, and serve as multifunctional agents in theranostics makes them invaluable in modern healthcare. As technology continues to evolve, the role of nanomaterials in MRI is expected to expand, offering even more precise and personalized diagnostic and therapeutic options for patients [132–136].

3.4.2 Positron emission tomography with radiolabeled nanomaterials

PET is a powerful imaging technique that provides high sensitivity and precision in detecting and monitoring diseases, particularly cancer. The use of radiolabeled nanomaterials in PET imaging has opened new avenues for enhancing its diagnostic capability, offering superior targeting, improved resolution, and more efficient imaging of tumors. By combining nanotechnology with radiolabeling, researchers have developed advanced contrast agents that can be specifically tailored for various biomedical applications, including tumor detection, drug delivery, and theranostics (combining diagnosis with therapy).

As shown in figure 3.18, after intravenous injection, the radiolabeled nanoparticles circulate through the bloodstream, where they accumulate in targeted tumor cells. PET scans taken at different time points demonstrate how these nanoparticles are distributed throughout the body. Early post-injection scans

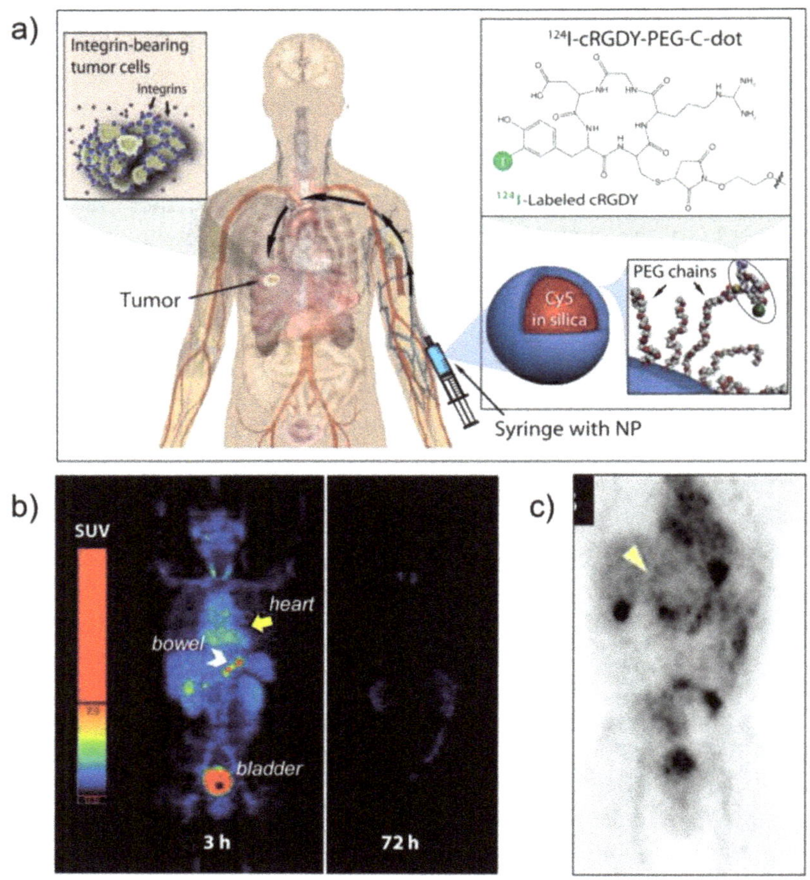

Figure 3.18. Figure showing targeted tumor imaging using 124I-labeled cRGDY-PEG-C-dots. Reprinted from [21], Copyright (2017), with permission from Elsevier.

show accumulation in organs like the heart, bowel, and bladder, which reflects the nanoparticles' initial biodistribution. Over time, the signal fades in non-target tissues as the nanoparticles are cleared, leaving a concentrated signal in the tumor site. This precise targeting enables real-time visualization of the tumor and the nanoparticles' behavior within the body [21].

This imaging approach offers several advantages for cancer diagnostics and therapy. It provides non-invasive, high-resolution images of the tumor's location and size, allowing clinicians to monitor disease progression or treatment response effectively. Furthermore, the versatility of radiolabeled nanomaterials extends beyond imaging, as they can be designed to carry therapeutic agents, making them useful for theranostic applications where diagnosis and treatment are combined in a single platform. The use of PET imaging with nanomaterials represents a significant advance in precision oncology, offering enhanced tumor detection and more personalized treatment strategies.

3.4.2.1 Nanomaterials in positron emission tomography imaging

Nanomaterials used in PET imaging provide several advantages over traditional imaging agents. These materials exhibit unique properties, such as high surface area, stability, and the ability to be easily functionalized. Their size enables them to navigate through biological systems effectively, reaching tumor sites and enhancing image contrast. Below are the primary types of nanomaterials that are widely used in PET imaging.

1. **Gold nanoparticles (Au NPs)**: **Au NPs** are among the most commonly used nanomaterials in PET imaging. Due to their biocompatibility, ease of surface modification, and ability to carry multiple functional groups, Au NPs can be radiolabeled with isotopes such as ^{64}Cu or ^{68}Ga. These particles enhance PET imaging by accumulating at tumor sites, providing high-contrast images. In addition, gold nanoparticles can be conjugated with therapeutic agents, making them suitable for theranostic applications. The combination of imaging and therapy allows real-time tracking of treatment efficacy, improving personalized medicine approaches [137, 138] (figure 3.19).

2. **Iron oxide nanoparticles**: iron oxide nanoparticles, particularly SPIONs, are used extensively in dual-modal imaging, including PET. When radiolabeled with isotopes like ^{68}Ga, these nanoparticles enable high-resolution imaging and, due to their magnetic properties, can also be used in MRI [140]. This dual functionality allows clinicians to use both anatomical and functional imaging simultaneously, improving the accuracy of tumor detection. SPIONs are also used for hyperthermia therapy, where localized heating destroys cancer cells, and their combination with PET allows for precise monitoring during treatment [141].
3. **QDs**: QDs are semiconductor nanomaterials with remarkable optical properties. Their fluorescence and small size make them ideal candidates for multimodal imaging. When combined with radionuclides, quantum dots provide not only fluorescent imaging capabilities but also high-contrast PET

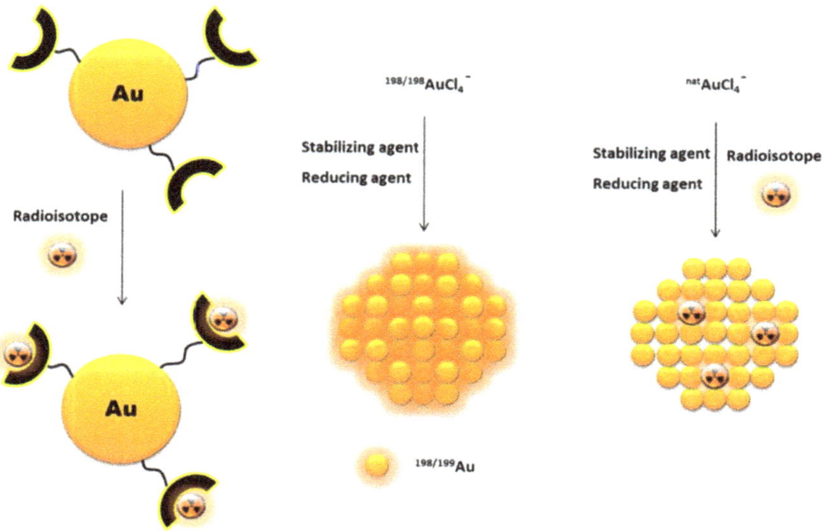

Figure 3.19. Different methods for synthesizing radiolabeled gold nanoparticles. Reproduced from [139]. CC BY 4.0.

imaging. Radiolabeled QDs are especially useful in cancer imaging, where they offer enhanced sensitivity in detecting tumors. For instance, QDs can be labeled with ^{64}Cu or ^{18}F, providing clear visualization of tumor margins and aiding in early diagnosis [142].

4. **CNTs**: CNTs are another class of nanomaterials employed in PET imaging. They are primarily used for drug delivery and PAI but have shown great promise in PET applications when functionalized with radionuclides. Radiolabeled CNTs can be designed to target specific tumor markers, allowing for precise imaging of cancerous tissues [143]. Due to their hollow structure, CNTs can also carry therapeutic agents, making them ideal for theranostic applications. Additionally, their large surface area enables multiple radiolabels or drugs to be loaded, enhancing both imaging resolution and treatment efficacy [144].
5. **Silica nanoparticles**: silica nanoparticles, often referred to as mesoporous silica nanoparticles (MSNs), are highly versatile due to their tunable pore sizes and biocompatibility. In PET imaging, silica nanoparticles are radiolabeled with isotopes like ^{68}Ga or ^{64}Cu, providing high-resolution images of tumors. Their porous structure allows for the encapsulation of therapeutic agents, enabling simultaneous drug delivery and imaging. The surface of silica nanoparticles can also be functionalized with targeting ligands, improving their specificity for cancer cells. These properties make silica nanoparticles highly effective for targeted drug delivery, multimodal imaging, and cancer treatment [145].
6. **Polymeric nanoparticles**: polymeric nanoparticles, made from biodegradable materials like poly(lactic-co-glycolic acid) (PLGA), are frequently used as

carriers for both drugs and imaging agents. In PET imaging, these nanoparticles can be radiolabeled with isotopes such as ^{18}F or ^{64}Cu and targeted to tumors using surface modifications. Their biocompatibility and ability to carry therapeutic agents allow them to be used for both diagnosis and treatment. Polymeric nanoparticles are particularly useful in targeted drug delivery systems, where they release their payload at the tumor site while simultaneously providing imaging feedback through PET [146].

7. **Liposomes**: liposomes are spherical vesicles composed of lipid bilayers that can encapsulate both hydrophilic and hydrophobic drugs. Radiolabeled liposomes are used in PET imaging for their ability to deliver imaging agents and therapeutics to tumors. Liposomes are commonly labeled with radionuclides like **^{18}F**, **^{64}Cu**, or **^{68}Ga**, which allow for detailed imaging of the tumor microenvironment. The flexible structure of liposomes also enables the delivery of chemotherapy drugs alongside imaging agents, making them suitable for theranostic applications [147, 148].
8. **Fullerenes**: fullerenes, a class of carbon-based nanomaterials, have shown potential in PET imaging due to their unique cage-like structure. Radiolabeled fullerenes can carry positron-emitting isotopes such as ^{18}F or ^{64}Cu, enhancing the visualization of tumor sites [149]. Their structure allows for the encapsulation of drugs or other therapeutic agents, enabling them to serve as both imaging and therapeutic platforms. Fullerenes are also being investigated for their antioxidant properties, which may reduce the side effects of chemotherapy when used in combination with PET imaging.

3.4.2.2 Advantages of radiolabeled nanomaterials in positron emission tomography [150]

Nanomaterials provide several benefits in PET imaging, including:

- **Enhanced targeting**: by functionalizing the surface of nanoparticles with ligands, antibodies, or peptides, radiolabeled nanomaterials can specifically target cancer cells, improving image contrast and reducing false positives.
- **Improved sensitivity**: nanomaterials can carry multiple radionuclides, increasing the signal strength and enhancing the sensitivity of PET scans, leading to more accurate diagnosis of early-stage tumors.
- **Multimodal imaging**: many nanomaterials, such as gold nanoparticles and SPIONs, allow for multimodal imaging by combining PET with other imaging techniques like MRI or FI. This enables comprehensive tumor mapping and better treatment planning.
- **Theranostic potential**: nanomaterials can be loaded with both imaging agents and therapeutic drugs, enabling real-time monitoring of treatment efficacy and reducing the need for separate imaging and therapy sessions.

3.4.2.3 Future directions and challenges

Despite their advantages, several challenges remain in the clinical translation of radiolabeled nanomaterials for PET imaging. The long-term safety and biocompatibility of these materials need further investigation, particularly concerning their accumulation in organs such as the liver and spleen. Additionally, manufacturing processes must be refined to ensure consistent particle size, shape, and surface properties for reproducibility in clinical applications. Nevertheless, ongoing research into biodegradable and non-toxic nanomaterials holds promise for overcoming these obstacles [151].

3.4.3 Computed tomography and nanocontrast agents

3.4.3.1 Nanoparticle contrast agents in computed tomography imaging

CT imaging has been a cornerstone of diagnostic medicine, especially in providing detailed anatomical data. However, the ability of CT to differentiate between soft tissues without a contrast agent is limited. This is where nanoparticle contrast agents come into play, offering enhanced contrast and clearer imaging in diverse medical applications, including cancer detection, cardiovascular disease, and tumor tracking. Nanoparticles, due to their size and modifiable surface, are increasingly being utilized as contrast agents in CT. They provide superior contrast compared to traditional iodine-based agents and offer more versatility in terms of functionalization with targeting molecules, enabling precise delivery to specific tissues or cell types [16].

3.4.3.2 Types of nanomaterials in computed tomography imaging

1. **Gold nanoparticles (Au NPs): Au NPs** are the most widely researched due to their high atomic number ($Z = 79$), which leads to enhanced x-ray attenuation. Their K-edge at 80.7 keV makes them excellent for generating strong contrast in CT imaging. Au NPs can be functionalized with ligands, peptides, or antibodies, allowing them to target specific tissues, such as tumors [152]. Their inert nature and stability in biological systems make them biocompatible for use in live subjects. Au NPs can also be used in multimodal imaging and therapy (theranostics), combining diagnostic imaging with therapeutic functions such as photothermal therapy [153].
2. **SPIONs:** SPIONs are also extensively studied as contrast agents. While primarily used in MRI, SPIONs can be utilized in CT by enhancing contrast when coated with materials that increase x-ray attenuation, such as gold or other high-Z elements. Additionally, SPIONs can be used in conjunction with magnetic fields for targeted drug delivery, combining diagnosis and treatment in one platform [154].
3. **Bismuth-based nanoparticles:** bismuth ($Z = 83$) is another high-atomic-number element that offers excellent attenuation properties. Bismuth-based nanoparticles provide higher contrast than traditional iodine agents and are more biocompatible. These nanoparticles are often used for imaging lymph nodes, tumors, and vascular diseases. Their stability and low toxicity profile make them a promising alternative to conventional contrast agents [155].
4. **Tungsten and tantalum nanoparticles:** tungsten and tantalum nanoparticles are high-density materials ($Z = 74$ and $Z = 73$, respectively) that offer

significant contrast enhancement in CT. These nanoparticles are particularly useful in imaging blood vessels, allowing for clearer visualization of vascular anomalies. Tungsten nanoparticles have been explored in combination with polymeric carriers to enhance circulation time in the bloodstream [156, 157].

5. **Iodine-encapsulated nanoparticles:** iodine remains a popular contrast agent in CT, and the development of iodine-encapsulated nanoparticles has shown improved bioavailability and reduced toxicity. By incorporating iodine into nanoparticle systems, researchers can enhance the distribution and retention of the contrast agent, allowing for more detailed imaging over extended periods. These nanoparticles can be engineered to target specific disease sites, such as cancerous tissues, enabling more effective diagnostics [158].
6. **Gadolinium-based nanoparticles:** gadolinium is commonly used in MRI but has applications in CT as well when incorporated into nanoparticle systems. These nanoparticles can combine both CT and MRI contrast properties, offering dual-modal imaging capabilities. The use of gadolinium nanoparticles helps in overcoming the limitations of poor contrast resolution, particularly in soft tissue imaging [159].

3.4.3.3 Applications in disease imaging

(a) **Cancer imaging:** nanoparticles such as gold and bismuth are particularly effective in cancer imaging. Their ability to enhance x-ray attenuation allows for precise visualization of tumors, even those located deep within tissues. Nanoparticles functionalized with cancer-targeting ligands enable more accurate detection of tumors and their metastases, aiding in early diagnosis and treatment planning [160].

(b) **Cardiovascular disease:** nanoparticles are also useful in vascular imaging, where they enhance the visibility of blood vessels and help in detecting anomalies such as plaque formation or blockages. Iron oxide nanoparticles, for instance, have been used to track the progression of atherosclerosis and monitor the efficacy of treatment [161].

(c) **Cell tracking:** CT imaging with nanoparticle contrast agents has shown promise in cell tracking, particularly in monitoring stem cell therapies. Au NPs have been used to label stem cells, allowing researchers to visualize their distribution, migration, and differentiation in real time, which is crucial for assessing the efficacy of regenerative treatments [162].

The advent of nanotechnology has revolutionized CT imaging by providing contrast agents that are not only more effective but also customizable for specific diagnostic needs. Nanoparticle-based contrast agents offer better contrast resolution, extended circulation time, and the ability to target specific tissues or disease sites. With ongoing advancements in nanomaterials, the future of CT imaging looks promising, with the potential for more precise, non-invasive diagnostics, and theranostic applications that combine imaging with targeted therapy.

3.4.4 Optical imaging with nanoprobes and fluorescence techniques

3.4.4.1 Hybrid nanomaterials and multi-modal imaging

(a) **Integration of nanoparticles for combined imaging techniques**

In recent years, nanotechnology has opened up significant advancements in medical imaging by enhancing the capabilities of various imaging modalities. Nanoparticles, due to their small size and unique physical and chemical properties, can serve as powerful imaging agents. The integration of nanoparticles for combined imaging techniques allows the convergence of multiple imaging modalities, thereby providing complementary information that significantly enhances diagnostic accuracy. This is particularly relevant in clinical scenarios where a single imaging technique may not be sufficient to provide a complete picture [131].

Nanoparticles, due to their ability to be functionalized with multiple imaging agents, enable multi-modal imaging. For instance, SPIONs are used extensively in MRI for enhanced contrast due to their magnetic properties, and they can also be utilized in PET by incorporating radioisotopes. Similarly, gold nanoparticles are often employed in CT due to their high atomic number, which leads to enhanced x-ray attenuation, while their surface can be functionalized to serve as contrast agents for fluorescence or PAI [131].

By utilizing nanoparticles in combined imaging techniques, such as MRI/PET, MRI/CT, and PET/CT, it becomes possible to obtain both anatomical and functional information, which enhances the precision of disease diagnosis. For example, gold nanoparticles conjugated with antibodies or aptamers can target specific tumor cells and provide real-time feedback through various imaging modalities. This enables detailed lesion characterization by offering superior resolution and tissue contrast compared to traditional imaging methods. Moreover, the EPR effect seen in tumor vasculature allows nanoparticles to accumulate at tumor sites, providing highly specific imaging capabilities [163].

(b) **Dual-function nanomaterials for imaging and therapy (theranostics)**

Theranostics, the concept of combining diagnostics and therapy within a single platform, has been made feasible through the development of dual-function nanomaterials. These nanomaterials are engineered to simultaneously act as imaging agents and deliver therapeutic agents to the targeted disease site. Nanoparticles, such as liposomes, micelles, and dendrimers, can encapsulate both imaging agents and drugs, providing real-time monitoring of drug delivery and therapeutic efficacy [133].

For example, QDs can serve as FI agents while delivering chemotherapeutic drugs to cancer cells. Similarly, SPIONs can be used to monitor drug delivery through MRI while also acting as carriers for targeted drug delivery systems. The theranostic approach provides a significant advantage in cancer treatment, as it allows clinicians to visualize the tumor, monitor the drug release, and assess the therapeutic response all in real-time. Gold nanoparticles, due to their plasmonic properties, have been used for both imaging and photothermal therapy. When exposed to NIR light, these nanoparticles can generate localized heat, which is useful in ablation therapy for cancer cells, while simultaneously being used as contrast agents in imaging modalities such as CT or PAI [57].

Another example is the use of nanomaterials in radiation therapy, where nanoparticles such as gadolinium or gold can enhance the radiotherapeutic effect due to their high atomic number, and their presence can be tracked through imaging techniques like MRI or CT. The integration of therapeutic agents with diagnostic capabilities enables precise, targeted treatments, reducing the damage to healthy tissues and improving patient outcomes [129, 163].

3.4.4.2 Case studies of multi-modal nanoplatform applications

One of the key applications of multi-modal nanoplatforms is in the early detection and treatment of cancer. For instance, researchers have developed nanoparticles that combine optical and magnetic properties for dual-modal imaging. These platforms can simultaneously provide FI and MRI for detailed tumor mapping. One study demonstrated the use of SPIONs conjugated with fluorescent dyes for the dual-modal imaging of tumors, showing both detailed anatomical information via MRI and real-time monitoring of drug delivery through FI. This dual-functionality enabled precise localization of the tumor and the ability to monitor the treatment progress [51, 151, 163].

Another case involved the use of gold nanoparticles in multi-modal imaging. Gold nanoparticles functionalized with targeting ligands for cancer cells were shown to enhance both CT and PAI. In preclinical studies, this nanoplatform provided high-resolution CT images for anatomical mapping and photoacoustic signals for functional imaging, allowing researchers to visualize the tumor's vascularization and oxygenation status. The high contrast provided by gold nanoparticles in both modalities allowed for better tumor delineation and real-time tracking of drug efficacy [164].

In addition to cancer, multi-modal nanoplatforms have been applied in cardiovascular diseases. Nanoparticles designed for MRI and US imaging have been used to track the progression of atherosclerotic plaques in real time. The combination of MRI's detailed anatomical resolution and US's ability to monitor blood flow dynamics provides a comprehensive view of plaque development, enabling more informed clinical decisions. These case studies highlight the potential of nanoparticles to revolutionize medical imaging by integrating multiple modalities into a single nanoplatform. This convergence allows for a comprehensive view of disease processes, leading to earlier diagnosis, better treatment planning, and improved patient outcomes [165].

3.5 Targeted imaging: precision at the cellular level

3.5.1 Nanoparticle-based targeting strategies for specific cancer biomarkers

Nanoparticles have become a transformative tool in the field of cancer imaging due to their ability to target cancer cells precisely based on molecular biomarkers. These biomarkers, which include proteins, receptors, and other molecules uniquely expressed or overexpressed in cancerous tissues, act as biological indicators that nanoparticles can be engineered to detect. Nanoparticle-based targeting offers a promising solution to some of the long-standing challenges in cancer imaging, such as distinguishing between healthy and malignant tissues and detecting tumors at an early stage [36, 51]. One of the key strategies in nanoparticle-based targeting is the exploitation of the EPR effect. This phenomenon is characterized by the leaky vasculature present in tumor tissues, which allows nanoparticles to accumulate preferentially at the tumor site. However, relying solely on passive targeting via the EPR effect can be insufficient due to the heterogeneity of tumors and their vascular structures, especially in smaller or less vascularized tumors. Therefore, active targeting strategies have been developed to enhance the specificity of nanoparticle delivery [160].

Active targeting involves the conjugation of nanoparticles with targeting moieties such as antibodies, peptides, or ligands that recognize specific cancer biomarkers. For instance, nanoparticles functionalized with ligands that bind to overexpressed receptors like HER2 (human epidermal growth factor receptor 2) in breast cancer or folate receptors in ovarian cancer can significantly improve the precision of tumor targeting. These ligand-functionalized nanoparticles not only enhance the accumulation of imaging agents at the tumor site but also provide more specific and localized signals, allowing for better detection and visualization of the cancerous tissue [160].

Gold nanoparticles, due to their tunable surface chemistry and optical properties, are widely used in imaging applications. When conjugated with antibodies that target specific cancer cell receptors, these nanoparticles can be used in combination with imaging modalities like CT or optical imaging to achieve high contrast and specificity. Similarly, SPIONs have been employed in MRI to target prostate-specific membrane antigen (PSMA), a marker for prostate cancer. By using SPIONs with a high affinity for PSMA, researchers have been able to enhance MRI contrast and detect prostate cancer with greater accuracy [166, 167].

In addition to targeting primary tumors, nanoparticle-based imaging has shown promise in detecting metastases. Nanoparticles functionalized with ligands that recognize circulating tumor cells (CTCs) can be used to track the spread of cancer throughout the body. This capability is crucial for early detection of metastasis, which often goes undetected until the disease has progressed to a more advanced stage. By targeting both the primary tumor and metastatic cells, nanoparticles can provide a more comprehensive view of cancer progression, enabling more timely and effective interventions [168, 169].

3.5.2 Role of antibodies, peptides, and ligands in targeted delivery

Antibodies, peptides, and ligands play a fundamental role in the targeted delivery of nanoparticles to cancer cells. These molecular agents serve as the 'homing devices' that guide nanoparticles to the specific biological markers associated with cancer. The precision of this targeting strategy is essential to the success of nanoparticle-based imaging, as it ensures that the nanoparticles accumulate predominantly in cancerous tissues, reducing the likelihood of false positives and minimizing damage to healthy tissues [170, 171]. Monoclonal antibodies have been one of the most widely used targeting agents in nanoparticle delivery systems. Their high specificity for particular antigens makes them ideal for use in imaging and therapeutic applications. For instance, monoclonal antibodies targeting the epidermal growth factor receptor (EGFR), commonly overexpressed in various cancers, have been conjugated to nanoparticles to improve the specificity of both imaging and therapeutic delivery. This approach has proven particularly effective in solid tumors, where nanoparticles can be directed to the tumor microenvironment via the overexpression of EGFR [171].

Peptides offer another versatile approach to targeting cancer cells. Small in size and highly flexible, peptides can penetrate tissues more easily than larger molecules such as antibodies. Peptides designed to bind specific receptors, such as integrins, which are overexpressed in angiogenic blood vessels of tumors, can be used to deliver nanoparticles to the tumor's blood supply [172]. This makes peptides highly effective for vascular targeting, ensuring that nanoparticles accumulate in the tumor's blood vessels and are subsequently taken up by cancer cells. Ligands, both natural and synthetic, also play a critical role in targeted nanoparticle delivery. Folic acid is an example of a small-molecule ligand that has been widely used to target folate receptors, which are overexpressed in several cancers, including ovarian, lung, and breast cancers. Folic acid-functionalized nanoparticles have been shown to enhance the uptake of imaging agents in folate receptor-positive tumors, thereby improving the sensitivity of diagnostic imaging [36, 160, 173].

The choice of targeting molecule—antibody, peptide, or ligand—depends largely on the tumor type, the expression profile of the target biomarker, and the imaging modality used. For example, monoclonal antibodies may provide higher specificity but may face limitations due to their large size and potential immunogenicity. Peptides, while smaller and less likely to induce an immune response, may not bind as tightly as antibodies. Therefore, researchers often optimize these targeting molecules by balancing their affinity, size, and potential for tissue penetration, depending on the clinical application.

3.5.3 Molecular imaging for precise tumor identification

Molecular imaging represents a paradigm shift in cancer diagnosis, providing a powerful tool for identifying tumors at the cellular and molecular levels with unprecedented precision. By integrating nanoparticles with imaging modalities such as PET, CT, MRI, and FI, molecular imaging enables real-time visualization of cancerous tissues and their microenvironments. One of the most significant

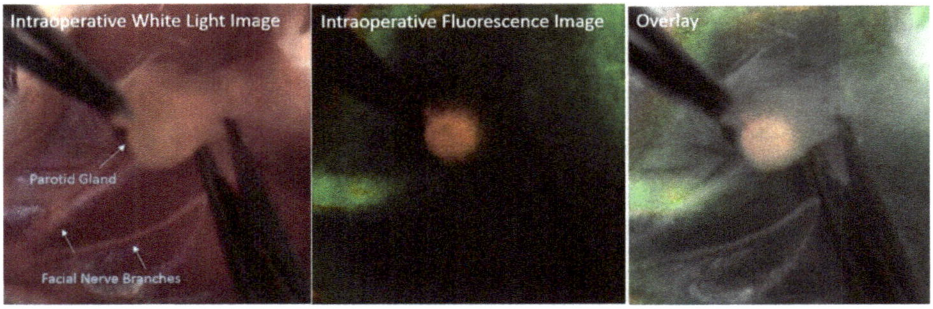

Figure 3.20. Fluorescent labeling facilitates intraoperative tumor identification. Reprinted from [174], Copyright (2017), with permission from Elsevier.

advantages of molecular imaging is its ability to detect tumors at an early stage, long before they become detectable by conventional imaging techniques. This early detection is achieved by exploiting the molecular characteristics of cancer cells—such as overexpression of certain proteins or genetic mutations—that distinguish them from normal cells. Nanoparticles functionalized with targeting molecules can be engineered to bind these molecular markers, allowing for the precise localization and characterization of tumors.

As shown in figure 3.20, intraoperative molecular imaging provides clear visualization of the tumor margins that may not be immediately apparent under traditional white light imaging. Fluorescent labeling, in particular, has proven to be an invaluable tool during surgeries, where real-time imaging helps guide the resection of tumors. In fluorescence-guided surgery, a fluorescent agent is administered to the patient before the procedure. Once bound to the tumor cells, it allows surgeons to identify the tumor's location and extent with much greater accuracy than with standard imaging techniques. This minimizes the risk of leaving residual tumor cells behind and reduces damage to adjacent healthy tissues [174].

In PET imaging, for example, radiolabeled nanoparticles can be used to track the biodistribution and accumulation of the imaging agent in cancerous tissues. By labeling nanoparticles with isotopes such as fluorine-18 or technetium-99m, researchers can visualize the metabolic activity of tumors in real time, providing valuable information about tumor growth, angiogenesis, and metastasis. This molecular-level insight is critical for planning and assessing treatment strategies, as it enables clinicians to tailor therapies based on the specific biological characteristics of the tumor [175]. Molecular imaging is also highly effective in guiding surgical interventions. Nanoparticles conjugated with fluorescent dyes can be used to delineate tumor margins during surgery, allowing surgeons to accurately remove cancerous tissues while sparing healthy tissue. This image-guided surgery reduces the likelihood of incomplete tumor resection and improves postoperative outcomes for patients [176].

Furthermore, molecular imaging can be combined with therapeutic strategies in a theranostic approach, where nanoparticles are used for both diagnosis and treatment. For instance, gold nanoparticles have been used in PAI to detect tumors while simultaneously serving as photothermal therapy agents. When exposed to NIR light, the gold nanoparticles generate heat that selectively destroys cancer cells. The ability to both visualize and treat tumors in real time represents a significant advancement in personalized cancer care [51, 164].

Targeted imaging at the cellular level has evolved significantly through the use of nanoparticles designed to exploit cancer biomarkers, the role of targeting agents like antibodies, peptides, and ligands, and the integration of molecular imaging techniques. These advances are paving the way for more precise, non-invasive cancer diagnostics, and personalized treatment strategies that are tailored to the unique molecular signatures of each patient's disease.

3.6 Theranostics: combining diagnosis and treatment

3.6.1 Nanoplatforms for simultaneous cancer diagnosis and therapy

The integration of nanotechnology in theranostics has opened new avenues for simultaneous cancer diagnosis and treatment. Theranostic nanoplatforms are multifunctional systems that deliver targeted therapies while also providing real-time diagnostic information, making them a cornerstone of personalized cancer treatment. These nanoplatforms are specifically designed to achieve a dual role—providing accurate imaging to identify tumors and delivering drugs to treat the disease—within a single system. Nanoplatforms such as gold nanoparticles, liposomes, dendrimers, and polymeric nanoparticles have been extensively developed for theranostic applications. Gold nanoparticles, for instance, have unique optical properties that make them ideal for both photothermal therapy and imaging applications such as CT scans and photoacoustic imaging. Their surface can be easily modified with targeting ligands, drugs, or imaging agents, making them highly versatile [52, 137].

Iron oxide nanoparticles are another example, primarily used for MRI due to their magnetic properties. When combined with chemotherapeutic agents or gene therapy payloads, these nanoparticles provide a dual functionality, enabling clinicians to visualize the location of the tumor while simultaneously delivering the therapy. For instance, in one study, magnetic iron oxide nanoparticles were functionalized with ligands specific to cancer cell receptors. Once accumulated at the tumor site, the magnetic properties of these nanoparticles allowed for both enhanced MRI contrast and heat generation for localized hyperthermia treatment, thereby killing cancer cells through a combined diagnostic and therapeutic approach [177].

Polymeric nanoparticles have gained considerable attention in theranostics due to their ability to encapsulate both drugs and imaging agents. These nanocarriers provide a stable platform for drug delivery while ensuring that imaging agents are protected until they reach the target tissue. Polymeric micelles and dendrimers are also widely used to co-deliver chemotherapeutic agents alongside imaging molecules, improving diagnostic sensitivity and therapeutic efficacy. One such example is the use of micelles loaded with paclitaxel and a NIR dye, which enables simultaneous tumor visualization through FI and drug delivery to treat breast cancer [178].

In addition to cancer detection, theranostic nanoplatforms are also being explored for other diseases such as cardiovascular conditions and neurodegenerative disorders, where early detection and timely treatment are crucial. These platforms allow for a non-invasive, highly sensitive approach to detect and treat diseases, thus revolutionizing the medical landscape.

3.6.2 Drug delivery and monitoring of treatment response via imaging

A crucial advantage of theranostics lies in its capacity to monitor drug delivery and treatment response in real time through advanced imaging technologies. This ability ensures that the therapeutic agents are delivered precisely to the target tissue and that clinicians can assess the effectiveness of the treatment immediately. This aspect is particularly valuable in the treatment of cancers, where variability in tumor microenvironments can affect drug uptake and efficacy. Nanoparticles that carry both therapeutic agents and imaging molecules can be tracked using modalities like MRI, PET, CT, or FI. This enables physicians to visualize the biodistribution of the drug and monitor its accumulation at the tumor site, helping to fine-tune the dosage and delivery schedule. For example, iron oxide nanoparticles conjugated with doxorubicin—a chemotherapy drug—can be monitored via MRI as they accumulate in the tumor tissue. This allows for real-time observation of how well the drug is being delivered and distributed, providing essential feedback to adjust the treatment plan if needed [38, 163, 178].

QDs, owing to their bright fluorescence, have been used in drug delivery systems where the therapeutic efficacy is monitored through changes in fluorescence intensity. This approach allows for a non-invasive way to track the tumor's response to treatment over time. Another strategy involves the use of gold nanoparticles functionalized with both anticancer drugs and imaging agents. These nanoparticles can be tracked using photoacoustic imaging, providing high-resolution images of the tumor vasculature while simultaneously delivering the drug directly to the tumor cells [179].

One innovative approach in theranostics is the use of radiolabeled nanoparticles for PET or SPECT imaging. These nanoparticles allow clinicians to monitor the pharmacokinetics of the drug and track its distribution within the body. Radiolabeled liposomes, for instance, have been shown to accumulate selectively in tumor tissues, offering valuable insights into drug delivery efficiency. This approach is highly beneficial in ensuring that the maximum concentration of the drug reaches the tumor site, minimizing systemic toxicity and improving patient outcomes. The capacity to monitor treatment response in real-time also enables early detection of drug resistance. By observing changes in tumor uptake of nanoparticles, clinicians can determine whether the cancer is responding to treatment or developing resistance. This timely information allows for immediate adjustments in the treatment protocol, preventing the progression of drug-resistant cancers [18, 133, 151].

3.6.3 Personalized medicine applications in oncology

Personalized medicine aims to tailor treatments to individual patients based on their unique genetic, molecular, and phenotypic characteristics. Theranostics plays a vital role in advancing personalized medicine, particularly in oncology, where patient variability can significantly affect treatment outcomes. With the integration of nanotechnology, theranostic platforms enable a more precise and individualized approach to cancer treatment by providing both diagnostic and therapeutic functions in one system. In oncology, the heterogeneity of tumors—both within a single tumor and across different patients—requires highly specific therapies that target the unique molecular markers of each cancer. Nanoparticles can be engineered to deliver drugs directly to cancer cells expressing certain biomarkers, such as HER2 in breast cancer or EGFR in lung cancer. By functionalizing nanoparticles with antibodies or ligands that bind to these receptors, the therapy can be tailored to the patient's specific tumor profile [160].

Furthermore, theranostic nanoplatforms can be used to assess the molecular and genetic makeup of a tumor through molecular imaging, providing a detailed picture of the tumor's characteristics before treatment begins. This level of precision ensures that the therapy is aligned with the unique biological behavior of the cancer, improving the chances of treatment success. For example, polymeric nanoparticles loaded with gene-silencing molecules and imaging agents can be used to silence specific oncogenes while simultaneously tracking the tumor's response through MRI or FI [163]. The real-time feedback provided by theranostic systems is invaluable in personalizing cancer treatment. By continuously monitoring how the tumor is responding to the therapy, clinicians can adjust the treatment plan to maximize efficacy and minimize side effects. This approach helps avoid the one-size-fits-all method of cancer treatment, ensuring that each patient receives the most effective therapy for their specific condition.

3.6.4 Nanoparticle toxicity and safety implications

Nanoparticles have demonstrated tremendous potential in advancing medicine, particularly in drug delivery, diagnostics, and imaging. However, their small size and unique physicochemical properties pose significant concerns related to toxicity. The potential health risks associated with nanoparticles largely stem from their ability to interact with biological systems at the molecular and cellular levels in ways that differ from larger particles [178].

The primary concern lies in their capacity to penetrate biological barriers and accumulate in organs, tissues, and cells, often leading to unintended toxic effects. Research has shown that nanoparticles can induce oxidative stress, inflammation, DNA damage, and mitochondrial dysfunction, all of which can contribute to long-term health consequences, including carcinogenicity and organ toxicity. Moreover, the surface properties, shape, and charge of nanoparticles can significantly influence their toxicity. For instance, certain nanoparticles may interact with proteins and enzymes in the body, leading to unpredictable immune responses. As a result, nanoparticles may trigger overactive immune responses or, conversely, suppress immune function, making the body vulnerable to infections [180].

Another area of concern is the route of exposure to nanoparticles—whether inhaled, ingested, or absorbed through the skin. Nanoparticles can easily enter the bloodstream and accumulate in vital organs such as the lungs, liver, kidneys, and brain, causing cytotoxic effects. This is particularly worrying for workers involved in the manufacture and handling of nanomaterials, as they may experience prolonged exposure that could lead to chronic health issues. Given the growing applications of nanoparticles in healthcare, it is imperative that their toxicological profiles are thoroughly investigated. This includes understanding how nanoparticles interact with different biological systems, their potential to accumulate in the body, and the long-term effects they may have on human health. Ensuring safety through comprehensive preclinical and clinical testing is essential to mitigate the risks associated with their use [181].

3.6.5 Ensuring biocompatibility and mitigating long-term health effects

For nanoparticles to be successfully integrated into clinical practice, their biocompatibility must be rigorously assessed. Biocompatibility refers to the ability of a material to perform its desired function within a biological environment without eliciting harmful effects. Nanoparticles intended for therapeutic use must not only demonstrate efficacy but also show that they do not induce adverse biological reactions [173].

One of the major challenges in developing nanoparticle-based treatments is predicting their long-term behavior in the human body. While some nanoparticles are designed to degrade and be cleared from the body over time, others may persist, leading to potential accumulation in tissues. This can cause prolonged exposure to nanomaterials, increasing the risk of chronic toxicity and tissue damage. Therefore, understanding how nanoparticles interact with biological tissues over extended periods is critical to evaluating their long-term safety [163, 178, 181].

Moreover, nanoparticles can induce immune responses that may complicate their use in medical treatments. For instance, certain nanoparticles can provoke inflammatory reactions or be recognized as foreign invaders by the immune system, leading to the release of pro-inflammatory cytokines. This immune activation can cause unwanted side effects, particularly when nanoparticles are used for drug delivery or in cancer therapies. Conversely, in some cases, nanoparticles may suppress immune responses, which could impair the body's ability to fight infections or cancers [182].

Furthermore, there are concerns about the potential for nanoparticles to cross critical biological barriers, such as the blood–brain barrier, leading to neurotoxicity. The effects of nanoparticles on the nervous system, as well as other critical systems like the respiratory, reproductive, and endocrine systems, need to be fully understood. To ensure the safe use of nanoparticles in medical applications, ongoing research is needed to develop strategies that enhance their biocompatibility and minimize their long-term effects. This includes refining nanoparticle designs to ensure they can be safely metabolized and cleared from the body without causing harm. Additionally, new testing models, such as three-dimensional organoids, are being explored to better predict the long-term effects of nanoparticles in human tissues [183].

3.6.6 Navigating regulatory and ethical challenges for clinical applications

The rapid advancement of nanotechnology in healthcare brings forth significant regulatory and ethical challenges. Nanoparticles, due to their novel properties and unique interactions with biological systems, require specialized frameworks for regulation to ensure their safe and effective use in clinical settings.

Regulatory bodies such as the US Food and Drug Administration (FDA) and the European Medicines Agency (EMA) face the challenge of establishing appropriate guidelines for nanoparticle-based therapies. The complexity of nanoparticles—ranging from their size and shape to their surface chemistry—demands that traditional regulatory approaches be adapted. Standard drug approval processes may not adequately capture the potential risks associated with nanoparticles, especially when considering long-term exposure, accumulation, and unknown interactions within the body [184]. Furthermore, there is a need for clearer guidelines regarding the environmental impact of nanoparticles. Once released into the environment, nanoparticles can persist and potentially harm ecosystems. Regulatory frameworks must address not only the human health risks but also the broader ecological consequences of nanoparticle use in both medical and industrial contexts [181].

In addition to regulatory challenges, the ethical considerations surrounding the use of nanoparticles in medicine must be carefully examined. One major concern is patient safety, particularly when nanoparticles are used in diagnostic tools or as drug carriers. There must be clear protocols for informed consent, ensuring that patients are fully aware of the potential risks and benefits of nanoparticle-based treatments. Another ethical issue is equitable access to nanoparticle therapies [185]. Given the high cost of developing and producing nanomedicines, there is a risk that these advanced treatments may not be accessible to all patients, particularly those in low-income regions. Addressing these disparities is crucial to ensuring that nanotechnology benefits a broad spectrum of the population.

Additionally, the use of nanoparticles raises questions about long-term monitoring and the responsibility of healthcare providers to track the effects of these treatments. Since nanoparticles can persist in the body for extended periods, long-term studies are necessary to understand their full impact. Healthcare systems must be prepared to monitor patients over time to detect any delayed adverse effects. To navigate these regulatory and ethical challenges, it is essential to foster collaboration between scientists, policymakers, and regulatory agencies. This will help establish robust frameworks that ensure the safe, effective, and equitable use of nanoparticles in healthcare while addressing the broader societal implications of nanotechnology [22, 181].

3.7 Artificial intelligence and machine learning in nanoplatform imaging

Artificial Intelligence (AI) has become a prominent focus in medical imaging research, both in diagnosis and treatment. In diagnostic imaging alone, the number of AI-related publications has surged dramatically—from around 100–150 papers annually in 2007–2008 to over 1000 per year by 2017–2018. AI is being applied to automatically recognize complex patterns in imaging data, facilitating quantitative assessments of radiographic features. In the field of radiation oncology, AI is being used across various imaging modalities at different stages of treatment, including tumor delineation and evaluating treatment effectiveness [186]. One particularly popular area of research is radiomics, which involves extracting large sets of imaging features from medical images in a high-throughput manner. AI has proven crucial in processing vast numbers of medical images, uncovering disease characteristics that might be missed by human analysis [187].

AI and nanotechnology are two key drivers behind the realization of precision medicine, which focuses on tailoring treatment to each cancer patient [187]. The convergence of these fields has enabled improved data acquisition and enhanced the design of nanomaterials for precision oncology. Diagnostic nanomaterials can create patient-specific disease profiles, which, when paired with therapeutic nanotechnologies, optimize treatment outcomes. However, the high degree of variability within tumors and between patients makes the design and analysis of diagnostic and therapeutic platforms challenging. Here, AI plays a pivotal role, using advanced pattern recognition and classification algorithms to improve diagnostic accuracy and therapeutic precision [188].

Each patient is unique, not just in obvious ways like age, gender, and physical appearance, but also in terms of molecular profiles. These molecular differences lead to varying phenotypic changes and responses to drugs. This diversity is especially prominent in cancer, where genetic mutations accumulate, resulting in differences within tumors and across patients. Such heterogeneity complicates both diagnosis and treatment. Precision medicine seeks to address these challenges by tailoring treatments to the individual, considering genetic and epigenetic factors [189].

Nanotechnology has been instrumental in advancing precision medicine across various stages of medical care. Breakthroughs in omics technologies, such as single-molecule nanopore sequencing, allow rapid and highly sensitive detection of genetic material, with the added benefit of longer sequence reads that preserve genetic context. Diagnostic assays based on nanosensors enable the detection of biomarkers at extremely low concentrations, while simultaneously scanning for multiple disease biomarkers in liquid biopsies (e.g. blood, urine, and saliva) or in cell cultures. In cancer treatment, nanomedicine has evolved from broad-spectrum approaches aimed at improving efficacy and reducing side effects to more precise systems that provide real-time data on drug activity inside the patient's body [29–31, 33].

Advancements in nanomedicine fabrication and a deeper understanding of cancer biology have led to the development of targeted therapies that utilize both internal and external stimuli for enhanced drug delivery. These advances have also supported the emergence of theranostic nanomedicines, which combine therapeutic agents with imaging capabilities to track treatment efficacy in real time. Despite these innovations, the clinical translation of nanosensors and targeted nanomedicines in cancer treatment has been limited [36, 190].

AI, particularly machine learning (ML)—a subset of AI where algorithms are trained on large datasets to identify patterns or optimize problem-solving—has found widespread application in medicine. From medical imaging to gene expression analysis, AI is transforming diagnostics and treatment planning. In the field of nanoinformatics, AI and computational techniques are being used to design and implement nanomaterials, pushing the boundaries of precision medicine [191]. By leveraging AI and nanotechnology, we are making significant strides towards a future where cancer treatment is highly personalized, allowing for more precise diagnosis and treatment tailored to the unique molecular makeup of each patient. These advances promise to improve outcomes and reduce side effects, setting the stage for a new era in cancer care [192].

While nanomedicine-based therapies offer significant advantages, they are not universally suitable for all patients or malignancies. A key challenge in this area is the variability of the EPR effect, which differs among patients and across cancer types. The majority of nanomedicines approved for clinical use rely on the EPR effect for effective delivery to the target site. However, this effect is highly heterogeneous among patients, as factors like vascular architecture and other physiological conditions vary. Consequently, different patients may exhibit different responses to the same treatment. This variability is also observed in the expression of targeting moieties in ligand-targeted nanoparticles. Therefore, it is critical to prescreen patients for their compatibility with specific nanomedicines before proceeding with such treatments [193].

The integration of AI into nanotheranostics offers exciting possibilities. Predictive ML algorithms can be applied to optimize nanomedicine formulation by predicting the encapsulation efficiency of imaging agents and drugs. For example, a quantitative structure–property relationship (QSPR) model has been used to predict the loading efficiency of molecules into liposomes with >90% accuracy, based on their chemical structure and the encapsulation conditions [194]. Algorithms such as support vector machines (SVM), decision trees, and iterative stochastic elimination (ISE) were implemented in this model. A similar approach has been used to predict the cytotoxicity of metal oxide nanoparticles. Expanding this method to other nanoparticles could help assess the biocompatibility of surface-labeled nanoparticles for imaging purposes [195, 196].

AI's contribution to medical imaging cannot be overstated. ML algorithms for tumor detection, characterization, and monitoring are constantly improving in accuracy and reproducibility, helping to save time and improve diagnostic precision. By integrating AI into nanotheranostic imaging, researchers can gain deeper insights into the bio-distribution of nanoparticles and their therapeutic efficacy, further advancing the field of precision medicine [193–196].

3.8 Future directions in nanotechnology and cancer imaging

3.8.1 Emerging nanomaterials for next-generation imaging

Over the past two decades, the advent of nanomaterials for biomedical applications has shown incredible potential, offering new possibilities for transforming all facets of disease management. These nanomaterials are particularly appealing due to their ability to be modularly customized, making them versatile systems capable of integrating functionalities that span across early diagnostics, drug delivery, treatment, and real-time patient monitoring. This review explores the diverse landscape of nanomaterials currently under development, focusing on their applications in medical diagnostics and imaging, as well as their role in the delivery of prophylactic vaccines and therapeutic agents like biologic drugs and small molecules. The discussion also highlights their vital contributions to the battle against COVID-19, especially in diagnostics and vaccination efforts [197].

Among the innovative approaches, one noteworthy example involves the work of Bardhan *et al* where engineered strains of the bacteriophage M13 serve as a biological scaffold. This scaffold not only facilitates the functionalization of nanoparticles—ranging from gold nanoparticles and carbon nanotubes to iron oxide particles and dyes—but also acts as a carrier for targeted delivery, enabled by peptide displays engineered on the virus's outer surface. Using this bio-template, they have successfully demonstrated M13-SWNT imaging probes for the non-invasive detection of deep tissue bacterial infections, as shown in figure 3.21(a), including an intramuscular model of infection and a model of *Staphylococcus aureus* endocarditis [198].

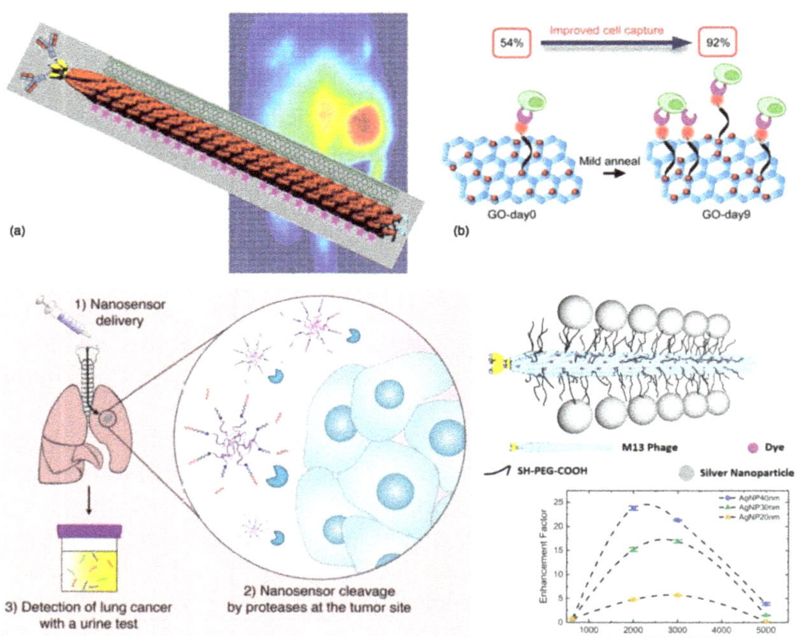

Figure 3.21. Various nanomaterial-based biomedical innovations for diagnostics and therapeutic applications. (a) A schematic representation of an engineered nanomaterial used for deep tissue bacterial infection imaging. (b) The improvement of cell capture efficiency by modifying graphene oxide (GO) over time through mild annealing. (c) The delivery of nanosensors for non-invasive lung cancer detection, where sensors cleaved by tumor-associated proteases are detected in urine samples. (d) The enhancement of dye fluorescence using M13 bacteriophage bio-scaffolds decorated with silver nanoparticles, with a graph illustrating the fluorescence enhancement factor based on nanoparticle size. Reproduced from [206]. CC BY 4.0.

Furthermore, this bacteriophage platform has been applied to enhance the fluorescence of Cy3 dye by a factor of 24×, achieved by decorating silver nanoparticles along the M13 bacteriophage backbone, as illustrated in figure 3.21(d). By adjusting the size and distance between the silver nanoparticles and fluorophore, the enhancement was optimized through plasmonic resonance effects. The incorporation of such bright, emissive nanomaterials has led to the development of cutting-edge imaging technologies. These systems are capable of detecting fluorophores in deep tissue up to 8 cm beneath the skin and allow real-time, non-invasive tracking of 0.1 mm-sized fluorophores through a living mouse's gastrointestinal tract. This pushes the boundaries of optical imaging, offering new opportunities for diagnostic applications, especially in early cancer detection and ensuring the efficacy of cancer treatments [198–201].

In addition to their imaging capabilities, nanomaterials are proving to be indispensable for the delivery of vaccines and therapeutics. These bio-templated systems hold great promise in revolutionizing cancer treatment, allowing for the targeted delivery of drugs and ensuring optimal treatment responses. As the field advances, nanomaterials will undoubtedly play a critical role in the future of personalized medicine, offering precise and efficient tools for both diagnostics and treatment. Bardhan *et al* have demonstrated the versatile nature of two-dimensional nanomaterials, particularly graphene and its derivatives like graphene oxide (GO) and reduced graphene oxide (rGO) by leveraging their capacity to easily modify surface functional groups. These materials have been used to create nanotemplates for bio-oriented applications, including the capture of cells directly from whole blood. Through a simple thermal annealing process, without the need for chemical treatments, they showed that the oxygen groups on the surface of GO can be redistributed via a phase transformation while maintaining the overall oxygen content [199].

This redistribution enables further functionalization, making it a highly adaptable material. A similar method can be applied to rGO, where the number of carbon and oxygen atoms removed during reduction can be controlled by manipulating oxygen clustering before the reduction step. Using this two-dimensional platform, researchers have developed a GO-based cell capture assay, coating the surface with nanobodies (single-domain antibodies) for efficient capture of white blood cells from small samples of whole blood. As depicted in figure 3.21(b), this microfluidic-free, planar device—constructed from these thermally-treated GO nanosheets—can enhance the density and reactivity of the cell capture agents, allowing for the efficient capture of MHC class-II-positive cells from blood without the need for fractionation. This example highlights the innovative use of nanomaterials to create scalable, cost-effective, and highly efficient bioanalytical assays, paving the way for low-cost diagnostics [200].

Additionally, other research groups are developing 'smart' nanomaterials capable of responding to specific stimuli to generate detectable signals. These stimuli may be endogenous, such as low pH, reduced oxygen levels (hypoxia), or other factors present in the local environment of tumors or infection sites. Alternatively, they may be exogenous, involving external triggers like light, heat, ultrasound, or magnetic fields. Delivered via the intrapulmonary route, these antibody-based nanoconjugates

(ABNs) work on the principle of protease-activated cleavage, providing a simple, urine-based diagnostic readout, as illustrated in figure 3.21(c). Building on this work, Hao and collaborators developed the PRISM (Protease-Responsive Imaging Sensors for Malignancy) platform, which combines the utility of ABNs with imaging agents for PET-CT scans, offering a precision diagnostic tool for various cancers. This dual-function system enables either urine-based diagnostics or imaging, significantly improving early cancer detection capabilities [202].

3.8.2 Innovative approaches in real time, *in vivo* imaging

In vivo imaging, which allows us to explore deep within living organisms, has unlocked extraordinary possibilities for both clinical diagnostics and research. Often, contrast agents are essential to enhance the visibility of physiological structures, providing a clear picture of their functional architecture. Recent advances in nanomaterials are revolutionizing this field by enabling the generation of high-resolution, high-contrast images, which are critical for precise diagnostic purposes. Nanomaterials have become key players in imaging by delivering large payloads that significantly improve sensitivity, enable multiplexing, and offer design flexibility. In fact, in some imaging modalities, nanomaterials are not just supplementary contrast agents—they are the primary source of image signal, making certain imaging techniques possible [203].

However, not all contrast agents, whether they are small molecules or nanomaterials, are universally advantageous for *in vivo* imaging. The choice of contrast agent should be guided by a detailed assessment of the desired outcome and associated risks. Even so, nanomaterials present several compelling benefits for *in vivo* imaging: (i) their small size (typically 1–100 nm), (ii) their high target-binding capacity, (iii) the ability to precisely control and tailor their physicochemical properties, including size, shape, material composition, density, and surface charge, (iv) their large payload delivery capability, (v) their multiplexing potential, and (vi) the possibility to combine imaging with therapeutic agents (theranostics) [178].

A key advantage of nanomaterials is their size, which allows them to carry significantly more contrast than small molecules, while remaining small enough to circulate through the bloodstream. Unlike larger structures, these nanomaterials can accumulate selectively in target areas, such as tumors, with greater specificity due to the EPR effect. The EPR effect allows nanomaterials to access disease sites and, when coupled with active targeting, bind to cancerous cells more effectively. Nanomaterials also stand out because their physical and chemical properties can be finely tuned, offering flexibility that small-molecule agents cannot match. For example, by adjusting the size, shape, or surface charge, researchers can customize a nanomaterial's behavior, optimizing its ability to target the unique pathophysiology of specific diseases [131].

3.8.3 Potential of nanotechnology to revolutionize cancer diagnostics

Nanomaterials designed for *in vivo* imaging must possess specific properties that enable them to function effectively within the body. A critical aspect of their design involves incorporating a suitable reporter structure tailored to the intended imaging application, alongside a biocompatible coating. This coating serves multiple purposes: not only does it help regulate the nanomaterial's toxicological and pharmacological characteristics, but it often also acts as a functional bridge that connects the reporter to other molecules, such as targeting ligands, additional imaging agents (for multimodality imaging), or therapeutic molecules. While the coating is crucial, this review focuses primarily on the nanomaterial itself rather than the chemistry of the coating, except when it directly affects imaging performance [131, 198].

Successful imaging nanomaterials typically exhibit several essential traits, largely dictated by their physicochemical properties. Among nanomaterials used for clinical diagnostics, non-toxicity is of the utmost importance, particularly because contrast agents for diagnostics are often administered to healthy individuals for screening purposes. This means that any adverse effects are unacceptable. For example, gadolinium-based (Gd^{3+}) nanomaterials have faced scrutiny in the MRI community because, under specific conditions, particularly in patients with advanced kidney disease, they can cause a condition known as nephrogenic systemic fibrosis, which can be fatal. Although this side effect only occurs in a small subset of the population, it has created a lingering stigma around Gd^{3+}-based contrast agents, reflecting the high safety standards required for diagnostic agents compared to therapeutic nanomaterials [204].

For nanomaterials used in imaging, it's essential that they efficiently target the desired site within a suitable time frame. In the case of cancer diagnostics, this typically involves specific size and shape constraints to ensure the material can extravasate into tumors via the EPR effect. Blood pool agents used for mapping blood vessels must circulate for a prolonged period, allowing for continuous imaging without missing crucial windows, such as during bolus injections. Additionally, nanomaterials designed for *in vivo* imaging need to be stable enough to generate a consistent signal over time, although they must eventually be cleared from the body to avoid long-term toxicity [6, 36, 198].

Interestingly, some nanomaterials are engineered to deliver a single, highly intense imaging signal before being deactivated, such as in nanodroplet vaporization for photoacoustic imaging. This approach allows for a one-time, high-contrast signal that enhances detection. Polydispersity, a common feature of nanomaterials, plays a significant role in their behavior and imaging capabilities. It refers to the distribution of particle sizes in a sample and is influenced by factors like aggregation, surface charge, shape, and coating [107]. Aggregation can have both positive and negative effects on imaging. For instance, aggregated QDs have been shown to improve targeting and circulation behaviors *in vivo*, particularly in targeting blood vessels, while aggregation of Raman-active nanomaterials can create 'hot spots' that amplify the Raman signal due to plasmonic coupling. However, aggregation can also disrupt biodistribution, increase the risk of capillary blockages, and lead to rapid clearance by the mononuclear phagocyte system (MPS), reducing the material's availability to reach the target tissue [203].

Recent studies have explored the relationship between nanomaterial aggregation, polydispersity, and the protein corona—a layer of proteins that forms around nanomaterials when exposed to biological fluids like blood. The protein corona significantly impacts how nanomaterials behave in the body, influencing their trafficking and biodistribution. For example, the surface chemistry of nanomaterials can dictate the type of protein corona that forms, affecting where the nanomaterials accumulate, whether in the liver, lungs, or skin. Furthermore, the protein corona and polydispersity influence each other, adding complexity to the design of nanomaterials for imaging applications [205].

Optimization of nanomaterials for *in vivo* imaging often involves a delicate balance between enhancing imaging properties and ensuring favorable *in vivo* behavior. Sometimes these two goals conflict, requiring compromises in design. For instance, QDs <5.5 nm are ideal for renal clearance while also providing efficient fluorescence emission. In other cases, larger nanomaterials are preferred for US imaging due to their better echogenic properties, but their size must be carefully controlled to allow them to extravasate into tumor tissues via the EPR effect [206].

The use of nanomaterials in medical imaging originated in parallel with the need to enhance MRI contrast, particularly through the use of iron oxide nanoparticles. These materials were initially developed for treating anemia but were later found to shorten water molecule relaxation times, making them effective MRI contrast agents. Breakthroughs in nanoparticle design, including the development of monodisperse, biocompatible iron oxide agents, have since paved the way for a wide range of nanoparticulate contrast materials used in modalities such as CT, PET, SPECT, and optical imaging. Today, nanomaterials are being utilized in a growing number of diagnostic applications, from cancer detection to cardiovascular imaging, offering new possibilities for improving the precision and effectiveness of medical diagnostics.

3.9 Conclusion: the future of cancer diagnosis with nanoplatforms

In recent years, remarkable progress has been made in the field of nanomaterial-based *in vivo* imaging, revolutionizing how we approach a wide range of diseases. Nanomaterials have demonstrated significant advantages over small-molecule imaging agents, filling a crucial gap between smaller and larger imaging systems. The unprecedented levels of sensitivity, penetration depth, and multimodality offered by these novel nanomaterials have transformed imaging capabilities, allowing for diagnostic insights that were scarcely possible just a decade ago. These innovations have led to high expectations within the medical community, and to meet these expectations, researchers must carefully balance several factors, such as safety, scalable production, and clinical utility. If nanomaterials continue to develop along these lines, they have the potential to revolutionize medical diagnostics.

Nanomaterials provide several features that small molecules cannot, offering unparalleled capabilities in medical imaging. For instance, nanomaterials can restrict the diffusion of contrast agents like gadolinium (Gd), boosting signal contrast and reducing toxicity. They are also being used to improve resolution and unlock novel imaging techniques like magneto-motive imaging, which requires MNPs. Furthermore, they open new avenues for theranostic applications—where diagnosis and treatment converge—pushing the boundaries of modern healthcare.

Despite these advances, the clinical integration of new nanomaterials remains slow but is gaining momentum, especially in therapeutic applications. Diagnostic nanomaterials face higher safety standards, given that they are often used in healthy individuals during disease screening, where long-term harm is not acceptable. Nonetheless, a diverse array of nanomaterials are currently in clinical trials, showcasing their enormous potential to detect and locate diseases at an earlier stage. As the field of nanotechnology advances, clinicians and scientists alike need to select the most appropriate nanomaterials for imaging applications, tailored to the specific demands of each disease. The properties of the nanomaterials—such as their anti-Stokes emission, which minimizes autofluorescence, or their ability to function in multiple imaging modalities like MRI or PET—are central to optimizing diagnostic information. These advances not only improve clinical imaging but also open the door to new biological discoveries through enhanced preclinical imaging.

Nanomaterials are fundamentally reshaping the landscape of medical imaging by offering greater sensitivity, spatial resolution, and contrast, as well as enabling multimodal imaging. Clinicians must stay informed about the latest developments in nanotechnology to make the best decisions for patient care. As nanomaterials evolve, they will allow the detection of increasingly smaller disease sites and earlier molecular signs of illness, ultimately improving diagnoses, prognoses, and patient outcomes. However, while these advances are promising, much work remains. The future of nanomaterials in diagnostics will depend on continued innovation and collaboration across disciplines to ensure that these materials meet the clinical and safety standards required to realize their full potential in transforming medicine.

References

[1] Umadevi K, Sundeep D, Vighnesh A R *et al* 2024 Current trends and advances in nanoplatforms-based imaging for cancer diagnosis *Indian J. Microbiol.* https://doi.org/10.1007/s12088-024-01373-9

[2] Umadevi K, Sundeep D, Latha A M *et al* 2024 Enhancement of diagnostic accuracy in endometrial carcinoma using CW-THz spectroscopy *Indian J. Gynecol. Oncolog.* **22** 100

[3] Umadevi K, Sundeep D, Varadharaj E K *et al* 2024 Precision detection of fungal co-infections for enhanced COVID-19 treatment strategies using FESEM imaging *Indian J. Microbiol.* **64** 1084–98

[4] Farkas D L 2021 Biomedical applications of translational optical imaging: from molecules to humans *Molecules* **26** 6651

[5] Pulumati A, Pulumati A, Dwarakanath B S, Verma A and Papineni R V 2023 Technological advancements in cancer diagnostics: improvements and limitations *Cancer Rep.* **6** e1764

[6] Khazaei M, Hosseini M S, Haghighi A M and Misaghi M 2023 Nanosensors and their applications in early diagnosis of cancer *Sens. Bio-Sens. Res.* **41** 100569

[7] Alrushaid N, Khan F A, Al-Suhaimi E A and Elaissari A 2023 Nanotechnology in cancer diagnosis and treatment *Pharmaceutics* **15** 1025
[8] Manson E N and Achel D G 2023 Fighting breast cancer in low-and-middle-income countries —what must we do to get every woman screened on regular basis? *Sci. Afr.* **21** e01848
[9] Fass L 2008 Imaging and cancer: a review *Mol. Oncol.* **2** 115–52
[10] Dawson L A and Ménard C 2009 Imaging in radiation oncology: a perspective *Oncologist* **15** 338–49
[11] Sullivan D C, Schwartz L H and Zhao B 2013 The imaging viewpoint: how imaging affects determination of progression-free survival *Clin. Cancer Res.* **19** 2621–8
[12] Paul S, Saikia A, Majhi V and Pandey V K 2022 *Introduction to Biomedical Instrumentation and its Applications* (New York: Academic)
[13] Demaerel P 2023 Calvarium *Imaging of the Scalp and Calvarium* (Cham: Springer)
[14] Patel N B, Bitners A C, Sin S and Arens R 2024 Imaging upper airway obstruction in obstructive sleep apnea *Snoring and Obstructive Sleep Apnea in Children* (New York: Academic) pp 165–203
[15] Lusic H and Grinstaff M W 2013 X-ray-computed tomography contrast agents *Chem. Rev.* **113** 1641–66
[16] Kim J, Chhour P, Hsu J, Litt H I, Ferrari V A, Popovtzer R and Cormode D P 2017 Use of nanoparticle contrast agents for cell tracking with computed tomography *Bioconjug. Chem.* **28** 1581–97
[17] Crişan G, Moldovean-Cioroianu N S, Timaru D-G, Andrieş G, Căinap C and Chiş V 2022 Radiopharmaceuticals for PET and SPECT imaging: a literature review over the last decade *Int. J. Mol. Sci.* **23** 5023
[18] Gupta D, Roy P, Sharma R *et al* 2024 Recent nanotheranostic approaches in cancer research *Clin. Exp. Med.* **24** 8
[19] Liu B, Zhou H, Tan L *et al* 2024 Exploring treatment options in cancer: tumor treatment strategies *Sig. Transduct. Target Ther.* **9** 175
[20] Zhu A, Lee D and Shim H 2011 Metabolic positron emission tomography imaging in cancer detection and therapy response *Semin. Oncol.* **38** 55–69
[21] Goel S, England C G, Chen F and Cai W 2017 Positron emission tomography and nanotechnology: a dynamic duo for cancer theranostics *Adv. Drug Deliv. Rev.* **113** 157–76
[22] Esze R, Balkay L, Barna S, Egeresi L S, Emri M, Páll D, Paragh G, Rajnai L, Somodi S, Képes Z *et al* 2024 Impact of fat distribution and metabolic diseases on cerebral microcirculation: a multimodal study on type 2 diabetic and obese patients *J. Clin. Med.* **13** 2900
[23] Salata O 2004 Applications of nanoparticles in biology and medicine *J. Nanobiotechnol.* **2** 3
[24] Umadevi K, Sundeep D, Jhansi R *et al* 2023 Effect of functionalization of 2D graphene nanosheets on oxidation stress of BEAS-2B cells *Bio. Nano. Sci.* **13** 1262–77
[25] Jhansi R, Reddy A V, Prasad K S, Kiran Y S and Sundeep D 2019 A comparative assessment of flexural bond strength of Ni–Cr metal–ceramic alloy on repeated castings *Int. J. Prosthodont. Restor. Dent.* **9** 70–6
[26] Jhansi R, Sundeep D, Umadevi K, Varadharaj E K, Sastry C C, Krishna A G, Raj N S and Patil S 2023 Mechanical and spectroscopic investigation of novel f-MWCNTS/g-C3N4/TiO_2 ternary nanocomposite reinforced denture base PMMA *Phys. Scr.* **98** 095930
[27] Venkatesan S, Jerald J, Sundeep D, Varadharaj E K and Sastry C C 2022 Evaluation of mechanical and corrosion properties of TiB_2-Y2O_3 nanocomposite fused bronze metal matrix composite *Surf. Topogr.: Metrol. Prop.* **10** 035003

[28] Ataide J A, Zanchetta B, Santos É M, Fava A L M, Alves T F R, Cefali L C, Chaud M V, Oliveira-Nascimento L, Souto E B and Mazzola P G 2022 Nanotechnology-based dressings for wound management *Pharmaceuticals* **15** 1286

[29] Sundeep D and K Varadharaj E 2022 Non-enzymatic electrochemical sensor based on ZIF-67 and MWCNTS-ZIF-67 nanocomposites for detection of uric acid in human urea *Electrochemical Society Meeting Abstracts 242* No. 61 pp 2237–7

[30] Sundeep D and K Varadharaj E 2022 (Digital presentation) super ultra-fast and highly-sensitive non-enzymatic electrochemical sensor to detect uric acid by electronic waste to MoS2 and functionalised MWCNT/MoS_2 coated high-performance aluminium electrode *Electrochemical Society Meeting Abstracts 241* No. 53 pp 2196–6

[31] Sundeep D and K Varadharaj E 2024 MoS2 modified aluminum electrode for detection of calcium oxalate through electrochemical oxidation *Electrochemical Society Meeting Abstracts 245* No. 8 pp 872–2

[32] Haleem A, Javaid M, Singh R P, Rab S and Suman R 2023 Applications of nano-technology in medical field: a brief review *Global Health J.* **7** 70–7

[33] Sundeep D, Varadharaj E K, Umadevi K and Jhansi R 2023 Role of nanomaterials in screenprinted electrochemical biosensors for detection of COVID-19 and for post-covid syndromes *ECS Adv.* **2** 016502

[34] Park S M, Aalipour A, Vermesh O *et al* 2017 Towards clinically translatable *in vivo* nanodiagnostics *Nat. Rev. Mater.* **2** 17014

[35] Baskar R, Lee K A, Yeo R and Yeoh K W 2012 Cancer and radiation therapy: current advances and future directions *Int. J. Med. Sci.* **9** 193–9 https://medsci.org/v09p0193.htm

[36] Chehelgerdi M, Chehelgerdi M, Allela O Q B *et al* 2023 Progressing nanotechnology to improve targeted cancer treatment: overcoming hurdles in its clinical implementation *Mol. Cancer* **22** 169

[37] Shi X, Wang X, Yao W *et al* 2024 Mechanism insights and therapeutic intervention of tumor metastasis: latest developments and perspectives *Sig. Transduct. Target Ther.* **9** 192

[38] Anitha K, Chenchula S, Surendran V, Shvetank B, Ravula P, Milan R, Chikatipalli R and Padmavathi R 2024 Advancing cancer theranostics through biomimetics: a comprehensive review *Heliyon* **10** e27692

[39] Yıldırım M, Acet B Ö, Dikici E *et al* 2024 Things to know and latest trends in the design and application of nanoplatforms in cancer treatment *Bio. Nano. Sci.* **14** 4167–4188

[40] Beaton L, Bandula S, Gaze M N *et al* 2019 How rapid advances in imaging are defining the future of precision radiation oncology *Br. J. Cancer* **120** 779–90

[41] Farajollahi A and Baharvand M 2024 Advancements in photoacoustic imaging for cancer diagnosis and treatment *Int. J. Pharm.* 124736

[42] Beh C Y, Prajnamitra R P, Chen L-L and Hsieh P C-H 2021 Advances in biomimetic nanoparticles for targeted cancer therapy and diagnosis *Molecules* **26** 5052

[43] Wang B, Hu S, Teng Y *et al* 2024 Current advance of nanotechnology in diagnosis and treatment for malignant tumors *Sig. Transduct. Target. Ther.* **9** 200

[44] Huang X *et al* 2024 Advances and applications of nanoparticles in cancer therapy *MedComm–Oncol.* **3** e67

[45] Suhag D, Kaushik S and Taxak V B 2024 Theranostics: combining diagnosis and therapy *Handbook of Biomaterials for Medical Applications, Volume 1. Biomedical Materials for Multi-functional Applications* (Singapore: Springer)

[46] Luengo Morato Y, Ovejero Paredes K, Lozano Chamizo L, Marciello M and Filice M 2021 Recent advances in multimodal molecular imaging of cancer mediated by hybrid magnetic nanoparticles *Polymers* **13** 2989
[47] Tempany C M, Jayender J, Kapur T, Bueno R, Golby A, Agar N and Jolesz F A 2015 Multimodal imaging for improved diagnosis and treatment of cancers *Cancer* **121** 817–27
[48] Yetisgin A A, Cetinel S, Zuvin M, Kosar A and Kutlu O 2020 Therapeutic nanoparticles and their targeted delivery applications *Molecules* **25** 2193
[49] Wang E C and Wang A Z 2014 Nanoparticles and their applications in cell and molecular biology *Integr. Biol.* **6** 9–26
[50] Pink R C, Beaman E M, Samuel P *et al* 2022 Utilising extracellular vesicles for early cancer diagnostics: benefits, challenges and recommendations for the future *Br. J. Cancer* **126** 323–30
[51] Raheem M A *et al* 2023 Advances in nanoparticles-based approaches in cancer theranostics *OpenNano* **12** 100152
[52] Haghighi F H, Binaymotlagh R, Mirahmadi-Zare S Z and Hadadzadeh H 2019 Aptamer/magnetic nanoparticles decorated with fluorescent gold nanoclusters for selective detection and collection of human promyelocytic leukemia (HL-60) cells from a mixture *Nanotechnology* **31** 025605
[53] Liu X, Jiang H and Wang X 2024 Advances in cancer research: current and future diagnostic and therapeutic strategies *Biosensors* **14** 100
[54] Cotta M A 2020 Quantum dots and their applications: what lies ahead? *ACS Appl. Nano Mater.* **3** 4920–4
[55] Walling M A, Novak J A and Shepard J R E 2009 Quantum dots for live cell and *in vivo* imaging *Int. J. Mol. Sci.* **10** 441–91
[56] Valizadeh A, Mikaeili H, Samiei M *et al* 2012 Quantum dots: synthesis, bioapplications, and toxicity *Nanoscale Res. Lett.* **7** 480
[57] Hamidu A, Pitt W G and Husseini G A 2023 Recent breakthroughs in using quantum dots for cancer imaging and drug delivery purposes *Nanomaterials* **13** 2566
[58] Badıllı U, Mollarasouli F, Bakirhan N K, Ozkan Y and Ozkan S A 2020 Role of quantum dots in pharmaceutical and biomedical analysis, and its application in drug delivery *TrAC, Trends Anal. Chem.* **131** 116013
[59] Yukawa H, Sato K and Baba Y 2023 Theranostics applications of quantum dots in regenerative medicine, cancer medicine, and infectious diseases *Adv. Drug Deliv. Rev.* **200** 114863
[60] Salvi A, Kharbanda S, Thakur P, Shandilya M and Thakur A 2024 Biomedical application of cabon quantum dots: a review *Carbon Trends* **17** 100407
[61] Jain S, Bharti S, Bhullar G K and Tripathi S K 2020 I–III–VI core/shell QDs: synthesis, characterizations and applications *J. Lumin.* **219** 116912
[62] Zhu Y J and Chen F 2014 Microwave-assisted preparation of inorganic nanostructures in liquid phase *Chem. Rev.* **114** 6462–555
[63] Marković Z M, Mišović A S, Zmejkoski D Z, Zdravković N M, Kovač J, Bajuk-Bogdanović D V, Milivojević D D, Mojsin M M, Stevanović M J, Pavlović V B *et al* 2023 Employing gamma-ray-modified carbon quantum dots to combat a wide range of bacteria *Antibiotics* **12** 919
[64] Alehdaghi H, Assar E, Azadegan B, Baedi J and Mowlavi A A 2020 Investigation of optical and structural properties of aqueous CdS quantum dots under gamma irradiation *Radiat. Phys. Chem.* **166** 108476

[65] Trofimova O Y, Meshcheryakova I N, Druzhkov N O, Ershova I V, Maleeva A V, Cherkasov A V, Yakushev I A, Dorovatovskii P V, Aysin R R and Piskunov A V 2024 Structural diversity of cadmium coordination polymers based on an extended anilate-type ligand *CrystEngComm* **26** 3077–3087

[66] Vasile Scaeteanu G, Maxim C, Badea M and Olar R 2024 An overview of various applications of cadmium carboxylate coordination polymers *Molecules* **29** 3874

[67] Hardman R 2006 A toxicologic review of quantum dots: toxicity depends on physicochemical and environmental factors *Environ. Health Perspect.* **114** 165–72

[68] Zhang T, Wang Y, Kong L, Xue Y and Tang M 2015 Threshold dose of three types of quantum dots (QDs) induces oxidative stress triggers dna damage and apoptosis in mouse fibroblast L929 cells *Int. J. Environ. Res. Public Health* **12** 13435–54

[69] Kays J C, Saeboe A M, Toufanian R, Kurant D E and Dennis A M 2020 Shell-free copper indium sulfide quantum dots induce toxicity *in vitro* and *in vivo Nano Lett.* **20** 1980–91

[70] Deng B *et al* 2021 Low temperature synthesis of highly bright green emission CuInS2/ZnS quantum dots and its application in light-emitting diodes *J. Alloys Compd.* **851** 155439

[71] Leach A D and Macdonald J E 2016 Optoelectronic properties of $CuInS_2$ nanocrystals and their origin *J. Phys. Chem. Lett.* **7** 572–83

[72] Oh S J, Yang J I, Kim O *et al* 2017 Human U87 glioblastoma cells with stemness features display enhanced sensitivity to natural killer cell cytotoxicity through altered expression of NKG2D ligand *Cancer Cell Int.* **17** 22

[73] Kim E M, Lim S T, Sohn M H *et al* 2017 Facile synthesis of near-infrared $CuInS_2$/ZnS quantum dots and glycol-chitosan coating for *in vivo* imaging *J. Nanopart. Res.* **19** 251

[74] Yadav P K, Chandra S, Kumar V, Kumar D and Hasan S H 2023 Carbon quantum dots: synthesis, structure, properties, and catalytic applications for organic synthesis *Catalysts* **13** 422

[75] Cui L, Ren X, Sun M, Liu H and Xia L 2021 Carbon dots: synthesis, properties and applications *Nanomaterials* **11** 3419

[76] Bhattacharya T, Shin G H and Kim J T 2023 Carbon dots: opportunities and challenges in cancer therapy *Pharmaceutics* **15** 1019

[77] Liang Z, Khawar M B, Liang J and Sun H 2021 Bio-conjugated quantum dots for cancer research: detection and imaging *Front. Oncol.* **11** 749970

[78] Gao G, Jiang Y W, Jia H R, Yang J and Wu F G 2018 On-off-on fluorescent nanosensor for Fe3+ detection and cancer/normal cell differentiation via silicon-doped carbon quantum dots *Carbon* **134** 232–43

[79] Shaheen S, Fatima B, Hussain D and Najam-ul-Haq M 2024 Carbon dots in cancer detection and therapy *Interdisciplinary Cancer Research* (Berlin: Springer Nature)

[80] Mishra S, Das K, Chatterjee S, Sahoo P, Kundu S, Pal M, Bhaumik A and Ghosh C K 2023 Facile and green synthesis of novel fluorescent carbon quantum dots and their silver heterostructure: an *in vitro* anticancer activity and imaging on colorectal carcinoma *ACS Omega* **8** 4566–77

[81] Zhang J, Zhao X, Xian M, Dong C and Shuang S 2018 Folic acid-conjugated green luminescent carbon dots as a nanoprobe for identifying folate receptor-positive cancer cells *Talanta* **183** 39–47

[82] Chung S, Revia R A and Zhang M 2021 Graphene quantum dots and their applications in bioimaging, biosensing, and therapy *Adv. Mater.* **33** 1904362

[83] Kurniawan D, Weng R J, Chen Y Y, Rahardja M R, Nanaricka Z C and Chiang W H 2022 Recent advances in the graphene quantum dot-based biological and environmental sensors *Sens. Actuat. Rep.* **4** 100130

[84] Iannazzo D, Pistone A, Salamò M, Galvagno S, Romeo R, Giofré S V, Branca C, Visalli G and Di Pietro A 2017 Graphene quantum dots for cancer targeted drug delivery *Int. J. Pharm.* **518** 185–92

[85] Bhattacharya T, Preetam S, Mukherjee S *et al* 2024 Anticancer activity of quantum size carbon dots: opportunities and challenges *Discov. Nano* **19** 122

[86] Semenov K N, Shemchuk O S, Ageev S V *et al* 2024 Development of graphene-based materials with the targeted action for cancer theranostics *Biochem. Moscow* **89** 1362–91

[87] Cui G, Wu J, Lin J *et al* 2021 Graphene-based nanomaterials for breast cancer treatment: promising therapeutic strategies *J. Nanobiotechnol.* **19** 211

[88] Prabhakar A K, Ajith M P, Ananthanarayanan A, Routh P, Mohan B C and Thamizhchelvan A M 2022 Ball-milled graphene quantum dots for enhanced anti-cancer drug delivery *OpenNano* **8** 100072

[89] Singh G, Kaur H, Sharma A, Singh J, Alajangi H K, Kumar S, Singla N, Kaur I P and Barnwal R P 2021 Carbon based nanodots in early diagnosis of cancer *Front. Chem.* **9** 669169

[90] Fernandes N B, Shenoy R U K, Kajampady M K *et al* 2022 Fullerenes for the treatment of cancer: an emerging tool *Environ. Sci. Pollut. Res.* **29** 58607–27

[91] Ye L, Kollie L, Liu X, Guo W, Ying X, Zhu J, Yang S and Yu M 2021 Antitumor activity and potential mechanism of novel fullerene derivative nanoparticles *Molecules* **26** 3252

[92] Bolskar R D 2016 Fullerenes for drug delivery ed B Bhushan *Encyclopedia of Nanotechnology* (Dordrecht: Springer)

[93] Gaur M, Misra C, Yadav A B, Swaroop S, Maolmhuaidh F Ó, Bechelany M and Barhoum A 2021 Biomedical applications of carbon nanomaterials: fullerenes, quantum dots, nanotubes, nanofibers, and graphene *Materials* **14** 5978

[94] Hamblin M R 2018 Fullerenes as photosensitizers in photodynamic therapy: pros and cons *Photochem. Photobiol. Sci.* **17** 1515–33

[95] Skivka L M, Prylutska S V, Rudyk M P *et al* 2018 C_{60} fullerene and its nanocomplexes with anticancer drugs modulate circulating phagocyte functions and dramatically increase ROS generation in transformed monocytes *Cancer Nano* **9** 8

[96] Paramasivam G, Palem V V, Meenakshy S, Suresh L K, Gangopadhyay M, Antherjanam S and Sundramoorthy A K 2024 Advances on carbon nanomaterials and their applications in medical diagnosis and drug delivery *Colloids Surf.* B **241** 114032

[97] Elsori D, Rashid G, Khan N A, Sachdeva P, Jindal R, Kayenat F, Sachdeva B, Kamal M A, Babker A M and Fahmy S A 2023 Nanotube breakthroughs: unveiling the potential of carbon nanotubes as a dual therapeutic arsenal for Alzheimer's disease and brain tumors *Front. Oncol.* **13** 1265347

[98] Khajuria A, Alajangi H K, Sharma A *et al* 2024 Theranostics: aptamer-assisted carbon nanotubes as MRI contrast and photothermal agent for breast cancer therapy *Discov. Nano* **19** 145

[99] Delogu L G *et al* 2012 Functionalized multiwalled carbon nanotubes as ultrasound contrast agents *Proc. Natl. Acad. Sci.* **109** 16612–7

[100] Naief M F, Mohammed S N, Mayouf H J and Mohammed A M 2023 A review of the role of carbon nanotubes for cancer treatment based on photothermal and photodynamic therapy techniques *J. Organomet. Chem.* 122819

[101] Qi K, Sun B, Liu S Y and Zhang M 2023 Research progress on carbon materials in tumor photothermal therapy *Biomed. Pharmacother.* **165** 115070
[102] Rastogi V, Yadav P, Bhattacharya S S, Mishra A K, Verma N, Verma A and Pandit J K 2014 Carbon nanotubes: an emerging drug carrier for targeting cancer cells *J. Drug Deliv.* **2014** 670815
[103] Hwang Y, Park S-H and Lee J W 2017 Applications of functionalized carbon nanotubes for the therapy and diagnosis of cancer *Polymers* **9** 13
[104] Liu Z, Chen K, Davis C, Sherlock S, Cao Q, Chen X and Dai H 2008 Drug delivery with carbon nanotubes for *in vivo* cancer treatment *Cancer Res.* **68** 6652–60
[105] Zhang W, Zhang Z and Zhang Y 2011 The application of carbon nanotubes in target drug delivery systems for cancer therapies *Nanoscale Res. Lett.* **6** 555
[106] Kateb B, Van Handel M, Zhang L, Bronikowski M J, Manohara H and Badie B 2007 Internalization of MWCNTs by microglia: possible application in immunotherapy of brain tumors *Neuroimage* **37** S9–17
[107] Rarokar N, Yadav S, Saoji S, Bramhe P, Agade R, Gurav S, Khedekar P, Subramaniyan V, Wong L S and Kumarasamy V 2024 Magnetic nanosystem a tool for targeted delivery and diagnostic application: current challenges and recent advancement *Int. J. Pharm.* X 100231
[108] Hosu O, Tertis M and Cristea C 2019 Implication of magnetic nanoparticles in cancer detection, screening and treatment *Magnetochemistry* **5** 55
[109] Materón E M, Miyazaki C M, Carr O, Joshi N, Picciani P H, Dalmaschio C J, Davis F and Shimizu F M 2021 Magnetic nanoparticles in biomedical applications: a review *Appl. Surf. Sci. Adv.* **6** 100163
[110] Sharma S K, Shrivastava N, Rossi F and Thanh N T 2019 Nanoparticles-based magnetic and photo induced hyperthermia for cancer treatment *Nano Today* **29** 100795
[111] Spoială A, Ilie C-I, Motelica L, Ficai D, Semenescu A, Oprea O-C and Ficai A 2023 Smart magnetic drug delivery systems for the treatment of cancer *Nanomaterials* **13** 876
[112] Wu M and Huang S 2017 Magnetic nanoparticles in cancer diagnosis, drug delivery and treatment *Mol. Clin. Oncol.* **7** 738–46
[113] Farzin A, Etesami S A, Quint J, Memic A and Tamayol A 2020 Magnetic nanoparticles in cancer therapy and diagnosis *Adv. Healthcare Mater.* **9** 1901058
[114] Londhe P V, Londhe M V, Salunkhe A B, Laha S S, Mefford O T, Thorat N D and Khot V M 2025 Magnetic hydrogel (MagGel): an evolutionary pedestal for anticancer therapy *Coord. Chem. Rev.* **522** 216228
[115] Hafiz M, Hassanein A, Talhami M, Maryam A E, Hassan M K and Hawari A H 2022 Magnetic nanoparticles draw solution for forward osmosis: current status and future challenges in wastewater treatment *J. Environ. Chem. Eng.* **10** 108955
[116] Rentzeperis F, Rivera D, Zhang J Y, Brown C, Young T, Rodriguez B, Schupper A, Price G, Gomberg J, Williams T *et al* 2024 Recent developments in magnetic hyperthermia therapy (MHT) and magnetic particle imaging (MPI) in the brain tumor field: a scoping review and meta-analysis *Micromachines* **15** 559
[117] Subhan M A 2022 Advances with metal oxide-based nanoparticles as MDR metastatic breast cancer therapeutics and diagnostics *RSC Adv.* **12** 32956–78
[118] Kami D, Takeda S, Itakura Y, Gojo S, Watanabe M and Toyoda M 2011 Application of magnetic nanoparticles to gene delivery *Int. J. Mol. Sci.* **12** 3705–22
[119] Sizikov A A, Kharlamova M V, Nikitin M P, Nikitin P I and Kolychev E L 2021 Nonviral locally injected magnetic vectors for *in vivo* gene delivery: a review of studies on magnetofection *Nanomaterials* **11** 1078

[120] Alromi D A, Madani S Y and Seifalian A 2021 Emerging application of magnetic nanoparticles for diagnosis and treatment of cancer *Polymers* **13** 4146

[121] Rahman M M *et al* 2022 Recent advancements of nanoparticles application in cancer and neurodegenerative disorders: at a glance *Biomed. Pharmacother.* **153** 113305

[122] Huang R Y, Liu Z H, Weng W H and Chang C W 2021 Magnetic nanocomplexes for gene delivery applications *J. Mater. Chem.* B **9** 4267–86

[123] Lapusan R, Borlan R and Focsan M 2024 Advancing MRI with magnetic nanoparticles: a comprehensive review of translational research and clinical trials *Nanoscale Adv.* **6** 2234–2259

[124] Caspani S, Magalhães R, Araújo J P and Sousa C T 2020 Magnetic nanomaterials as contrast agents for MRI *Materials* **13** 2586

[125] Sezer N, Arı İ, Bicer Y and Koc M 2021 Superparamagnetic nanoarchitectures: multimodal functionalities and applications *J. Magn. Magn. Mater.* **538** 168300

[126] Nguyen M D, Tran H V, Xu S and Lee T R 2021 Fe3O4 nanoparticles: structures, synthesis, magnetic properties, surface functionalization, and emerging applications *Appl. Sci.* **11** 11301

[127] Qiao R, Fu C, Forgham H, Javed I, Huang X, Zhu J, Whittaker A K and Davis T P 2023 Magnetic iron oxide nanoparticles for brain imaging and drug delivery *Adv. Drug Deliv. Rev.* **197** 114822

[128] Stephen Z R, Kievit F M and Zhang M 2011 Magnetite nanoparticles for medical MR imaging *Mater. Today* **14** 330–8

[129] Smith L, Byrne H L, Waddington D *et al* 2022 Nanoparticles for MRI-guided radiation therapy: a review *Cancer Nano* **13** 38

[130] Yin X, Russek S E, Zabow G *et al* 2018 Large T_1 contrast enhancement using superparamagnetic nanoparticles in ultra-low field MRI *Sci. Rep.* **8** 11863

[131] Liu R *et al* 2023 Nanotechnology for enhancing medical imaging ed N Gu *Nanomedicine. Micro/Nano Technologies* (Singapore: Springer)

[132] Niculescu A-G and Grumezescu A M 2022 Novel tumor-targeting nanoparticles for cancer treatment—a review *Int. J. Mol. Sci.* **23** 5253

[133] Hosseini S M, Mohammadnejad J, Salamat S, Zadeh Z B, Tanhaei M and Ramakrishna S 2023 Theranostic polymeric nanoparticles as a new approach in cancer therapy and diagnosis: a review *Mater. Today Chem.* **29** 101400

[134] Szwed M and Marczak A 2024 Application of nanoparticles for magnetic hyperthermia for cancer treatment—the current state of knowledge *Cancers* **16** 1156

[135] Lee J H, Kim J W and Cheon J 2013 Magnetic nanoparticles for multi-imaging and drug delivery *Mol. Cells* **35** 274–84

[136] Hosseingholian A, Gohari S D, Feirahi F, Moammeri F, Mesbahian G, Moghaddam Z S and Ren Q 2023 Recent advances in green synthesized nanoparticles: from production to application *Mater. Today Sustain.* **24** 100500

[137] Kus-Liśkiewicz M, Fickers P and Ben Tahar I 2021 Biocompatibility and cytotoxicity of gold nanoparticles: recent advances in methodologies and regulations *Int. J. Mol. Sci.* **22** 10952

[138] Apostolopoulou A, Chiotellis A, Salvanou E-A, Makrypidi K, Tsoukalas C, Kapiris F, Paravatou-Petsotas M, Papadopoulos M, Pirmettis I C, Koźmiński P *et al* 2021 Synthesis and *in vitro* evaluation of gold nanoparticles functionalized with thiol ligands for robust radiolabeling with ^{99m}Tc *Nanomaterials* **11** 2406

[139] Silva F, Cabral Campello M P and Paulo A 2021 Radiolabeled gold nanoparticles for imaging and therapy of cancer *Materials* **14** 4
[140] Nelson N R, Port J D and Pandey M K 2020 Use of superparamagnetic iron oxide nanoparticles (SPIONs) via multiple imaging modalities and modifications to reduce cytotoxicity: an educational review *J. Nanotheranostics* **1** 105–35
[141] Ai F *et al* 2023 Carbon quantum dots: preparation, optical properties, and biomedical applications *Mater. Today Adv.* **18** 100376
[142] Calatayud D G, Lledos M, Casarsa F and Pascu S I 2023 Functional diversity in radiolabeled nanoceramics and related biomaterials for the multimodal imaging of tumors *ACS Bio. Med. Chem Au* **3** 389–417
[143] Zhang Y, Wu M, Wu M, Zhu J and Zhang X 2018 Multifunctional carbon-based nanomaterials: applications in biomolecular imaging and therapy *ACS Omega* **3** 9126–45
[144] Zheng S, Tian Y, Ouyang J, Shen Y, Wang X and Luan J 2022 Carbon nanomaterials for drug delivery and tissue engineering *Front. Chem.* **10** 990362
[145] Xu B, Li S, Shi R *et al* 2023 Multifunctional mesoporous silica nanoparticles for biomedical applications *Sig. Transduct. Target Ther.* **8** 435
[146] Krekorian M, Sandker G G, Cortenbach K R, Tagit O, van Riessen N K, Raavé R, Srinivas M, Figdor C G, Heskamp S and Aarntzen E H 2021 Characterization of intrinsically radiolabeled poly (lactic-co-glycolic acid) nanoparticles for *ex vivo* autologous cell labeling and *in vivo* tracking *Bioconjug. Chem.* **32** 1802–11
[147] Low H Y, Yang C-T, Xia B, He T, Lam W W C and Ng D C E 2023 Radiolabeled liposomes for nuclear imaging probes *Molecules* **28** 3798
[148] Nsairat H, Khater D, Sayed U, Odeh F, Al Bawab A and Alshaer W 2022 Liposomes: structure, composition, types, and clinical applications *Heliyon* **8**
[149] de Barros A B, Tsourkas A, Saboury B *et al* 2012 Emerging role of radiolabeled nanoparticles as an effective diagnostic technique *EJNMMI Res.* **2** 39
[150] Liu R *et al* 2022 Nanotechnology for enhancing medical imaging ed N Gu *Nanomedicine. Micro/Nano Technologies* (Singapore: Springer)
[151] Najdian A, Beiki D, Abbasi M *et al* 2024 Exploring innovative strides in radiolabeled nanoparticle progress for multimodality cancer imaging and theranostic applications *Cancer Imaging* **24** 127
[152] Mutreja I, Maalej N, Kaushik A, Kumar D and Raja A 2023 High atomic number nanoparticles to enhance spectral CT imaging aspects *Mater. Adv.* **4** 3967–88
[153] Dong Y C, Hajfathalian M, Maidment P S N *et al* 2019 Effect of gold nanoparticle size on their properties as contrast agents for computed tomography *Sci. Rep.* **9** 14912
[154] Lassenberger A, Scheberl A, Stadlbauer A, Stiglbauer A, Helbich T and Reimhult E 2017 Individually stabilized, superparamagnetic nanoparticles with controlled shell and size leading to exceptional stealth properties and high relaxivities *ACS Appl. Mater. Interfaces* **9** 3343–53
[155] Xie J, Zhou Z, Ma S *et al* 2021 Facile fabrication of BiF_3: Ln (Ln = Gd, Yb, Er)@PVP nanoparticles for high-efficiency computed tomography imaging *Nanoscale Res. Lett.* **16** 131
[156] Ahmad M Y, Liu S, Tegafaw T, Saidi A K A A, Zhao D, Liu Y, Nam S-W, Chang Y and Lee G H 2023 Heavy metal-based nanoparticles as high-performance x-ray computed tomography contrast agents *Pharmaceuticals* **16** 1463
[157] Gupta D, Roy I and Gandhi S 2023 Metallic nanoparticles for CT-guided imaging of tumors and their therapeutic applications *OpenNano* **12** 100146

[158] Zhang P, Ma X, Guo R, Ye Z, Fu H, Fu N, Guo Z, Zhang J and Zhang J 2021 Organic nanoplatforms for iodinated contrast media in CT imaging *Molecules* **26** 7063
[159] Shariati A, Ebrahimi T, Babadinia P *et al* 2023 Synthesis and characterization of Gd^{3+}-loaded hyaluronic acid-polydopamine nanoparticles as a dual contrast agent for CT and MRI scans *Sci. Rep.* **13** 4520
[160] Sun L, Liu H, Ye Y *et al* 2023 Smart nanoparticles for cancer therapy *Sig. Transduct. Target Ther.* **8** 418
[161] Xu H, Li S and Liu Y S 2022 Nanoparticles in the diagnosis and treatment of vascular aging and related diseases *Sig. Transduct. Target Ther.* **7** 231
[162] Huang J, Bao H, Li X and Zhang Z 2022 *In vivo* CT imaging tracking of stem cells labeled with Au nanoparticles *View* **3** 20200119
[163] Al-Thani A N, Jan A G, Abbas M, Geetha M and Sadasivuni K K 2024 Nanoparticles in cancer theragnostic and drug delivery: a comprehensive review *Life Sci.* **352** 122899
[164] Luo D, Wang X, Burda C and Basilion J P 2021 Recent development of gold nanoparticles as contrast agents for cancer diagnosis *Cancers* **13** 1825
[165] Bejarano J *et al* 2018 Nanoparticles for diagnosis and therapy of atherosclerosis and myocardial infarction: evolution toward prospective theranostic approaches *Theranostics* **8** 4710–32
[166] Siddique S and Chow J C L 2020 Gold nanoparticles for drug delivery and cancer therapy *Appl. Sci.* **10** 3824
[167] Kong F-Y, Zhang J-W, Li R-F, Wang Z-X, Wang W-J and Wang W 2017 Unique roles of gold nanoparticles in drug delivery, targeting and imaging applications *Molecules* **22** 1445
[168] Gu X, Wei S and Lv X 2024 Circulating tumor cells: from new biological insights to clinical practice *Sig. Transduct. Target Ther.* **9** 226
[169] Das U, Banik S, Nadumane S S, Chakrabarti S, Gopal D, Kabekkodu S P, Srisungsitthisunti P, Mazumder N and Biswas R 2023 Isolation, detection and analysis of circulating tumour cells: a nanotechnological bioscope *Pharmaceutics* **15** 280
[170] Milewska S, Sadowska A, Stefaniuk N, Misztalewska-Turkowicz I, Wilczewska A Z, Car H and Niemirowicz-Laskowska K 2024 Tumor-homing peptides as crucial component of magnetic-based delivery systems: recent developments and pharmacoeconomical perspective *Int. J. Mol. Sci.* **25** 6219
[171] Kateb B *et al* 2011 Nanoplatforms for constructing new approaches to cancer treatment, imaging, and drug delivery: what should be the policy? *Neuroimage* **54** S106–24
[172] Wang L, Wang N, Zhang W *et al* 2022 Therapeutic peptides: current applications and future directions *Sig. Transduct. Target Ther.* **7** 48
[173] Mitchell M J, Billingsley M M, Haley R M *et al* 2021 Engineering precision nanoparticles for drug delivery *Nat. Rev. Drug Discov.* **20** 101–24
[174] Kircher M F, Hricak H and Larson S M 2012 Molecular imaging for personalized cancer care *Mol. Oncol.* **6** 182–95
[175] Mushtaq S, Bibi A, Park J E and Jeon J 2021 Recent progress in technetium-99m-labeled nanoparticles for molecular imaging and cancer therapy *Nanomaterials* **11** 3022
[176] Olson M T, Ly Q P and Mohs A M 2019 Fluorescence guidance in surgical oncology: challenges, opportunities, and translation *Mol. Imaging Biol.* **21** 200–18
[177] Israel L L, Galstyan A, Holler E and Ljubimova J Y 2020 Magnetic iron oxide nanoparticles for imaging, targeting and treatment of primary and metastatic tumors of the brain *J. Control. Release* **320** 45–62

[178] Patra J K, Das G, Fraceto L F *et al* 2018 Nano based drug delivery systems: recent developments and future prospects *J. Nanobiotechnol.* **16** 71
[179] Le N and Kim. K 2023 Current advances in the biomedical applications of quantum dots: promises and challenges *Int. J. Mol. Sci.* **24** 12682
[180] Abbasi R, Shineh G, Mobaraki M *et al* 2023 Structural parameters of nanoparticles affecting their toxicity for biomedical applications: a review *J. Nanopart. Res.* **25** 43
[181] Xuan L, Ju Z, Skonieczna M, Zhou P and Huang R Nanoparticles-induced potential toxicity on human health: applications, toxicity mechanisms, and evaluation models *MedComm* **4** e327
[182] Liu J, Liu Z, Pang Y *et al* 2022 The interaction between nanoparticles and immune system: application in the treatment of inflammatory diseases *J. Nanobiotechnol.* **20** 127
[183] Zia S, Islam Aqib A, Muneer A, Fatima M, Atta K, Kausar T, Zaheer C N, Ahmad I, Saeed M and Shafique A 2023 Insights into nanoparticles-induced neurotoxicity and cope up strategies *Front. Neurosci.* **17** 1127460
[184] Rodríguez-Gómez F D, Penon O, Monferrer D and Rivera-Gil P 2023 Classification system for nanotechnology-enabled health products with both scientific and regulatory application *Front. Med.* **10** 1212949
[185] Elumalai K, Srinivasan S and Shanmugam A 2024 Review of the efficacy of nanoparticle-based drug delivery systems for cancer treatment *Biomed. Technol.* **5** 109–22
[186] Pesapane F, Codari M and Sardanelli F 2018 Artificial intelligence in medical imaging: threat or opportunity? Radiologists again at the forefront of innovation in medicine *Eur. Radiol. Exp.* **2** 35
[187] Skepu A *et al* 2023 AI and nanomedicine in realizing the goal of precision medicine: tailoring the best treatment for personalized cancer treatment ed Z Dlamini *Artificial Intelligence and Precision Oncology* (Cham: Springer)
[188] Kovuri U *et al* 2024 Predictive analysis of breast cancer metastasis and identification of genetic markers using machine learning *JCO* **42** 4
[189] Nguyen H L, Geukens T, Maetens M *et al* 2023 Obesity-associated changes in molecular biology of primary breast cancer *Nat. Commun.* **14** 4418
[190] Fan D, Cao Y, Cao M *et al* 2023 Nanomedicine in cancer therapy *Sig. Transduct. Target Ther.* **8** 293
[191] Alowais S A, Alghamdi S S, Alsuhebany N *et al* 2023 Revolutionizing healthcare: the role of artificial intelligence in clinical practice *BMC Med. Educ.* **23** 689
[192] Najjar R 2023 Redefining radiology: a review of artificial intelligence integration in medical imaging *Diagnostics* **13** 2760
[193] Hare J I, Lammers T, Ashford M B, Puri S, Storm G and Barry S T 2017 Challenges and strategies in anti-cancer nanomedicine development: an industry perspective *Adv. Drug Deliv. Rev.* **108** 25–38
[194] Sarkar C, Das B, Rawat V S, Wahlang J B, Nongpiur A, Tiewsoh I, Lyngdoh N M, Das D, Bidarolli M and Sony H T 2023 Artificial intelligence and machine learning technology driven modern drug discovery and development *Int. J. Mol. Sci.* **24** 2026
[195] Adir O, Poley M, Chen G, Froim S, Krinsky N, Shklover J, Shainsky-Roitman J, Lammers T and Schroeder A 2020 Integrating artificial intelligence and nanotechnology for precision cancer medicine *Adv. Mater.* **32** 1901989
[196] Das K P 2023 Nanoparticles and convergence of artificial intelligence for targeted drug delivery for cancer therapy: current progress and challenges *Front. Med. Technol.* **4** 1067144
[197] Mabrouk M, Das D B, Salem Z A and Beherei H H 2021 Nanomaterials for biomedical applications: production, characterisations, recent trends and difficulties *Molecules* **26** 1077

[198] Bardhan N 2022 Nanomaterials in diagnostics, imaging and delivery: applications from COVID-19 to cancer *MRS Commun.* **12** 1119–39
[199] Dang X, Bardhan N M, Qi J *et al* 2019 Deep-tissue optical imaging of near cellular-sized features *Sci Rep.* **9** 3873
[200] Bardhan N M, Kumar P V, Li Z, Ploegh H L, Grossman J C, Belcher A M and Chen G Y 2017 Enhanced cell capture on functionalized graphene oxide nanosheets through oxygen clustering *ACS Nano* **11** 1548–58
[201] Kumar P, Bardhan N, Tongay S *et al* 2014 Scalable enhancement of graphene oxide properties by thermally driven phase transformation *Nat. Chem.* **6** 151–8
[202] Hao L, Rohani N, Zhao R T *et al* 2021 Microenvironment-triggered multimodal precision diagnostics *Nat. Mater.* **20** 1440–8
[203] Smith B R and Gambhir S S 2017 Nanomaterials for *in vivo* imaging *Chem. Rev.* **117** 901–86
[204] Martino F, Amici G, Rosner M, Ronco C and Novara G 2021 Gadolinium-based contrast media nephrotoxicity in kidney impairment: the physio-pathological conditions for the perfect murder *J. Clin. Med.* **10** 271
[205] Akhter M H, Khalilullah H, Gupta M, Alfaleh M A, Alhakamy N A, Riadi Y and Md S 2021 Impact of protein corona on the biological identity of nanomedicine: understanding the fate of nanomaterials in the biological milieu *Biomedicines* **9** 1496
[206] Corbo C, Molinaro R, Parodi A, Toledano Furman N E, Salvatore F and Tasciotti E 2016 The impact of nanoparticle protein corona on cytotoxicity, immunotoxicity and target drug delivery *Nanomedicine* **11** 81–100

IOP Publishing

Nanoplatforms for Cancer Imaging

Nanasaheb D Thorat and Sandeep B Somvanshi

Chapter 4

Clinical advancements in cancer Diagnosis: the role of nanotechnology in cancer imaging and drug delivery

Raje Sengar, Swati Dubey and Harshit Dubey

Cancer continues to be a worldwide medical concern, demanding ongoing advances in diagnostic tools to allow for early and precise identification. As per the latest world cancer statistics report, the number of new cancer cases will increase to more than 25 million by 2040. Nanotechnology offers the capability to revolutionize cancer diagnosis and treatment. Nanotechnology has a significant influence on disease examination, earlier identification, assessment, and prediction through improvements to medically applicable technologies. Thus the field of nanotechnology has shown tremendous potential in cancer imaging, providing new avenues for improvement of the sensitivity, specificity, and accuracy of diagnostic techniques. In this chapter we briefly discuss the introduction of cancer, its classification depending on different modes and the general mechanism of action of cancer drugs, which will inform readers about cancer. It also illustrates the various routes of delivery of certain drugs. The different methods of delivery have an impact on the accessibility of the medication existing in the body tissues. Further, it includes the classification of different administrative routes, as well as their key characteristics, benefits, drawbacks, and examples.

The chapter later focuses on currently available imaging modalities for the diagnosis, prevention, and treatment of cancer. We address the most frequently utilized nanomaterials in the detection and treatment of cancer. We emphasize the potential benefits of these nanoplatforms for cancer therapy depending upon their physical, chemical, and biological characteristics. In recent decades, tumor scanning has progressed dramatically, with nanotechnology arising as an essential aid for improving accuracy in diagnosis and treatment success. This chapter intends to provide full knowledge of the contribution of nanoplatforms in the alteration of cancer imaging's landscape and its future prospects, through a comprehensive assessment of the existing literature, experimental research, and clinical trials.

doi:10.1088/978-0-7503-5864-4ch4

4.1 Introduction

4.1.1 Cancer

Cancer is an important and increasing cause of morbidity and mortality worldwide. Nearly 10 million deaths worldwide were caused by cancer in 2020, making it the second largest cause of mortality globally [1]. The latest world cancer statistics report that the number of new cancer cases will increase to more than 25 million by 2040 [2]. Apart from its high mortality rate, it also imposes a heavy financial cost on society and the families of cancer patients. The development of cancerous cells is the sole factor causing the death of the majority of cancer patients. As a result, efforts to prevent, diagnose, and treat cancer are crucial. According to molecular and cellular investigations, cancerous cells shows uncontrolled development, maturation, and cell survival [3]. There are more than a hundred different varieties of cancer, which can vary greatly in behavior and responsiveness to treatment. Cancer can be caused by erroneous proliferation of any of the multiple kinds of cells in the body. The overall anomalies in cancer cells result in lost control of growth, which is reflected by a number of characteristics of cancerous cells that differ from those of their normal counterparts [4]. Cell division is normal, but when this process is uncontrolled, a mass of tissue (called a growth or tumor) forms, which is clearly shown in figure 4.1. Cancer is a hereditary disease that mostly develops as a result of the suppression of physiological apoptosis [5], DNA damage, induction of senescence, and p53 mutation [6]. Some tumors have the capacity to spread beyond the area of their genesis and invade different body regions. We refer to this process as metastasis [7].

The most difficult problem in cancer pathology is differentiating benign from malignant tumors. Both benign and malignant tumors are classified according to the type of cell from which they arise. Tumors develop from benign to malignant lesions through a series of changes. Malignant tumors actively release cells that spread to nearby tissues and distant organs, whereas benign tumors are restricted to the site of the cancer.

4.1.1.1 Classification of cancer

The World Health Organization (WHO) and the Union for International Cancer Control (UICC) designed classification of malignant tumors on the grounds of their

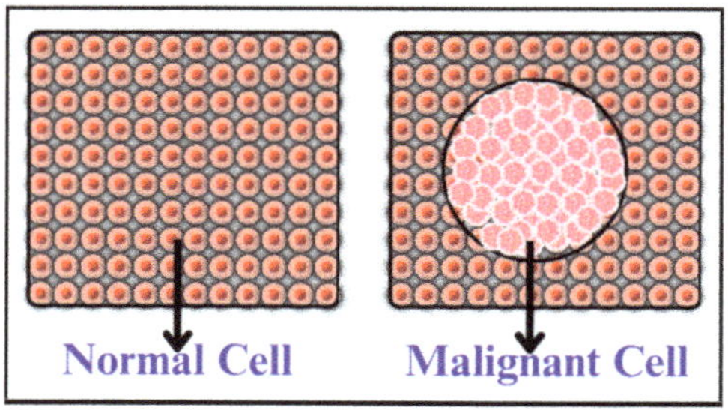

Figure 4.1. Image showing a normal cell versus a cancerous cell.

malignancy, site of origin, cytology, structural grade, and metastasis. The above mentioned characteristics are helpful in the diagnosis and management of tumors. These categories, which are based on physiological, morphological, epidemiological, and clinical data, in particular indicate agreement among pathologists, radiologists, and clinical oncologists, and aid in management choices.

According to the site of origin, cancer is chiefly classified into five main types: carcinoma, sarcoma, leukemia, lymphoma, and brain and spinal cord cancers. Carcinomas, which include approximately 90% of human cancers, begin in the skin or in tissues that line or cover internal organs. They are further subcategorized into adenocarcinomas, basal cell carcinomas, squamous cell carcinomas, and transitional cell carcinomas [8]. The majority of carcinomas attack glands or organs that may secrete, including the breasts, which produce milk, the lungs, which releases mucus, the colon, the prostate, and the bladder. Sarcoma is a term for cancer that develops in connective and supporting tissues, including bone, tendons, cartilage, muscle, fibrous tissues, and fat [9]. The most typical sarcoma often develops as a painful lump on the bone that usually affects young individuals. Sarcoma tumors frequently mimic the tissue in which they develop. Leukemia refers to the malignancy of the white blood cells, which originates in the tissues that make blood cells such as the bone marrow [10]. There are different types of leukemias, such as acute lymphocytic leukemia, chronic lymphocytic leukemia, acute myeloid leukemia, and chronic myeloid leukemia. Lymphoma arises from the cells of the immune system. Hodgkin lymphoma and non-Hodgkin lymphoma are the two main types of lymphomas, respectively. Tumors growing in the tissue inside the brain or spinal cord are classified as central nervous system (CNS) cancers. Gliomas, chordomas, etc are CNS cancers. Another classification of cancer is based on the organ of origin, according to which cancers are named on the basis of the targeted organ, such as lung, colon, breast, head and neck, kidney, bladder, prostate, ovary, etc [11], as depicted in figure 4.2.

A crucial factor in assessing the severity of cancer is 'staging'. Patients may receive prescriptions that are suitable and appropriate for their current stage of cancer. Depending upon unique characteristics and signs, cancer is subdivided into four stages as:

Stage 1: this is the first stage of cancer, with no outward signs. The tumor is not yet fully developed. A normal physical examination can aid in identifying the presence of early-stage cancer. It will be simpler to treat cancer if it is discovered at this stage.

Stage 2: this is the secondary stage, which has few apparent signs and ultimately relies solely on scan results for diagnosis.

Stage 3: this is the tertiary stage with clearly detectable signs. The tumor is benign in nature and fully grown at this stage.

Stage 4: this is the last stage of cancer with zero recovery chance as the tumor has totally migrated to other biological structures. At this stage symptoms such as cachexia (sudden significant weight loss), patches on skin, etc become clearly apparent.

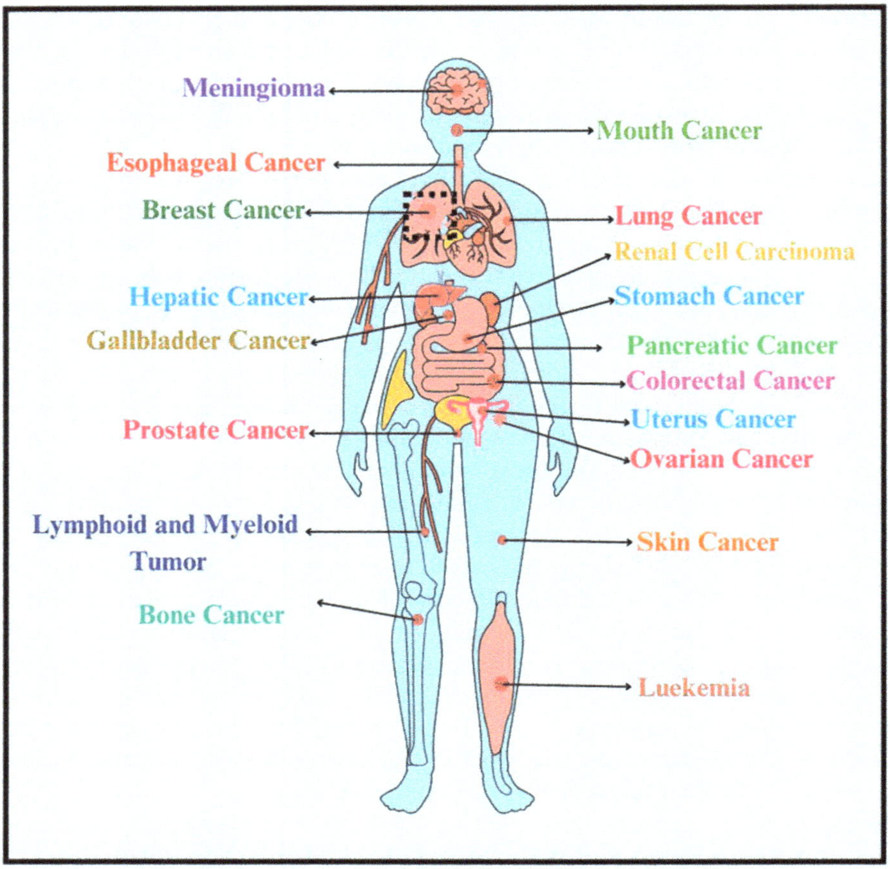

Figure 4.2. Types of cancer on the basis of targeted organs.

Another classification system is based on the extent and severity of the cancer, according to which it is classified as: T cancer, N cancer, and M cancer [12]. T cancer is classified as a primary stage cancer, the severity of which relies on how far the tumor has migrated from its initial site. N cancer is classified as a secondary stage cancer when the tumor spreads from its primary site to lymph nodes. M cancer is classified as a third stage cancer with zero chance of recovery; at this time the tumor has completely spread to other biological organs.

4.1.2 Anticancer drugs

As discussed in an earlier section, cancer is a general term applied to unregulated growth of abnormal cells affecting different parts of body and continues until the organism's death if not arrested in time. The three primary treatment modalities for advanced cancer in people are surgery, radiation, and medication (cancer chemotherapeutic agents). Chemotherapeutic treatments for cancer can frequently offer momentary symptom alleviation, life extension, and occasionally cures [13].

The synthesis of possible anti-cancer medicines has received much attention recently. The recognized class of cancer chemotherapeutic drugs has thousands of chemical variations, but they all show greater adverse effects. A potent anti-cancer drug should be capable of destroying or paralyzing cancer cells without adversely impacting healthy cells. This objective is extremely challenging and almost practically unattainable, which is one of the reason why cancer patients frequently encounter adverse side effects while under therapy [14].

4.1.2.1 Plants as a source of anti-cancer compounds

Plant-derived compounds, which are an important source of clinically useful anti-cancer drugs, have been shown to have potential for treatment or prevention of cancer in humans. Plants have a long history in the treatment of cancer; more than 3000 plant species have been reported by Hartwell to be used in the treatment of cancer [15]. Plants as well as plant-derived compounds have played a significant role in the development of a number of clinically used anti-cancer agents. Chemotherapy, a major treatment used for the control of advanced stages of malignancies and a prophylactic against possible metastasis, exhibits severe toxicity on normal tissues. Plants have been used for treating various diseases of human beings and animals. They maintain the health and vitality of individuals and also cure diseases, including cancer, without causing toxicity. More than 50% of all modern drugs in clinical use are natural products, many of which have the ability to control cancer cells [16]. Table 4.1 lists a few plants and derived chemicals responsible for anti-cancer activity.

4.1.2.2 Mode of action

The goal of chemotherapy is to inhibit cell proliferation and tumor multiplication, thus avoiding invasion and metastasis. But this results in toxic effects from chemotherapy due to the effects on normal cells. Inhibition of tumor growth can take place at several levels within the cell and its environment.

Conventional chemotherapeutic medicines generally disrupt cancerous cell macromolecular production or activity by interference with DNA, RNA, or protein production, or by inhibiting the normal operation of the prefabricated molecule. When a chemotherapeutic substance interacts with macromolecular production or function sufficiently, it causes cell death either directly or by inducing apoptosis. Conventional medications may prolong apoptosis because a percentage of cells

Table 4.1. List of anti-cancer plants.

S. No.	Plant name	Family	Chemical responsible for anti-cancer activity
1	Turmeric	*Zingiberaceae*	Curcumin
2	Vinca	*Apocynaceae*	Vinblastine, vincristine, vinorelbine, vindesine
3	Wheat grass	*Grasses*	Chlorophyll, selenium and lactrile
4	Neem	*Meliaceae*	Flavonoids (rutin and quercetin)
5	Taxus	*Taxaceae*	Paclitaxel
6	Aloevera	*Xanthorrhoeaceae*	Aloeemodin, emodin

perish as a result of a particular therapy. As a result, the drug may need to be repeated in order to produce a reaction. Cytotoxic medicines are most dangerous during the S stage of the cell cycle, which is where DNA is synthesized [17]. Drugs like vinca alkaloids and taxanes inhibit mitotic spindle development during the M phase [18].

The mechanism of cancer therapy involves the inhibition of cancer cell production directly by stimulating macrophage phagocytosis, enhancing natural killer cell activity, and promoting apoptosis of cancer cells by increasing production of interferon-I, interleukin2, immunoglobulin, and complement in blood serum and so enforcing the necrosis of tumor and inhibiting its translocation and spread by blocking the blood source of tumor tissue.

This results in enhancement of the number of leukocytes and platelets by stimulating the hemopoietic function, which promotes the reverse transformation from tumor cells into normal cells, causing promotion of metabolism and prevention of carcinogenesis of normal cells. Thus treatment finally results in the stimulation of appetite, improved quality of sleep, and pain relief, ultimately benefiting the patient's health.

4.1.2.3 Classification of anti-cancer drugs

Chemotherapeutic drugs are widely used to treat cancer in order to kill cancer cells, prevent tumor growth, and reduce pain. The delivery of chemotherapy is possible in neoadjuvant, adjuvant, combination, and metastatic situations. The treatment given prior to primary treatment is classified as neoadjuvant therapy. Adjuvant therapy is a form of treatment used in conjunction with the primary therapy to slow or stop the growth of hidden cancer cells. It is becoming increasingly common for cancers of the ovary, colorectal, breast, and lung. While treating tumors of the head and neck, lung, or anus, combined therapy including chemotherapy and radiation is utilized to reduce the tumor size prior to surgery or other curative procedure. In the majority of cancer therapies, multitargeted therapy or combination therapy is more effective than single-agent therapy. According to their pharmaceutical mechanism of action, anti-cancer medications can be categorized as alkylating agents, plant alkaloids, DNA-interactive agents, antimetabolites, monoclonal antibodies, antitubulin agents, topoisomerase inhibitors, corticosteroids, hormones, molecular targeting agents, or other biological agents [19].

(i) **Alkylating agents**

These substances damage genetic material and halt mitosis when they interact with nucleophilic sites present in nucleic acid bases and proteins. This interaction results in the creation of the R-CH_2^+ group, which is unstable in nature. They are utilized for the treatment of cancers like lung, breast, and ovarian, as well as leukemia, lymphomas, multiple myeloma, and sarcoma [20]. This class of medications includes nitrogen mustards such as cyclophosphamide, bendamustine, and ifosfamide; nitrosoureas, including lomustine and carmustine; triazenes, such as temozolamide, dacarbazine, and procarbazine; alkyl sulfonates such as busulfan; platinum analogs like cisplatin, oxaliplatin, and carboplatin; and ethyleneimines like thiotepa [21].

(ii) **Antimetabolites**

These chemicals impede cell replication and proliferation by disrupting the synthesis of nucleic acids due to substitution of structural replicas of pyrimidine or purine into cell components. These are used to treat leukemia and cancers of the breast and ovary. 5-fluorouracil (5-FU), 6-mercaptopurine (6-MP), cytarabine, capecitabine, fludarabine, gemcitabine, methotrexate, pemetrexed, pentostatin, and thioguanine are a few examples of medications in this family [22].

(iii) **Antimicrotubular agents**

There are different types of antimicrotubular agents, such as topoisomerase inhibitor I and II, taxanes, and vinca alkaloids. Topoisomerase inhibitors include irinotecan and etoposide compounds. These agents inhibit the responsible enzyme, which would usually help in the detangling and relaxation of supercoiled double-stranded DNA strands for replication [23]. They are used to treat leukemia, lung, ovarian, and gut cancer. This class, which includes doxorubicin, daunorubicin, idarubicin, and epirubicin, is responsible for inhibiting RNA and DNA synthesis. Taxanes like paclitaxel, docetaxel, cabazitaxel, etc bring about apoptosis because of aberrant cellular activity and replication disruption and so inhibit microtubule assembly. Vinca alkaloids such as vincristine, vinblastine, vinorelbine, etc bind tubulin, causing inhibition of microtubule formation in the metaphase, resulting in cell cycle senescence and thus blocking mitotic spindle formation [24].

(iv) **Antibiotics**

The term 'antibiotics' describes the types of secondary metabolites that are derived either from microscopic species or higher plant or animal species during their lives. These compounds may possess anti-pathogenic or other properties that might impede the growth of other biological cells. Antibiotics are classified into two types based on their activity against microbiological cells as bactericidal and bacteriostatic antibiotics. These compounds typically attack bacteria by one of four mechanisms: suppression of microbial cell membrane development, increased cell membrane penetrability, disruption of protein formation, and hindering of microbial DNA multiplication and transcription. Antibiotics includes those classes of drugs that inhibit RNA and DNA synthesis, producing single- and double-strand DNA strand scission at the binding site. Actinomycin D, bleomycin, and daunomycin are antibiotics that are used as chemotherapy agents. Lee *et al* in their study investigated the impact of salinomycin, both on its own and in conjunction with paclitaxel on ovarian cancer cells [25].

4.2 Traditional methods of drug administration

The route of administration is as important as the drug itself for therapeutic success. The choice of a delivery route is driven by patient acceptability, the properties of the drug (such as its solubility), access to a disease location, or effectiveness in dealing

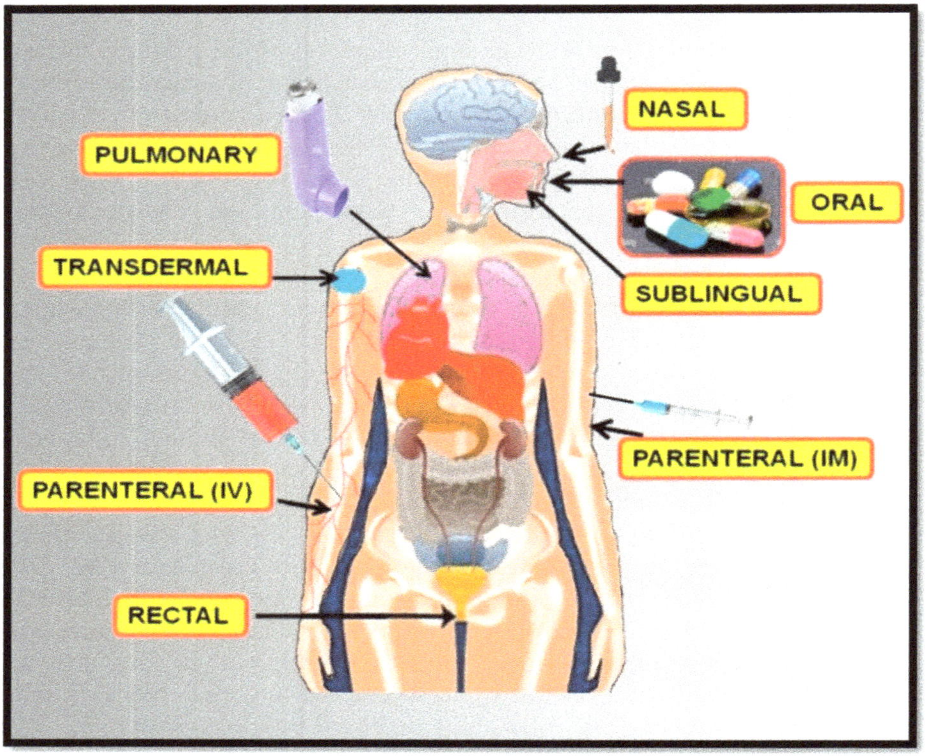

Figure 4.3. Routes of administration.

with the specific disease. Drugs are administered through various routes, such as injection, mouth, transdermal, and mucous membrane. Different type of administration routes are shown in figure 4.3.

(i) **Oral administration**

The oral route is a well-established means of drug introduction into the systemic circulation due to patient acceptability and convenience [26]. Although it promotes quicker medication release, it also causes local toxicity in the body. Therefore orally delivered medicines show restricted dissolution and slow permeability across the intestinal epithelium [27]. Unfortunately, the drug types that can be introduced by this route are limited, due to the harsh conditions encountered in the system. The present approaches to addressing these challenges emphasize a variety of systems in which medications are inserted into oral magic bullet transporters. Because of the possibility that nanoparticles may shield enzymatic breakdown of sensitive medications in acidic media these nano-agents have been developed as oral distribution vehicles for large molecules like proteins, polynucleotides, etc [28]. This strategy was investigated in detail in research demonstrating that insulin encapsulated nanoparticle intake by mouth lowered blood glucose levels in diabetic rats [29]. The oral administration route is being studied most extensively since it offers benefits such as easy and simple administration inside the body and reduction in manufacturing costs, etc. Thus, it could be employed as a future route for the delivery of sensitive drugs loaded in different nanocarriers.

(ii) **Pulmonary administration**

Due to their vast surface areas and low levels of intrinsic and extrinsic enzyme decomposition, large-molecular-weight drugs can potentially be delivered through the respiratory and olfactory routes. In light of this, it may be that medicine-loaded nanoformulations transportation through the nasal route do not require the same level of protection in acidic media as in the oral route. In order to extend the duration of interaction among the nanoparticulate composition and nostril tissue, medication can be supplied in the form of a powder or solution containing an uptake-boosting element, resulting in retardation of the congenital safety mechanism of the lung. Pulmonary drug delivery offers both local targeting for the treatment of respiratory diseases and increasingly appears to be a viable option for the delivery of drugs systematically. Nanoparticle-based devices that deliver drugs can be used as gene delivery vehicles in pulmonary medication and to stabilize therapeutic compounds that might decay prematurely [30].

The distribution of medications through the olfactory and sublingual channels may be made more effective by using nanostructured drug vehicles since they avoid first-pass metabolism. By coupling active pharmaceutical giant molecules with nanoparticles, it has become feasible to administer proteins and vaccinations effectively via the nasal route [31]. In recent years, the healthcare sector has shown intense curiosity about the utilization of nasal approaches for medication administration. To boost the uptake of polar medicines, many uptake boosters have been researched. For instance, compositions comprising chitosan particles were previously investigated for nasal delivery of insulin and morphine [32].

(iii) **Parenteral administration**

Intravenous, intramuscular, and subcutaneous administration routes are collectively known as the parenteral administration route. It has been shown that anti-cancer medicines are the most promising medications to be administered in this manner. The easiest and quickest way to get a medication into the circulatory system is by an intravenous dose. Since the capillary's diameter is about 4 μM, intravenous administration of nanoparticles produces efficient distribution throughout the body unlike conventional drugs. The particle's dimensions and surface charge, and the lipophilicity of the nanoplatforms significantly impact the biodistribution of nanoparticles.

(iv) **Transdermal administration**

Therapeutic substances being injected into the circulatory system via skin cells is classified as the topical route of drug administration [33]. Drug distribution can be induced actively by applying a voltage (iontophoresis) or passively, depending on pharmaceutical dispersion through the dermis. Compared to other means of drug delivery, the transdermal route offers the potential advantages of avoiding hepatic first-pass metabolism, maintaining constant blood levels for longer periods of time, decreased side effects, decreased gastrointestinal effects that occur due to local contact with gastric mucosa, and improved compliance [34]. It is appropriate for individuals who are not conscious. The dosage regimen can be made simpler and the discomfort associated with conventional medication intake can be reduced by using sustained distribution of medicinal products in transdermal drug delivery systems. Furthermore, topical distribution systems also enable appropriate regulation of medication dosage and delivery pace by regulating the electric field. Thus, drug content and the pH of the medium, which affects the solubility and skin permeability of the drug, are the two main factors that influence the rate of therapeutic delivery through the skin [35]. Slow absorption rates, a shortage of dose adjustability and/or accuracy, and limited access to a comparatively small quantity of medications are its limitations.

4.3 Cancer imaging

Cancer is a complex disorder resulting from several alterations in biological processes and signaling pathways. Complicated metabolic development and signaling tracks can change in many different ways, leading to cancer. The major factor behind the failure of conventional therapies and uncontrolled growth of tumor cells is the physiological and structural diversity inside the cancerous cell. Yet, the full scope of cancer biology and the role of cancer diversity in particular cancer types are still topics that researchers are just beginning to explore. Because of the aberrant proliferation of diseased cells to different body parts, it is a major cause of mortality and thus efficient treatment of cancer requires early identification. In the example of lung and bronchus cancer, when the malignancy becomes apparent at an early stage before proliferation to distant parts of the body the survival chance of patients is about 53%. The survival percentage, however, drops sharply to 4% when cancer is discovered late and has spread into other body parts [36].

The creation of an entirely novel class of treatment options that target particular molecular entities, such as receptors, genes, or signaling cascades, has been made possible by a greater knowledge of the genetic profile of cancer. However, the findings of research investigations employing targeted medicines and DNA microarray-based sickness screening have amply illustrated the inherent variety of human cancers, both genetically and phenotypically [37]. Even when receiving the same therapy, patients with comparable cancer types frequently respond very differently. The introduction of imaging techniques that enable an early evaluation of therapy response in specific individuals, therefore, could aid considerably in the development of these revolutionary targeted medicines [38]. These might be applied in initial studies to offer a quick indication of therapeutic efficiency. The integration of the detecting and medicinal aspects of treating numerous diseases with a single tool has been made possible by novel and promising uses of nanomedicine, which are referred to using the term theranostics [39]. This incorporates a number of approaches to produce thorough diagnosis, *in vivo* molecular imaging, and a customized treatment plan. For instance, preliminary investigations of tumor permeability were performed using dynamic contrast agent-enhanced magnetic resonance imaging (DCE-MRI) in a phase I trial of combretastatin A4 3-O-phosphate (an anti-vascular agent) [40].

The adoption of these imaging techniques in the clinic would thereafter enable clinicians to quickly evaluate a new therapy's efficacy in specific patients. It may be possible to cease inefficient therapy early and switch to more beneficial ones, which would benefit the well-being of the patient and save money for the healthcare system. Delivering medications and imaging agents to the target site effectively is one of the most important needs for both diagnosis and therapy. Many imaging modalities, including positron emission tomography (PET), computed tomography (CT), magnetic resonance imaging (MRI), and fluorescent optical imaging, have been created and employed in medical research for accurate diagnosis of illness [41].

4.3.1 New technologies for molecular imaging in oncology: imaging modalities

Molecular imaging is a multidisciplinary field that combines *in vivo* imaging with molecular biology to provide visual representations of the interior parts of the body at the molecular and cellular levels for therapeutic and scientific study [42]. Molecular imaging needs the intravenous delivery of an imaging agent that interacts with a specific environment to reveal biological processes [43]. These vary in terms of how complicated they are for the user to operate, how sensitive they are, and whether they require external contrast agents or utilize intrinsic molecular signatures and processes to produce signals. Contrast agents have been developed for the purpose of enhancing applications of cellular scanning and producing better results. An additional material known as contrast material can be used in conjunction with the scanning technique to strengthen the signal across the area of interest and starting point, improving the quality of the picture. This precise description conceals the enormous progress over the past 20 years in implementing molecular imaging concepts across a wide range of domains, from fundamental and clinical research to cutting-edge disease detection and treatment. Therefore, any improvements in this field of study will benefit the medical sector. The following are examples of biological imaging techniques and current advancements, as shown in figure 4.4, from the standpoint of nanotechnology instruments.

4.3.1.1 Optical imaging

Using laboratory equipment and methods in real-world scenarios where the capacity to distinguish across cellular and anatomical frameworks is essential for timely detection and therapy is one of the goals of molecular imaging. Non-harmful and non-intrusive imaging techniques enable medical professionals and scientists to observe organisms without the need for tissue removal or permanent changes [44]. This allows them to investigate cells and tissues in their novel position, without

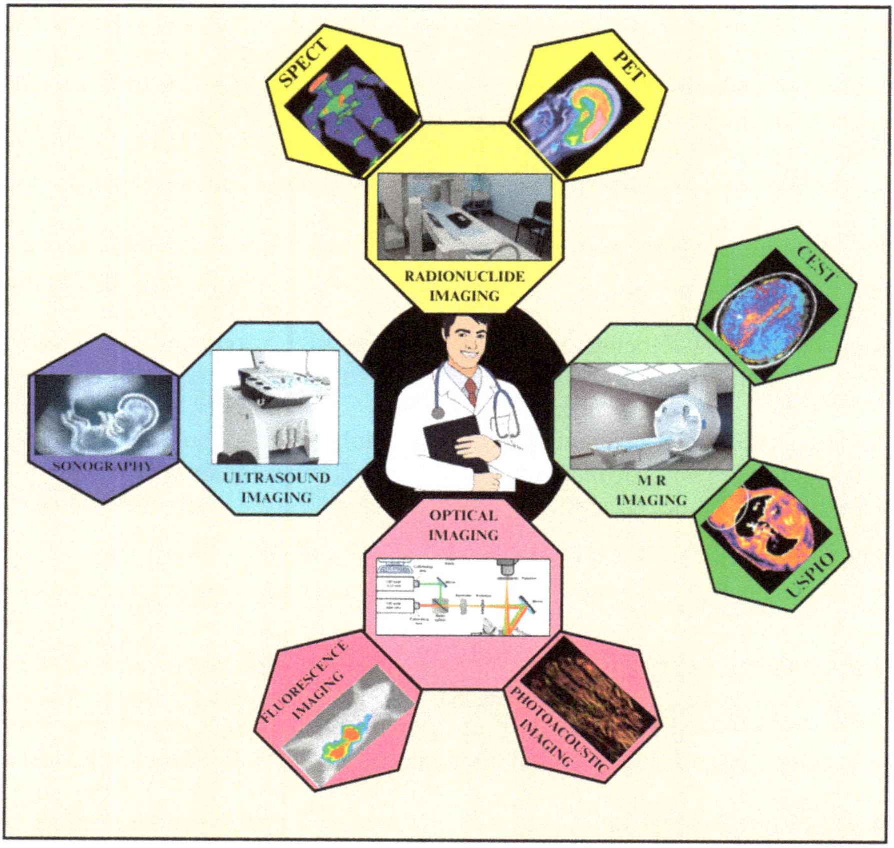

Figure 4.4. Molecular imaging modalities.

affecting their interactions with the surrounding environment. Additionally, the use of real-time scanning allows for vibrant studies of target biology, which can offer a more comprehensive and insightful depiction. An optical technique in cellular scanning provides non-invasive visual observation, comprehension, and occasionally measurement of microscopic cellular structures and processes in clinical settings [45]. Optical imaging methods are largely effective due to non-ionizing radiations. Thus, this approach is used for therapy surveillance, viewpoints, and lengthy, recurring procedures [46].

Optical imaging utilizes harmless radiation that does not ionize and relies on photons interacting with biological structures to obtain detailed scans of soft tissues. In order to create pictures, this technique stimulates electrons to record several aspects of cells, including their absorption, reflection, dispersion, emission, coherence, polarization, and fluorescence of visible, ultraviolet, and infrared light [47]. Optical imaging is not only known for its diagnosis method; it is also well known for its ease of carrying, compact size, portability, and affordable design possibilities.

Different forms of optical imaging include endoscopy, fluorescence imaging, bioluminescence imaging, photoacoustic (PA) imaging, diffuse optical tomography, Raman spectroscopy, and super-resolution microscopy [48]. Optical imaging can be used to identify gastrointestinal issues, skin cancer, the formation of blood vessels leading to tumors, the functioning of neurons, and the analysis of individual cells, due to its distinctive characteristics [49]. Optical probes that are produced through genetic engineering, like fluorescent protein and luciferase, have the ability to mark the cell membrane, organelles, and even specific molecules related to tumor metabolism. The most widespread use is to create a model of tumors by using tumor cells that contain luciferase or fluorescent protein. This allows for the non-invasive tracking of tumor size and the spread of tumors through the use of optical imaging.

4.3.1.1.1 Flourescence imaging

Fluorescence imaging is a flexible method that offers various advantages, including affordability and the ability to conduct multiple imaging tasks simultaneously. The fluorescent process involves absorbing light from various sources in tissues and then releasing some of this light a few nanoseconds afterward, which is captured using a collection of detectors. The objective is to distinguish the emitted radiations from the absorbed radiations. A model that considers the scattering and excitation characteristics of light is employed to simulate its propagation. The experimental intensity measurements from the entire source are then evaluated and compared to this model [50]. Hence achieving effective imaging using contrast agents relies heavily on the development and arrangement of optical filters, filter cubes, and dichroic mirrors.

Nevertheless, the effectiveness of fluorescent imaging is reduced because the tumor cells have lower levels of fluorescent substances and slower uptake rates. The depth of light penetration is restricted when absorbed by molecules like hemoglobin, resulting in limited angiogenesis that usually indicates increased blood vessel formation in cancerous tissue. Thus, there are numerous external fluorescent probes available to label different parts of biological systems. These probes can be small molecules, peptides, antibodies, substrates, or activity-based compounds, as explained in detail by Koch and Ntziachristos [51] in their work. Atreya and coworkers [52] demonstrated that the specific visualization of vascular endothelial growth factor (VEGF) can be accomplished utilizing a fluorescent-labeled antibody that targets VEGF receptor (VEGFR). Utilizing imaging in conjunction with a reporter gene, like the gene responsible for green fluorescent protein (GFP), offers a non-intrusive method for tracking genetic activity. Fluorescent proteins consist of proteins that have different spectral properties, typically emitting short wavelengths of light and having a high efficiency in converting absorbed energy into emitted light. Fluorescent protein typically has a molecular weight ranging from 25 to 30 kDa. Its fluorescence primarily relies on the chromophore produced internally and is not influenced by other cofactors. Various fluorescent probes have been developed to enable tumor imaging and potentially even tumor treatment, with the help of fluorescent proteins extensively used in imaging techniques. For instance, by incorporating GFP genes into the genetic makeup of cancer cells, it becomes possible to not only visually track tumors spreading through fluorescence, but also identify individual cancer cells [53]. These have the potential to make the histopathological procedure less complex. Furthermore, after the identification of GFPs derived from aequorin, researchers have extensively incorporated and modified fluorescent proteins through genetic encoding for various purposes, spanning from studying the brain to visualizing cancer [54]. As it is commonly understood, when removing tumors through surgery, the use of imaging guidance is necessary to obtain information about the edges of the tumor tissue, presence of metastases, and similar details.

Likewise, in the near-infrared (NIR) range, significant progress has been achieved in the enhancement of probe development, ensuring high efficiency in maximum quantum yield, enabling large Stokes shifts, and effectively addressing issues related to bleaching. Sakuda and colleagues [55] conducted a research study and created a method for introducing a virus into cells using vesicular stomatitis virus (VSV) that carries a plasmid with an NIR fluorescent protein called Katushka (rVSV-K). Katushka possesses NIR wavelength ranges that have peak excitation and emission spectra at 588 and 635 nm, respectively. It has the capability to penetrate several millimeters. After the viral transfection system was introduced into mice with osteosarcoma, the tumor was surgically excised using fluorescent imaging as a guiding tool. In laboratory tests, it was confirmed that rVSV-K only causes infection in osteosarcoma cells, in contrast to the conventional surgical method. The use of rVSV-K in NIR fluorescence bioimaging makes it simpler to identify the boundaries of the main tumor and remove it during surgery.

4.3.1.1.2 Bioluminescence imaging

Certain organisms have the ability to transform chemical energy into light. This occurrence in nature led to the development of a scientific field known as bioluminescence imaging (BLI). The method is based on detecting the photons emitted by cells or tissues within a living organism. BLI emits light at a longer wavelength without the need for absorbing light, unlike fluorescence. Bioluminescence is a natural occurrence in living organisms that necessitates the presence of an enzyme named luciferase, a material called luciferin, and oxygen.

Bioluminescence is the term used to describe the emission of visible light by living organisms [56]. Bioluminescent displays, though occasionally hidden by widespread artificial lighting, are sufficiently bright for other animals to see. These displays do not involve the extremely faint light emitted by certain cells, which can be detected by modern sensitive instruments. This displays chemiluminescence, which can occasionally be caused by active oxygen species reactions. Bioluminescence, although similar to chemiluminescence, is different because it is triggered by enzymes called luciferases and can be observed visually. Bioluminescence is not produced by or reliant on light that is absorbed by the organism. This suggests that there is a chemical reaction that produces a lot of energy. Instead of all of this energy being lost as heat, some of it is converted into light energy. Hence, when a substance reacts with molecular oxygen, one of the resulting products is created with an excited electronic state, leading to the emission of a photon ($h\nu$). The reflected spectrum maximum of luciferase generally ranges between 400 and 620 nm [57]. There are three main types of luciferase that are most commonly used in tumor imaging, including luciferases, the *Renilla* and *Gaussia* luciferases, firefly and click beetle luciferases, and bacterial luciferases [58].

Bioluminescence imaging is an imaging method that is used in experimental stages to observe biological processes in living organisms. The conventional form of luciferase is able to sustain a bioluminescence signal within the tumor for a duration of 10–20 min, leading to improved consistency in imaging and simplification of the operational process. Nevertheless, there are still obstacles that need to be overcome in tumor imaging for traditional luciferases. Traditional luciferase imaging is still hindered in its ability to penetrate tissue due to various external factors. For instance, changes in basic intracellular metabolism can affect imaging signals, and the brightness of imaging is restricted when it comes to deep tissue. Hence, it is of the utmost importance to create a new luciferase reporter gene for effective tumor imaging. A new type of luciferase called NanoLuc was discovered by Coralie and colleagues from a deep sea shrimp [59]. In experiments involving glioblastoma cell lines and tumors, NanoLuc was evaluated and found to have better chemical stability, lower background autoluminescence, and higher photon yield compared to traditional bioluminescence imaging probes like Fluc and Rluc. NanoLuc was found to be more appropriate for *in vivo* imaging of deep tumor bioluminescence due to its high brightness [60]. Furthermore, NanoLuc possesses distinct substrates compared to firefly luciferase, making it compatible with Fluc for detecting sequences, thereby allowing effective subimaging with dual-report capabilities. This compatibility enables the observation of multicellular events in a single imaging procedure [61].

While bioluminescence imaging manages to prevent the dispersion of lasers, some of the signal produced by activated luciferase is still soaked up and scattered by tissues, leading to a reduction in the sensitivity and resolution of images. To tackle this issue, Mezzanotte *et al* [62] modified a human hepatoblastoma cell line (HepG2) by introducing a reporter gene that produces a red-shifted thermostable luciferase. The green bioluminescent signal was absorbed for approximately 75% ± 8%, while only around 20% ± 6% absorption was observed for the red signal in liver cancer xenograft models. These findings indicate that compared to the normal green luciferase, a shift towards red fluorescence can decrease the absorption and scattering of signals for imaging through tissues and skin [63]. As a result, this leads to improved specificity in imaging. Furthermore, the scientists utilized two reporter genes concurrently to demonstrate two distinct physiological occurrences in one image, thereby expanding the potential applications of bioluminescence imaging technology.

Bioluminescence imaging has been employed to evaluate the molecular and cellular occurrences that precede the development of cancer, the progression of tumors, and the actions of cells after being implanted into animal models. The sensitivity of molecular tumor imaging can be enhanced by continuously improving and optimizing luciferase probes [64]. This improvement can aid greatly in detecting the mechanisms of protein–protein interaction and ligand–receptor interaction. Luciferase-based reporter systems have been utilized for the purpose of observing the manifestation of the tumor-associated gene [65]. CXCL12 is a type of tumor chemotactic cytokine that has a significant impact on both the growth and spread of tumors [66]. Luker and colleagues created a novel imaging system called the dual-luciferase imaging system, in which they fused CXCL12 with *Gaussia* luciferase (CXCL12-GL). This system uses the luciferase gene to monitor and measure the amount of CXCL12 expression. Furthermore, firefly luciferase was employed to indicate the overall quantity of breast cancer cells [67]. The researchers examined the relationship between CXCL12 and CXCR7 in tumors using a fluorescence ratio, specifically by comparing the serum GL (green fluorescence) to the tumor FL (fluorescence). Based on the findings, they effectively achieve the monitoring of the chemokine scavenging process by CXCR7 using dual-luciferase imaging. They also measured the impact of CXCR7 on the growth and spread of breast cancer cells expressing CXCR4. This provides a valuable imaging technique for quantifying the role of tumor chemokines and assessing the progress of tumor development [68].

4.3.1.1.3 Photoacoustic imaging

PA tomography technology provides a fresh opportunity for biomedical imaging. It is a hybrid imaging technique that merges optical excitation with ultrasonic detection to enhance spatial resolution compared to traditional ultrasound imaging [69]. This combination helps surpass the conventional depth constraints of optical imaging, thus offering a new perspective for studying biological tissues. PA investigation using strong penetration, high spatial resolution, and absence of ionizing radiation is well-suited for accurately monitoring physiological, anatomical, metabolic and pathological processes in the body [70]. It can generate three-dimensional images of cell culture framework at different scales and contrasts ranging from individual cells to organoid cultures, additionally, utilizing a laser of one or multiple wavelengths allows for acquiring both structural and functional data.

The technique of PA imaging relies on combining optical irradiation and ultrasonic detection physically. When using a short-pulse laser on light-absorbing materials, it causes an increase in pressure by expanding due to the transfer of heat. The pressure waves that occur can be understood as waves transmitted to us when the pressure wavefront moves through the area that absorbs light. The US waves, which are also called PA waves, can be identified by ultrasound transducers to generate electric signals. After amplification, digitalization, decoding, and transfer, these signals are sent to a computer to create an image [71]. The size of the PA response is directly related to the amount of the absorbing material, the light absorption capacity of the substance, and how much the substance expands when heated. The difference in PA imaging between imaging samples inside a living organism or in laboratory conditions can be enhanced by using different substances that absorb light as contrast agents, like hemoglobin and gold nanoparticles [72].

Traditional optical imaging relies on contrast agents that emit fluorescence or bioluminescence. These agents can usually be visualized with high spatial resolution and imaging capabilities at the micrometer or sub-micrometer scale. Using the principles of laser-based PA, it is possible to convert photons into ultrasonic waves within biological samples. PA imaging techniques can overcome the depth limitation of optical imaging systems by using advanced external chromophores to improve the scanning contrast [73]. Thus, this technique can be utilized for the detection and treatment of cancerous cells as it utilizes electromagnetic radiations in the visible and NIR range for producing acoustic signals [74].

In general, a contrast agent that is considered praiseworthy should possess various characteristics. These characteristics include having a low quantum yield, a high extinction coefficient, a peak absorption in the NIR window, excellent photostability, a strong affinity towards the intended target, specificity, and biocompatibility [75]. In recent times, there have been numerous advancements in genetically encoded PA probes that show promising potential in the field of oncology applications. PA imaging has successfully addressed the problem of limited depth and resolution in imaging, making it an effective tool for detecting cellular and molecular activities in the deep tissues of organisms. Fluorescent proteins are frequently used as probes for tumor scanning in PA imaging. However, the poor thermal conversion efficacy of fluorescent proteins restricts the production of a PA signal, which is a drawback of amplification for the specific region of interest [76]. The GFP-like protein synthesized by the team of Ogunlade [77] using E2 crimson fluorescent protein resulted in a reporter protein that emits greater PA signal. The Verkhusa group [78] used low-dose 880 nm two-photon excitation (6.5 mW) to conduct two-color imaging of EGFP and iRFP680. They were able to capture detailed images of neurons within living organisms, focusing on structures within cells. These images were taken at a considerable depth (285 μm) beneath the surface of the brain.

Yang and colleagues [79] discussed a lanthanide complex probe (Nd-DOTA) that operates in the NIR range II (NIR-II) and has the ability to be quickly eliminated from the body. Over 50% of the probe can be eliminated through the kidneys within a period of 3 h after being injected. The probe has a very low molecular weight of only 0.54 kDa. In terms of resistance to light and ability to penetrate tissues, the new probe's NIR-II imaging quality surpasses that of the clinically approved ICG. Further, they reported that this lanthanide complex probe achieve a remarkable ratio of tumor to normal tissue, which helps in accurately identifying micro-tumors during abdominal metastatic ovarian cancer surgeries.

Guo and colleagues [80] employed NIR-II fluorescence and PA imaging techniques to investigate and accurately distinguish the vascular system and micro-tumors. The timely treatment of patients with nervous system diseases is largely reliant on the accurate diagnosis of cerebrovascular structures with an intact blood–brain barrier and micro-tumors, which is a widely acknowledged fact. The use of both NIR-II fluorescence and PA imaging (PAI) for diagnosis and treatment is expected to enhance performance, such as better ability to distinguish spatial and temporal information, deeper tissue penetration, high signal-to-noise ratio (SNR), and precise brain diagnosis.

4.3.1.2 Magnetic resonance imaging

MRI is one of the most frequently utilized imaging modalities in clinics. It is a non-invasive method employed in medicine to provide images of the architecture and biological functions of one's body in genuine three-dimensional data sets. The MRI machine employs powerful magnetic domains, electric field, and radio signals to produce images of organs and the body's structure. MRI is based on the same fundamental scientific principles as nuclear magnetic resonance (NMR), a spectroscopic method that acquires physicochemical information about the structure of a molecule using radio waves [81]. MRI employs a powerful magnetic area to produce spatial variations in the phase and frequency of radiofrequencies (RFs) that are being absorbed and emitted by the imaged object.

The basic principle of the MRI technique is based on measurements of energy emitted from hydrogen nuclei such as 31P, 23Na, 19F, 1H, or 13C, following their stimulation by RF signals. The energy emitted varies according to the tissues from which the signals emanate. This allows MRI to draw different images that are generated due to discrepancies raised in protonic signals of different tissues [82]. As we know, biological animals such as human beings have tissues that are predominantly made up of water molecules (accounting for up to 63% of the total weight of the human body). These particles possess unique magnetic moment stimulus by showing variation in alignment in the absence and presence of applied magnetic field. Depending on the kind and amount of nuclei present in each tissue, MRI generates high-resolution anatomical pictures of the human body with great sensor resolution [83].

MRI imaging in sufferers does not need to employ ionizing radiation. It is primarily utilized for cell monitoring, blood vessel development, apoptosis, assessment of illness, monitoring after therapy, multiple sclerosis, CNS malignancies, brain and spine infections, stroke, ligament and tendon injuries, muscle deterioration, bone tumor, and blood artery blockage etc.

Clinicians have been utilizing the MRI technique extensively for the identification of metabolic alterations in both malignant and healthy tissues. For instance, 1 H MRS is frequently utilized to track metabolic modifications in cancer tissue [84], and 19F (fluorine) [85], 31P (phosphorus) [86], 23Na (sodium) [87], 13C (carbon) [88], and other active nuclei are also used to track biological energies and metabolic processes in cancer.

The MRI technique is advantageous over other imaging modalities as it gives very high spatial resolution due to its multi-planar scanning potential and improved soft tissue contrast resolution [89]. Despite this, the fundamental disadvantage of MRI for medical purposes is its extremely poor sensitivity, which has been demonstrated to be significantly lower than that for nuclear imaging procedures like PET and SPECT [90]. Present MRI methods employed in clinical application are restricted by its modest sensitivity for molecular diagnosis. The incorporation of contrast materials in MRI enables signal augmentation for specific kinds of tissues, organs, or components by varying the radial and horizontal relaxation times (T1 and T2) of H_2O protons inside these systems.

4.3.1.2.1 MRI contrast agents

As has been noted, a tissue's ability to relax depends greatly on its immediate surroundings. Since contrast chemicals alter this milieu, they are now a critical component of the majority of medical scanning investigations. Based on the incorporation of exogenous compound the MRI agents are classified into two types as positive (paramagnetic agents) or chemical exchange saturation transfer and negative (superparamagnetic) compounds [91]. The contrast agents present in the human body alter the magnetic properties of nearby water molecules, and are thus responsible for enhancing the quality of the images, improving the sensitivity and specificity of the diagnostic images.

4.3.1.2.2 Chemical exchange saturation transfer magnetic resonance imaging

Chemical exchange saturation transfer (CEST) MRI is an MRI technique that uses CEST to detect and measure the exchange of protons between molecules in the body such as proteins, lipids, and metabolites. CEST MRI has the potential to provide molecular information for treatment and identification of diseases at the cellular and molecular level [92]. The ability to offer molecular imaging has sparked intense study on adapting CEST MRI techniques for use in contemporary radiology clinics. It provides a substitute for the conventional MRI method that enhances signal by boosting water proton relaxation. CEST is a type of MRI technique that can be used to detect and quantify compounds at low concentrations. It works by exploiting the chemical exchange between a compound of interest and the surrounding water protons. The exchange of protons between the compound and the water creates a signal that can be detected and quantified using MRI. CEST can be used to detect compounds at very low concentrations, making it a useful tool for measuring them [93].

CEST agents are also known as positive contrast agents. Small molecules with a single lanthanide chelate are examples of positive contrast agents serving as the signal-producing ingredient (e.g. gadolinium-DTPA) [94]. CEST frequently uses the magnetic qualities of Gd^{3+}-derived contrast molecules (GBCAs) to improve image contrast because they shorten the water proton relaxation periods of specific tissues [95]. It is widely used methodology in finding the concentration of glucose, glycogen, glycosaminoglycan (GAG), amide protein, and pH in diseased organs [96]. Longo *et al* reported that using this process considerably enhanced renal pH values in a mouse model of acute kidney injury [97].

4.3.1.2.3 Ultrasmall superparamagnetic iron oxide magnetic resonance imaging

Another type of MRI contrast compounds are known as negative contrast materials, which specifically reduce the signal in T2-weighted images. They are also known as superparamagnetic materials due to the presence of hydrogen atoms in biological molecules. Superparamagnetic iron oxide (SPIO) and ultrasmall superparamagnetic iron oxide (USPIO) are widely used negative contrast agents [98].

USPIO contrast agents are injected into the bloodstream and the nanoparticles are engulfed by immune cells called macrophages. These macrophages then move into the spaces between cells and are eventually absorbed by the lymph nodes [99]. After entering the lymph nodes, macrophages filled with iron stay for a few days until the iron is gradually converted into storage units. Because iron oxide exhibits superparamagnetic properties, it becomes highly magnetic in the powerful magnetic field of an MRI. This magnetization causes the spinning of particles to become out of sync and leads to susceptibility effects, ultimately resulting in a loss of signal. Therefore, the signal intensity is significantly decreased in regular lymph node tissue because of the impact of magnetic susceptibility and T2 shortening effects caused by USPIO particles [100]. On the other hand, in regions where malignant cells have replaced the normal lymph nodes, there is a lower absorption of USPIO particles. As a result, these portions of the lymph nodes maintain the same signal intensity on T2-weighted imaging (T2 WI) and T2*-weighted imaging (T2*WI) for 24–48 h after the USPIO is injected intravenously [101].

It has been reported that ferumoxide is one illustration of an SPIO agent. It is coated with dextran to ensure biocompatibility. It is accumulated in the bone marrow, spleen, and liver cells immediately after absorption by the reticuloendothelial system [102]. Almost 80% but uneven accumulation takes place in liver cells. It has been observed that poor absorption occurs in liver fibrosis regions having fewer Kupffer cells and so less accumulation of iron oxide takes place. This gives higher signal intensities. By contrast, low signal intensities are seen in normal parenchymal cells due to an increased buildup of iron oxide contrast agents [103].

MRI can be used to evaluate specific molecular events by utilizing targeted contrast agents made of SPIO. Akhtar and colleagues [104] linked a VCAM-1 monoclonal antibody to iron oxide microparticles measuring 1 micron in size. They then observed and characterized the spatial distribution of VCAM-1 expression in a rat kidney injury caused by ischemia–reperfusion. Sargsyan and colleagues [105] attached a modified version of a protein called complement-receptor-2 (CR2) that can bind to C3d to a 70-nm SPIO particle. They then observed the presence of C3 protein in the kidney's cortex, outer medulla, and inner medulla in the MRL/lpr mouse model of lupus nephritis.

Overall, MRI is one of the most important molecular imaging research methods, which can be used for non-invasive monitoring and early diagnosis of diseases at the cellular and molecular level. In recent years, the use of magnetic resonance molecular imaging has increased and it is mainly employed for cell tracking, angiogenesis, apoptosis, and *in vivo* tissue gene imaging. Although the techniques still have some problems that need an urgent solution, their unique advantages make their application of great potential use in clinical medicine and basic research.

4.3.1.3 Radionucleotide imaging

Another imaging technique gaining popularity as a secure and efficient targeted strategy for treating a wide range of cancers is radiopharmaceutical treatment (RPT). It utilizes radiopharmaceuticals that irradiate cancer-associated cellular lesions as part of a treatment plan designed to treat, reduce, and manage an illness, such as thyroid, lymphoma, or bone metastases. It can be applied to specific locations or to the whole body [106]. It is a type of non-invasive method that is capable of conquering the limitations associated with traditional biopsy-based diagnostics, like restricted quantity of specimens, inability to collect specimens from particular sites, diversity in object expression, and modifications in conveyance over the course of time [107], etc. This imaging technique assists medical personnel in the detection of cancer and the assessment of its level by providing supplementary data, as well as helping in the formulation of therapy regimens and the monitoring of an object's response as per the applied treatment [108].

Strongly binding radiopharmaceuticals or vehicles having a high affinity for tumors are appropriate for successful therapeutic use. They have the ability to deliver appropriate radiation amounts to tumors and their metastases while protecting surrounding healthy tissue. The molecule that delivers the radiation to the tumor is selected on the basis of its binding affinity for the target structures of the tumor, such as antigens or receptors [109]. Ionizing radiation released by radionuclide coupled to the carrier kills cancer cells by inducing DNA damage, leading to tumor shrinkage [110]. These radionuclides emit photons, Auger electrons (AEs) (4–26 keV μm^{-1}) and α-particles (50–230 keV μm^{-1}) or beta (β)-particles (0.2 keV μm^{-1}) [111]. X-rays and γ-rays are two types of photons. X-rays have lower energy than γ-rays and are derived from orbital electron transitions.

PET and single-photon emission computed tomography (SPECT) are the two primary nuclear medicine imaging modalities. Nuclear medicine tomography and biologically imprinted cellular imaging sensors are frequently employed together for tumor imaging, primarily for measuring cell levels, tracking the spread and development of cancer, and assessing the effectiveness of chemotherapy for cancer. For instance, the DNA makeup of the type 1-herpes simplex virus thymidine kinase (HSV1-TK) was created to specifically ingest ^{18}F in order to find and monitor treatments in gliomas [112]. Sodium iodide symporter (NIS) is one of the most used radioactive gene markers in experimental and clinical investigations, and it has been applied extensively in tumor detection and therapy. Thyroid follicular cells are known to express NIS, which can facilitate iodide ion absorption. In order to achieve radionuclide imaging, Zhang *et al* engineered the oncolytic vesicular stomatitis virus (VSV) to code for NIS by controlling the absorption of I^{125} [113].

4.3.1.3.1 Single-photon emission computed tomography

SPECT is a sophisticated method of imaging that uses gamma rays to produce very accurate three-dimensional images of things. Kuhl and Edwards [114] published the first report on SPECT in 1963. Modification with new equipment such as computer-linked devices and revolving gamma cameras gradually leads to the creation of a unique SPECT technique. It analyses an object's three-dimensional data by generating a succession of small sections using tomographic pictures. These vital tomographic pictures may assist doctors to locate deeper and extremely small injuries in individuals. SPECT uses high-energy gamma rays to evaluate numerous three-dimensional pictures from various perspectives. The computing device evaluates the detector's data and generates an accurate depiction of the body area wherein radiation tracers are administered. These vital tomographic pictures may assist doctors to locate deeper and extremely small injuries in individuals [115]. The SPECT imaging technology is less costly than imaging tiny animals alone. It is capable of monitoring target bone metabolism [116], cardiac problems, and cerebral blood flow.

4.3.1.3.2 Positron emission tomography

PET is a diagnostic and therapeutic method that uses crisp pictures to show the overall amount of radioactively tagged components in the body. It is particularly useful in (a) distinguishing between malignant and benign tumors based on precise site identification; (b) recognizing primary tiny or unidentified malignancies among individuals with malignant illness; and (c) assessing tumor aggressiveness depending on marker intake measurement [117].

There are a number of PET radiotracers that are capable of recognizing cancer cells based on higher biotransformation (e.g. glucose, fatty acids, and lactate); the preparation of protein, DNA, and cell membrane as cellular expansion indicators; and the appearance of several receptors, enzymes, and tumor-associated antigens. 2-[^{18}F] fluoro-2-deoxy-D-glucose (FDG) and 3- deoxy-3-[^{18}F] fluorothymidine (FLT) are the two most frequently used PET radiotracers to image cancer. FDG is a derivative of ^{18}F-labeled glucose that is utilized to detect disorders by altering the breakdown of glucose in cardiac ailments, Alzheimer's disease, and different types of cancers like gliomas, prostate cancer (PCa), lung cancer (LC), and hepatocellular carcinomas (HCC), etc [118]. FLT is a derivative of F-18-labeled thymidine that is widely utilized for estimating activities such as cell growth and copying of DNA through phosphorylation and thymidine mobility studies. As a result, FLT and FDG are regarded as the best potential tracers for molecular scanning [119].

In PET technology a computer system creates three-dimensional pictures of positron-emitting radionuclides within the body. Three-dimensional imaging is achieved in PET-CT scanners via the same procedure and on the same instrument using the assistance of a CT x-ray scan performed on the patient. The advancement of PET imaging allows for the examination of initial and malignant disorders using precise full-body pictures [120]. For example, breast cancer, especially invading and inflamed cancers, is one of the main prevalent reasons for ^{18}F-FDG PET imaging, which is mostly used for grading [121].

4.3.1.4 Theranostic imaging

Many illnesses, such as cancer, are diverse from birth, therefore clinical therapies should be tailored per the patient's features as well as the disease progression level. This realization has led to the demand for personalized medicine. Current research scholars expect that logically structured clinical therapies that are best for each individual patient may be produced by coupling treatment and diagnostics. Thus to achieve customized treatment, the term 'theranosis' was established to represent contemporary biomedical attempts to unite diagnostic and therapeutic modalities in a single unified material and to generate individually designed remedies against diverse illnesses [122].

Theranostics involve nano- or molecular-scale substances that can be used for both medical diagnosis as well as treatment. Theranostics are gaining popularity by providing concurrent processing of medical diagnosis and real-time medication impact analysis. This combination therapy can give patients optimum treatment as well as aiding in the early diagnosis of many ailments [123].

Nanotechnology has had a tremendous impact on imaging, early detection, diagnosis, and prognosis of diseases by improving upon existing clinically relevant technologies [140]. Theranostic probes are employed for effective image diagnosis and treatment so as to achieve selective identification of biological targets, medicinal chemicals, and scanning markers. The primary challenge associated with this technique is even delivery and release of theranostic agents into tumors or significant bystander effects of treatment. In clinical research, nano-theranostics utilizes an extensive spectrum of different types of scanning modalities, namely magnetic resonance imaging, PA, optical, ultrasound, and tomography (PET and SPECT) techniques, for diagnosis and therapy assistance. Table 4.2 summarizes the interrelationship between nanoplatforms, imaging modalities and therapeutics, which are collectively known as nano-theranostics.

Yordanova *et al* [141] reported various radiolabelled theranostic agents like iodine-131 and lutetium-177. Both are capable of emitting beta and gamma rays and are thus used for identification, tracing, and killing of cancer cells. Duan and Lagaru [142] highlight the fundamental ideas of theranostics. They claim that theranostics limit the collateral harm to healthy tissues by targeting tumor-specific biomarkers. They propose that molecular imaging, which screens patients based on the presence of tumor-specific markers, offers an initial glimpse into the infected cell. The same molecular marker will later, in the second stage, use radionuclide treatment to target the tumor cell by employing radioactive compounds that may deliver tumoricidal dosage of radiations.

In another study Solnes *et al* [143] give a summary of agents that have previously received approval as well as those that may soon be available. In the clinical trial of NETTER-1 it was found that use of theranostic agents significantly enhances disease-free survival in patients with metastatic gastroenteropancreatic neuroendocrine tumors [144]. In another clinical trial study it was observed that patients with prostate cancer respond significantly to ^{177}Lu-labeled medicines that target prostate-specific membrane antigen. Out of numerous ^{177}Lu-labeled medicinal trials, there are now at least two possible clinical trials employing ^{177}Lu-PSMA medicines underway, which will probably facilitate clearance by the US Food and Drug Administration (FDA).

Therefore, it would not be incorrect to state that a crucial element in the treatment of severe illnesses is nanotheranostics. They use a variety of methods to provide *in vivo* molecular pictures, thorough diagnostics, and a customized therapy plan, as shown in figure 4.5.

4.4 Nanoplatforms for cancer imaging

Nanotechnology is the process of modifying matter at a size close to the atomic level to create innovative structures, materials, and technological advances. The technique promises to enhance science in a variety of fields, including nanomedicine, targeted drug delivery, molecular imaging, diagnostics, and invasive therapy of various diseases like cancer [145].

Table 4.2. Interrelationship between nanoplatforms, imaging modalities, and therapeutics: nano-theranostics.

Nanoplatforms	Imaging modalities	Therapeutics	References
		Organic nanoplatforms	
Polymeric nanoparticles	PET, MRI, optical imaging	Chemotherapy (paclitaxel, docetaxel, camptothecin, doxorubicin, cisplatin), Biotherapeutics (pDNA, siRNA, protein), Photodynamic therapy	[124]
Polymeric micelles	MRI, ultrasound imaging	Chemotherapy (doxorubicin, platinum-based drugs)	[125]
Liposomes	MRI	Biotherapeutics (peptide, siRNA)	[126]
Dendrimers	MRI	Gene delivery vehicles (docetaxel), chemotherapy (paclitaxel), biotherapeutics (pDNA, siRNA, protein)	[127]
Polymersomes	MRI	Chemotherapy (doxorubicin)	[128]
Nanoemulsion	MRI, optical imaging, ultrasound and PA imaging	Chemotherapy (paclitaxel), photodynamic therapy (methylaminolevulinate)	[129]
		Inorganic nanoplatforms	
Quantum dots	MRI, optical imaging, PET	Photodynamic therapy, chemotherapy (doxorubicin)	[130, 131]
Magnetic nanoparticles	MRI, optical imaging (NIR fluorescence imaging)	Chemotherapy (doxorubicin MTX, curcumin, cisplatin), biotherapeutics (pDNA, siRNA, protein), hyperthermal therapy	[132]
Silica nanoparticles	Optical imaging (photoluminescence imaging)	Chemotherapy (doxorubicin) biotherapeutics (siRNA, protein), photodynamic therapy	[133]
Gold nanoparticles	Optical imaging (photoluminescence imaging)	Photothermal therapy	[134]
Carbon-based nanoparticles	Optical imaging (photoluminescence imaging), Raman spectroscopy, microwave detection	Photothermal therapy, hyperthermal therapy, chemotherapy (platinum-based drug)	[135]
Gold nanorod	Optical imaging (photoluminescence imaging)	Photothermal therapy	[136]
Gold nanoshell	Optical imaging, ultrasound, MRI	Photothermal therapy	[137]
		Hybrid nanoplatforms	
Lipid–polymer hybrid nanoparticles	Optical imaging (photoluminescence imaging), MRI	Photothermal therapy, photodynamic therapy, chemotherapy	[138]
Organic–inorganic hybrid nanoparticles	MRI, optical imaging (photoluminescence imaging)	Photothermal therapy, photodynamic therapy, chemotherapy	[139]

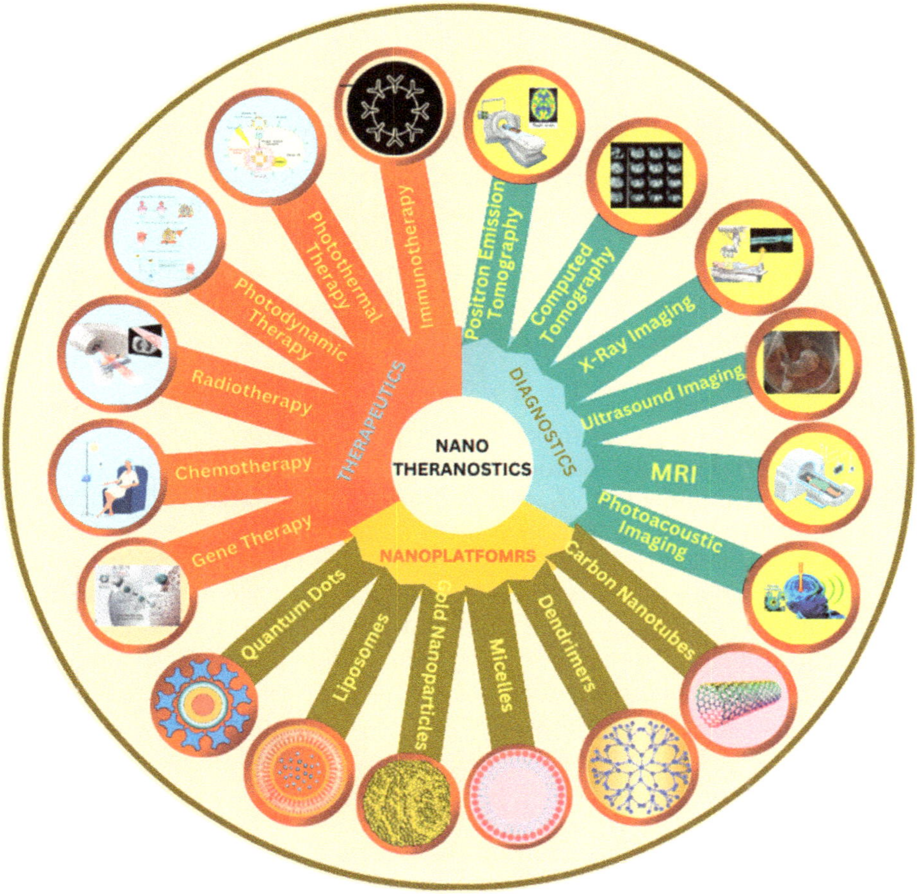

Figure 4.5. Relation between therapeutics, diagnostics and nanoplatforms.

Nanotechnology brought a new and revolutionary technique to the identification and treatment of cancer. The scientific community and engineers have been continuously working to achieve significant advances in the creation of clinically approved nanotechnology-based cancer medicines and diagnostics. The study of nanomedicine, an emerging discipline that combines the biological sciences with nanoscience, nanoengineering, and nanotechnology, has produced some intriguing findings for both society and the medical industry [146]. Currently, the most fascinating area of research includes nanoplatform-based targeted drug delivery and imaging nano-agents [147]. Nanoplatforms hold great potential in cancer diagnostics and therapeutics due to unique physicochemical properties dependent upon size, shape, and surface chemistry. Over 20 years ago, the FDA approval of DoxilR [148] for the treatment of breast and ovary cancer, Kaposis' sarcoma, etc became a turning point in cancer treatment. Thereafter, a sudden boom occurred in the number of research and clinical studies committed to cancer nanotechnology.

Despite this, the transformation of nanotherapeutics has been challenging to move from the lab to the clinic [149].

4.4.1 Applications of nanotechnology for human health

Batteries that can survive for a longer time, microprocessors that run more quickly while using fewer calories, solar energy systems that produce multiple times as much electricity, and microscopic particles that kill cancerous cells are just a few of the numerous applications for nanotechnology, a field that has all the makings of a coming industrial revolution. The various examples of nanotechnology are representative of current, developing, and futuristic applications which relate to human health. These are:

(i) **Device technology**

Device technology makes extensive use of nanotechnology. Instances of device technology include: (i) DNA machines with moving components and programmed DNA that can carry replicable electrical devices and have the potential to function as nanochemical sensors, switches, and tweezers [150]; (ii) nanopatterns that can be molded or printed using soft lithography techniques on both curved and flat surfaces [151]; (iii) batteries with fast recharging capabilities that are less hazardous [152]; (iv) photovoltaic cells for trapping IR radiations [153]; (v) solar cell technology using less material and cheaper processes [154]; (vi) optical/holographic tweezers for performing non-invasive surgery, purifying pharmaceuticals, building nanocomputers using nanotubes, and producing spinning liquid vortices that can serve as miniature pumps [155].

(ii) **Medical**

Many treatments and medications for chronic illness, including cancer, brain tumors etc cause major adverse effects in patients. Instead of treating the entire body, the medicine will be directed to the afflicted cells using nanoparticles [156]. The effectiveness of imaging systems is also being increased by the use of various nanomaterials [157]. The uses of nanotechnology in medicine go beyond those listed above and also encompass topics like gene therapy, molecular imaging, targeted drug delivery, and wound care.

(iii) **Medical imaging**

In vivo uses for superparamagnetic iron oxide nanoparticles include MRI, tissue repair, biological fluid detoxification, drug administration, and hyperthermia therapy [158]. Medical imaging employs semiconductor quantum dots for the fluorescent labeling of living cells, receptors, and oncologic markers [159].

(iv) **Drug delivery**

One of the most important technologies for the implementation of nanomedicine is nanoplatform-based drug delivery, which has the ability to improve the bioavailability of pharmaceuticals, the controlled release of therapeutic molecules, and precise medication targeting [160]. Particle size has a direct impact on how well drugs are delivered to different sites of affected areas. Due to inconsistent or loose vascular boundaries, which generally comprise holes with a diameter of 100–1000 nm, nanoscale drug transport structures can penetrate tumors [161]. In bronchial therapy, nanoscale drug delivery devices can be employed as gene delivery vectors, and in the stabilization of therapeutic molecules that would otherwise degrade too quickly [162].

(v) **Food additives**

To improve the overall quality of food containers and lengthen their shelf lives, polymers and nanostructures like silver are combined, making food more flavorful and longer lived. One of the important uses of nanotechnology is 'smart packaging,' which allows for the detection of biological modifications taking place in food items [163]. Numerous uses of nanotechnology have been employed in the farming and agricultural sectors with the goal of ensuring the safety of food. When evaluating the significance of nanomaterials in food processing, one should consider how they have improved food items in terms of their texture, appearance, flavor, nutritional content, and durability [164].

(vi) **Chemical sensors**

To detect potentially the lowest amounts of hazardous components, many sensors have been created by employing nanomaterials such as palladium nanoparticles, carbon nanotubes (CNTs), zinc oxide nanowires, etc [165]. This is plausible given that these materials' electrical properties are better at the nanoscale.

(vii) **Environment**

Nanomaterials are widely employed to address the global problem of air quality decline [166]. On the one hand, air pollution is being removed using membranes embedded with nanoparticles such as graphene oxide. The effectiveness of catalysts, which may assist in reducing the impact of air pollution from factories, commercial vehicles, air conditioning systems, etc, is being researched. On the other hand, efforts are also being made to increase their efficiency. These nanoparticle-based catalysts offer a large contact area for chemical reactions to take place. Additionally, some of their eco-friendly uses include heavy metal nanofiltration systems and wastewater cleaning utilizing nanobubbles. There are also nanocatalysts available to improve the effectiveness and reduce the pollution of chemical processes [167].

4.4.2 Characteristics of nanoplatforms

Nanoparticles offer a variety of characteristics that enable improved pharmacologic activities when compared to bigger particles. As a result, numerous studies are being performed to alter the size, shape, surface area, and surface chemistry of nanoparticles in order to optimize their benefits for medicinal applications. The characteristics of compounds are affected when they are reduced to small size

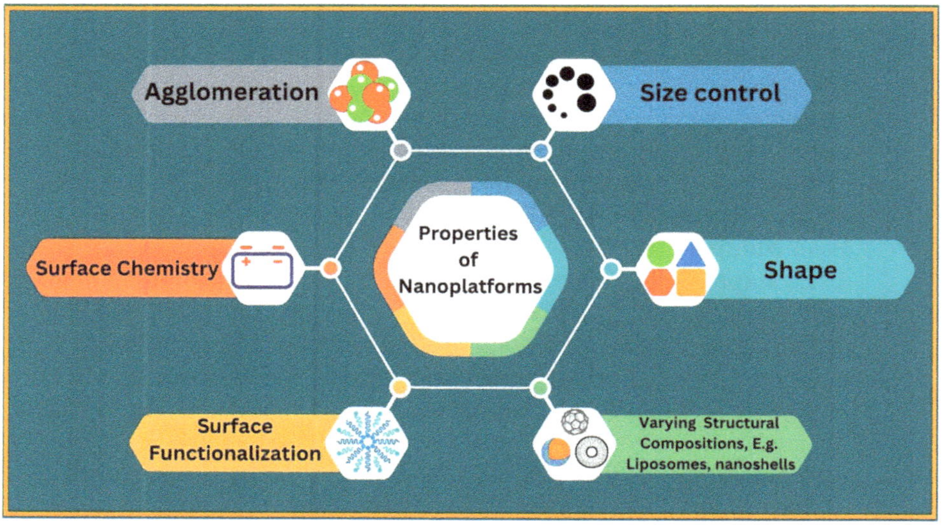

Figure 4.6. Physiochemical properties of nanoparticles.

because this frequently results in modifications to the molecular architecture of the material. A robust relationship is established in between their dimensionality, and optoelectronic and physicochemical characteristics. This can be attributed to the fact that quantum limitations become evident at nanoscale levels. Different physico-chemical characteristics of nanoparticles, such as charged surfaces, the capacity to aggregate, the potential for binding different species to the surfaces, as well as controlled synthesis, etc (figure 4.6), make it possible to create them in a variety of forms and sizes. Due to these characteristics, nanoparticles are more reactive than ordinary particles in the biological world. A few important properties are discussed below.

4.4.2.1 Surface area and size of nanoparticles

Nanoparticles are those tiny particles having dimensions between 1 and 100 nm. These particles are well known for their large surface-area-to-volume ratio. Due to this feature, certain typically inert particles, such as gold, become reactive in the nanometer range. Nanoplatforms offer higher surface area of contact per mass unit than massive particles [168]. The nano size of the particles permits easy penetration inside soft tissues and fluid, which is normally difficult in the bulk form. Essentially, the dimensions and surface area of nano-sized particles affect how quickly they are endocytosed, disseminated, maintained, and removed by biological processes [169]. The detailed investigation of nanoparticle motions into healthy and cancerous cells has demonstrated that they are infused through endocytotic methods in a size-dependent manner since nano-sized particles do not simply penetrate across the cell membrane. Clathrin-coated vesicles can internalize nanoparticles with dimensions smaller than 200 nm, but caveolae-mediated endocytosis can internalize larger nanoparticles [170].

Similarly, like size, nanoparticles' surface area plays a significant role in their biological action. For instance, it has been demonstrated that PEGylated nano-sized particles show increased stability and stay in the blood vessels longer. PEGylated nanoparticles possess a larger surface area because of adsorption of polyethylene glycol (PEG) over the nanoparticulate surface [171].

4.4.2.2 Shape

The usefulness of nanoparticles is also thought to be significantly influenced by their shapes [172]. Numerous morphologies, including tubes, fibers, and spheres, might be achieved while creating nanoparticles. According to study findings, nanoparticle shape has a significant impact on cellular absorption, blood flow, anti-cancer efficacy, and biologic distribution [173]. When considering bio–nano interactions, it is important to describe how the shape of the nanoparticles affects these. One factor to consider is the arched structure of different nanoparticle shapes. An illustration of this is that rod-shaped nanoparticles possess a greater area of interaction for cellular surface receptors than spherical nanoparticles. As a result, the number of receptor areas accessible for binding may be reduced.

One reason why elongated particles are preferred over spherical ones, such as cylindrical ones, is because they have a higher membrane wrapping time. Therefore, spherical nanoparticles can be internalized more quickly and easily through endocytosis than other types [174]. Additionally, research has shown that spherical nanoparticles are often less hazardous compared to other shapes [175]. Furthermore, the shape of nano-sized particles of iron oxide (Fe_2O_3) also plays a significant role in their cytotoxicity. Studies have demonstrated that using rod-shaped nanoparticles of Fe_2O_3 can cause more harm to membranes, necrosis, and generation of reactive oxygen species.

Li and collegues [176] reported that spherical nanoparticles are more readily absorbed than other shapes of nanoparticles. Previous studies have compared nanoparticles with the same surface area, ligand–receptor bonding strength, and implanting frequency as polyethylene glycol. The results showed that spherical nanoparticles have the fastest internalization rate, followed by cubic, rod- and disk-like nano-sized particles.

4.4.2.3 Surface modification of nanoparticles

The surface characteristics of nanoparticles have a large influence on their behavior with cellular parts. Among various characteristics, the density and the potential difference between the external and internal surface of the nanoparticles have an impact on the degree of cellular absorption as well as the particles' interaction with biomolecules [177]. In order to give the nanoparticles enough durability in the physiological media, chemical modification of the surface is required [178]. Nonetheless, nanoparticles have the ability to affect biological responses in living organisms because of their highly reactive surface. Additionally, chemical modification of the surface is required to prevent undesirable cell absorption and inhibit the phenomenon of aggregation in nanoparticles. Moreover, adopting a safe-design approach that is critical to the prospective uses of nanoparticles and reducing their hazardous effects requires chemical surface modification [179].

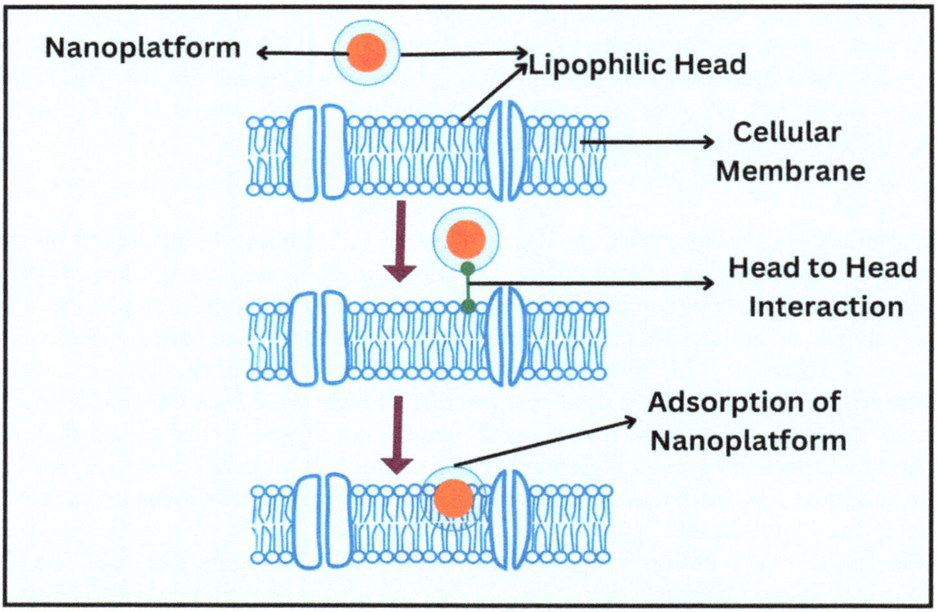

Figure 4.7. Incorporation of hydrophobic surfaced nanoplatforms into the lipophilic membrane.

4.4.2.4 Hydrophilic and hydrophobic properties of nanoparticles
Other crucial elements that significantly influence nanoparticles' capacity to interact with cells and biomolecules include their hydrophilic and hydrophobic characteristics. According to several studies [180], the hydrophobic surface of hydrophobic nanoparticles prefers to interact with lipid tails, which favors surface membrane absorption, as shown in figure 4.7.

4.4.3 Types of nanoplatforms for cancer imaging

The dimensions, shape, surface area, surface charge, and hydrophilic/hydrophobic properties are among the physical and chemical characteristics of nanoplatforms that influence how readily they are taken in by cells, how long they propagate, and their ultimate degree of toxicity. These characteristics help to determine which nanoplatforms are best for a particular malignancy. Furthermore, in biological and clinical fields, including cancer diagnosis, biomedical imaging, genetic variation exposure, and targeted therapeutic treatment directed at both cells and within cells, nanoparticles with the appropriate surface transformations have considerable advantages [181]. Therefore, the target substance can be customized with nanoplatforms to create medications that have targeted internalization, prolonged circulation, and accumulations. Nanoplatforms employed in nanotherapeutics are widely classified into three sections, namely organic, inorganic, and hybrid nanoparticles, which are further sub-classified into different types, as depicted in figure 4.8.

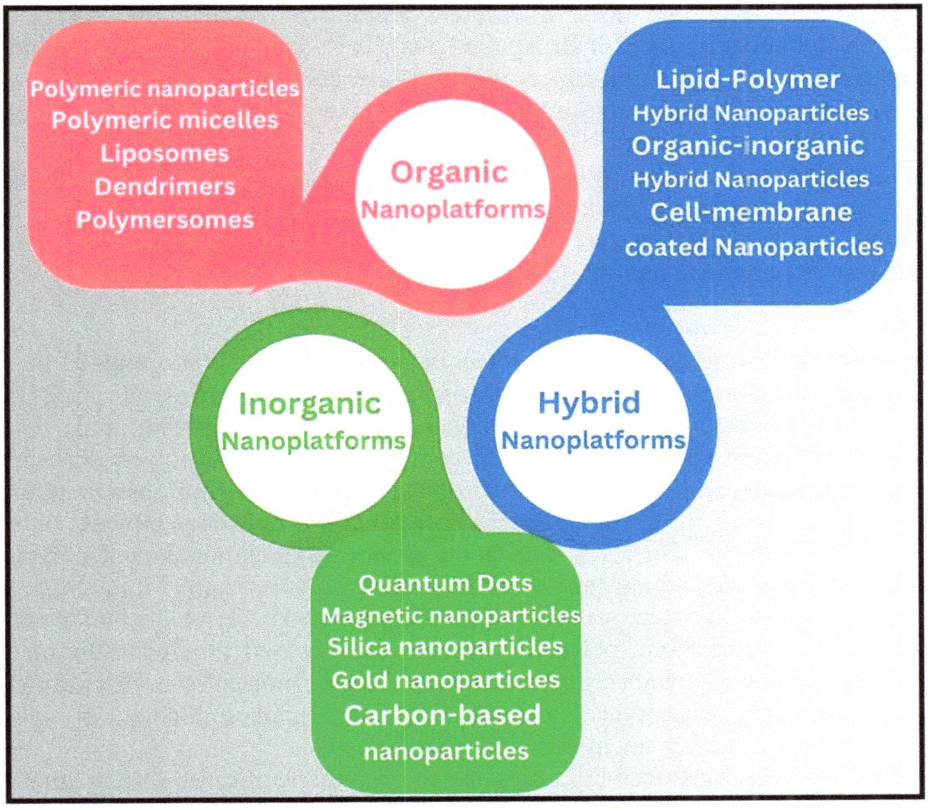

Figure 4.8. Types of nanoplatforms.

4.4.3.1 Organic nanoparticles

The macromolecules present in the biological system, such as lipids (or fats), proteins, and synthetic organic molecules, are responsible for the production of organic nanoparticles. The key benefits of employing organic nanoparticles are their complete safety, biocompatibility, and ease of transformation due to the presence of functional groups [182]. Different types of organic nanoparticles are discussed below.

4.4.3.1.1 Polymeric nanoparticles

Polymer-based nanoplatforms are made by the combination of different monomer units and have distinct molecular configurations for delivering medicines. These nanoplatforms having particle dimensions in the range of 10–1000 nm are known as polymeric nanoparticles (PNPs) [183]. PNPs are further classified as nanospheres, nanocapsules, polymeric micelles, dendrimers, liposomes, and polymersomes on the basis of their structures. PNPs are generally spherical in shape and are composed of either natural or human-made polymers. They are widely used in drug delivery applications, such as for delivering vaccines, biomolecules, lipophillic and lipophobic drugs, protein drugs, etc through different administraton channels. Bajpai and Chouhan synthesized poly (2-hydroxyethyl methacrylate) nanoparticles and studied the release kinetics of the anti-cancer drug 5-flurouracil. Their study suggested that polymeric nanosystems having sorption quality have emerged as dependable materials in drug release technologies [184].

Li *et al* [185] reported that polymeric nanoparticles conjugate or encapsulate anti-cancer drugs and release drugs targeted at a cancer's site of action. They also reported their responsive nature, specifically their pH and temperature sensitivity, which moves polymeric nanoparticles one step ahead.

4.4.3.1.2 Polymeric micelles

Polymeric micelles are type of nanoparticles having dimensions in the range of 10–100 nm. In their structure a hydrophobic center is surrounded by a hydrophilic shell [186]. Several hydrophobic medicinal products, including paclitaxel, camptothecin, doxorubicin, and cisplatin, can be bound in their hydrophobic core. The polyethylene glycol is one of the main components of the hydrophilic shells. One major obstacle to using polymeric micelle as medication carriers is crossing the reticuloendothelial barrier. The polyethylene glycol helps in preventing macrophage elimination of polymeric micelles and provides ample time to remain in the bloodstream. Thus, drugs will passively aggregate in cancerous tissue due to the enhanced permeability and retention (EPR) effect. Furthermore, polymeric micelles can be used to proactively aim at tumors by binding the outer layer with small biological molecules, such as proteins, glucose molecules, nucleotide ligands (like aptamer), and antibodies, as well as different cancer-targeting assemblies.

This can further enhanced by combining the polymeric micelles with magnetized nanoparticles. Thus, employing polymeric micelles in drug distribution activity can lower the harmful and adverse consequences of medications while also greatly increasing their biological availability and anti-cancer efficacy [187]. A clinical trial using styrene-maleic anhydride (PSMA) copolymer-targeted polymeric nanoparticles featured the first micelle to be used for active targeting of an anti-cancer drug. Currently, numerous strategies have been investigated for anti-cancer medications to improve cytoplasmic diffusion and cellular uptake. The key concept is to modify corresponding micelles to boost their chemotherapeutic efficiency.

4.4.3.1.3 Liposomes

Another of the most researched polymeric nanodelivery vehicles used in the healthcare and cosmetics sectors are liposomes. These are sphere-shaped vessels that are typically between 50 and 450 nm in size [188]. The cellular surface of a liposome is composed of two distinct layers of phosphate and lipid molecules, with the hydrophobic lipid end pointing inside and the hydrophilic phosphate side projecting outward. They are known for their sophisticated technology in delivering active compounds to the precise location of operation, and some of their formulations are now being used in clinical settings.

In order to decrease penetration and improve the structural integrity of the phospholipid bilayer frameworks both *in vivo* and *in vitro*, cholesterol is introduced

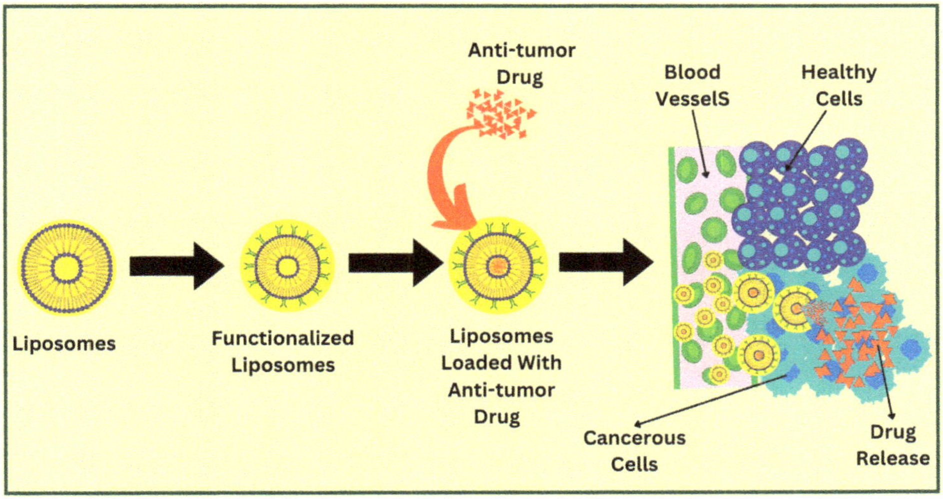

Figure 4.9. Schematic representation of liposome-based anti-tumor drug delivery.

to liposomes' phospholipid layer. This phospholipid-based bilayer model of liposomes offers the administration of both hydrophobic and hydrophilic medicines. Liposomes are utilized as efficient drug transporters because of their structural resemblance to cell membranes, which eases the incorporation of pharmaceuticals into them [189]. A schematic representation of liposomal based anti-tumor drug delivery is presented in figure 4.9.

4.4.3.1.4 Dendrimers

Another type of nanoscale polymeric particles that has been used in targeted drug delivery is dendrimers. These are adaptable, sustainable and environmental friendly giant molecules with a three-dimensional multifaceted globular branched structure [190]. Additionally, targeting moieties like proteins or antibodies can be added to the dendrimers' surface to modify them and increase their selectivity for a particular target identified in the living system, such as cancerous cells. The ability of dendrimers to hold a significant quantity of medicine within their internal or outer surface is one of their principal benefits as a drug delivery mechanism. This makes it possible for the drug to be released gradually and in a controlled manner, which results in increased therapeutic benefit and reduced adverse consequences [191].

The use of dendrimers for drug distribution presents certain difficulties in spite of their possible advantages. A primary obstacle is the intricacy of managing dendrimer morphology and size, as this influences their physiological effects and dispersion within the living system [192]. Furthermore, dendrimers have cytotoxicity and immune system-interacting properties that restrict their use in specific applications. Clinical trials are now being conducted on a number of dendrimer-based therapeutics like transdermal hydrogels, transfection reagents, contrast dye, and agents for theranostic substances. Dendrimers like poly(propyleneimine) (PPI), polyamidoamine

(PAMAM), polyethyleneimine, etc are a few of the most studied nano-based drug carriers for biological uses [193]. The inclusion of amine groups in dendrimers limits their therapeutic use. These amine groups are responsible for the poisonous character of dendrimers and possess positive charge. Thus, cationic dendrimers require alteration in their structure to lessen or completely remove toxicity.

4.4.3.1.5 Polymersomes

Polymersomes, self-assemblies of block co-polymers, are being used as promising nanomedicines for targeted drug delivery. They have a spherical structure consisting of single or double layers, similar to cell membranes [194]. One may simply tailor the characteristics of polymersomes like drug loading discharge potential, etc by using environmentally friendly block co-polymers having multiple responsive properties (e.g. pH, temperature, magnetic, etc) [195].

Polymersomes employed as drug vehicles have the capability to modulate drug distribution rates, prohibit pharmaceutical destruction, and prolong release rates, as well as minimizing unwanted side effects [196]. Due to these benefits, polymersomes rank among the most promising self-assembled structures for potential outcomes in the rapidly developing fields of biomedical and healthcare systems, such as for delivering drugs, genetic codes, and peptides, etc, as well as being used in theranostics. They have the ability to deliver both hydrophilic and hydrophobic types of drugs. Furthermore, polymersomes' hydrophilic layer exhibits improved penetrability, retention, and durability.

4.4.3.2 Inorganic nanoparticles

The materials which are synthesized from inorganic chemical substances having dimensions in the nanorange are called inorganic nanoparticles. For example, silica and gold nanoparticles, magnetic (iron, nickel, cobalt) nanoparticles, and quantum dots, etc are included under inorganic nanoplatforms [197]. These specifically designed inorganic nanoparticles have a broad range of dimensions, shapes, surface areas and geometrical patterns. Inorganic nanoparticles are mainly formed by the combination of two different components. The inner component comprising metals like iron oxide, gold nanoparticles, and quantum dots, etc is called the core. The outer components are made up of organic substances or metallic particles that shield the core region from chemical transformation and act as a carrier block for association with biological molecules.

Some important characteristics, such as physicochemical, magnetic, mechanical, radioactive, and optoelectronic one, make inorganic nanoparticles best suited for use in scanning and photothermal treatments [198]. Most inorganic nanoparticles are stable and biocompatible in nature, and they satisfy specialized applications that organic nanomaterials are unable to offer. Nevertheless, their insoluble nature and safety problems, particularly in formulations containing toxic substances, hinder their clinical applicability.

4.4.3.2.1 Quantum dots

Quantum dots are extremely small metal-based particles, ranging from 1.5 to 10.0 nm in size. They are made up of semiconductor elements such as InAs, GaAs, ZnS, ZnSe,

ZnO, CdS, CdSe, and CdTe [199]. The photostability behavior of quantum dots can be enhanced by integrating two different types of semiconductor materials. One atom is situated in the core region and another with a higher spectral bandgap forms the protective layer, which helps in boosting their photostability. Because of their unique optical characteristics (bright and steady illumination for a longer duration), quantum dots have a variety of applications in biosensors for tumor diagnosis and biological scanning [200].

In order to track cancerous cell migration in a living animal, Voura *et al* employed inorganic nanoparticle-based quantum dots with multiphoton microscopic imaging. Further, the quantum dot-labeled cells were introduced intravenously into rodents, and their lung tissue dissemination was monitored. By employing multiphoton laser stimulation, it was observed that quantum dots and spectral scanning enabled the selection of five distinct tumor cell colonies [201].

4.4.3.2.2 Magnetic nanoparticles

Inorganic nanoparticles possessing magnetic, radioactive, and optoelectronic characteristics are often referred to as magnetic nanoparticles. These nanoparticles are especially suited for uses in targeted drug delivery, scanning, photothermal treatments, and diagnostics. Multifunctional nanoparticles are frequently encased with organic compounds, such as polymers and triglycerides, to enhance their durability and biological compatibility. These magnetic nanoparticles are found to be highly effective in treating tumors using genetic therapy and chemotherapy [202]. Additionally, thermal destruction of malignant cells can be accomplished via hyperthermia using alternative magnetic fields employing magnetic nanoparticles, providing an alternative method of treating malignant tumors [203].

The most frequently studied material for magnetic nanoparticles production is iron oxide. These FDA-permitted inorganic-based nanoparticles are used in medicines for cancer treatment. Magnetized iron oxide nanoparticles are made of magnetite (Fe_3O_4) or maghemite (Fe_2O_3) and exhibit superparamagnetic characteristics at specific sizes. They have demonstrated efficacy in use as contrast media, drug carriers, and thermal-based treatments. However, poor solubility and toxicological issues, particularly in formulations containing toxic metals [204], limit the practical applicability of magnetized nanoparticles.

4.4.3.2.3 Silica nanoparticles

Mesoporous silicon- and silica-based nanostructures are attracting increasing attention from the scientific and medical communities for potential use in gene delivery and medicine. Large pores located inside the cell and a supramolecular structure situated outside that functions as an envelope enable the absorption and ejection of significant amounts of anti-cancer drugs [205]. Mesoporous silica nanoparticles have been identified as one of the best drug carriers owing to their improved pharmacokinetics, durability, and therapeutic efficiency [206]. Furthermore, because of their immunoadjuvant qualities, which include promotion of antigen cross-display, polarization of lymphocytes, and secretion of interferon-γ (IFN-γ), mesoporous silica nanoparticles have demonstrated significant promise in immune therapy [207]. Numerous researchers are investigating the potential uses of these silica nanostructures for oral, intramuscular, and parenteral transportation of medicinal drugs due to their excellent *in vivo* biocompatibility as well as their biodegradable properties [208].

4.4.3.2.4 Gold nanoparticles

Another extensively researched type of inorganic nanoparticles is gold nanoparticles, which are employed in a variety of configurations, including nanoshells, nanospheres, nanorods, nanocages, and nanostars [209]. Because of the characteristics of the parent metal itself, these nanoparticles have distinctive physiological, electromagnetic, and luminescent capabilities. For instance, gold nanoparticles have photothermal qualities because of the free electrons that are constantly oscillating at a frequency that varies according to their dimensions and shape [210]. Due to their superior properties over other nanovehicles, including polymeric nanoparticles, polymeric micelles, liposomes, and dendrimers, gold nanoparticles are particularly useful in surface plasmon resonance (SPR) investigation. These materials exhibit high biocompatibility and multifaceted/adaptibility on subsequent surface functionalization. The expulsion and distribution of medicines to the desire location can be regulated via biological or environmental stimuli when gold nanoparticles combine with pharmaceuticals through either physical penetration or ionic and covalent interaction [211]. Additionally, it is believed that gold nanoparticles are engaged in immuno, radiation, and gene therapy as part of multimodal tumor treatment [212]. In a recent study, *Fusarium solani* ATLOY-8, an endophytic strain isolated from the plant species *Chonemorpha fragrans*, was used by Clarance *et al* to create gold nanoparticles. They investigated the anti-cancer potential of gold nanoparticles in their study and found that the nanoparticles effectively inhibit HeLa cells *in vitro* by causing destruction of DNA and cell death in the G2/M stage [213].

In another investigation, it came to light that gold nanoparticles coated with doxorubicin had more potent anti-cancer action against HeLa than free doxorubicin [214]. Additionally, gold nanoparticles have been employed as drug delivery vehicles to deliver these particles into developing tumor sites in mice, and it has been shown that this complex may be efficiently transported to eliminate the malignant tissues in rodents [215]. Because of their low cytotoxicity and great tomography attenuation efficiency, gold nanoparticles are expected to find future applications as imaging agents and antibiotics [216].

4.4.3.2.5 Carbon-based nanoparticles

Carbon-based nanostructures, including carbon nanotubes, fullerenes, nanodiamonds, and graphene, have been found enormous application in the biomedical and healthcare sectors, particularly in the field of nanotheranostics [217].

(i) **Carbon nanotubes**

These exhibit a tubular structure that holds great potential for use in the drug transportation sector. Due to the presence of distinctive physicochemical and biological properties these nanotubes have been employed as nanovehicles for anti-cancer drugs such as methotrexate, doxorubicin, gemcitabine, and paclitaxel for treating a wide range of malignancies [218]. On the other hand, they also show thermal ablation behavior [219] due to heat release after bombardment with NIR radiations over carbon nanotubes.

(ii) **Fullerenes**

Fullerenes are an interesting subject of several research fields, notably in cancer theranostics, due to their unique cage-like framework and electron-deficit character, which confer distinct and remarkable characteristics. Although fullerenes show promise in cancer treatment methods like PDT, PTT, radiation, and chemotherapy, in spite this they are also used in the diagnosis of tumor cells [220]. Huang *et al* [221] developed a carboxyl group-grafted luminescent fullerene containing 60 carbon atoms (C_{60}). The synthesized nanoparticles exhibit excellent fluorescent behavior, dispersibility in water, and biological compatibility. Additionally, scientists loaded the controlled-release medication cisplatin. This innovative nanoplatform has the potential to be an appealing nanotheranostic because of its biomedical imaging and regulated drug distribution capabilities. Nonetheless, additional *in vivo* research ought to be performed to validate these findings.

(iii) **Nanodiamonds**

Nanodiamonds are a new class of carbon-based nanoparticles possessing a diameter of 2 to 8 nm and exhibiting truncated octahedral morphology. These nanoparticles showcase remarkable durability, rigidity, toughness, and chemical stability, in addition to their tiny size, vast surface area-to-volume ratio, and excellent potential for adsorption [222]. Nanodiamonds possess a luminescent property that is utilized in magnetic monitoring of multipotential stromal cells developed in the choriodecidual film of placenta in guinea pigs quantitatively [223].

(iv) **Graphene and graphene oxide**

These are characterized as two-dimensional nanostructures consisting of an sp^2 hybridized carbon skeleton arranged in a hexagonal lattice forming a monolayer. Due to their simple preparation and unique framework, which allows for facile conjugation with active compounds or polymers, it is categorized as a significant sector of theranostics [224]. However, tracking them *in vivo* is highly difficult. In order to successfully achieve drug absorption, distribution and elimination of graphene oxide *in vivo*, Liang *et al* designed a unique dual-element labeling technique utilizing lanthanum and cerium, as labeled on the surface of polyvinylpyrrolidone (PVP)-modified graphene oxide (La/Ce-GO-PVP). It was discovered that these altered graphene oxide nanosheets penetrated inside the kidney, liver, spleen, and lung following systemic administration; however, they were gradually removed from the accumulating organs, with some expelled through urine [225]. Additionally, prior research demonstrated that following intravenous treatment, I-labeled nanographene sheets mostly gather in the reticuloendothelial membrane, which includes the liver and spleen, and can be progressively eliminated through excreta [226].

4.4.3.3 Hybrid nanoparticles

Both inorganic and organic nanoparticles have benefits and drawbacks of their own. Blending both the components together constitutes a hybrid drug distribution platform which gives a multifaceted carrier optimized biological characteristics that can improve clinical outcomes and lower resistance to therapeutic agents [227].

4.4.3.3.1 Lipid–polymer hybrid nanoparticles

The lipid–polymer hybrid nanoparticle framework contains two major regions: the internal core region is made up of polymeric material and the outer shell is made up of multilayers of lipid molecules. These lipid-based hybrid nanostructures are potentially effective for drug distribution systems for treating a variety of cancers, including breast [228], pancreatic [229], and metastatic prostate cancer [230]. Because these hybrid nanoparticles integrate the high biological compatibility of lipids with the architectural stability offered by polymeric nanoparticles, they can effectively encapsulate water-soluble and water-resistant medicines for improved therapeutic [231] outcomes. Su *et al* [232] demonstrated that tumor cells can efficiently internalize this system, preventing it from being quickly cleared by the reticuloendothelial film [233].

4.4.3.3.2 Organic–inorganic hybrid nanoparticles

The utilization and advancement of hybrid nanostructures, which integrate the blended characteristics of distinctive nanoparticles, has propelled this kind of drug-carrier system to new heights. In this regard, researchers have manufactured liposomal–silica-based hybrid (LSH) nanoparticles, which have a core center made up of silica that is surrounded by multilayers of lipid molecules. These LSH nanoparticles were demonstrated to be effective nanocarriers in delivering medications to destroy prostate and breast tumor cells [234]. As per the clinical trial reports of a rodent suffering from pancreatic cancer, the LSH nanoparticles provide a vehicle for the dual administration of paclitaxel and gemcitabine [235]. By integrating large liposomal and mesoporous silicon nanoparticles onto a microfluidic membrane, Kong *et al* [236] developed a novel nano-in-micro system. It has been demonstrated that co-delivering medication and developed DNA nanostructures using this system substantially boosts the disintegration of doxorubicin-resistant tumor tissues.

Furthermore, poly(lactic-co-glycolic acid) (PLGA) hybrid nanoparticles have shown improved potential applications in drug distribution and hyperthermia, which lead to enhanced tumor cell ablation when combined with multilayer gold and manganese half-shells. Additionally, without harming healthy tissue, the carbon nanotubes and chitosan hybrid nanoparticles function as a vehicle to deliver methotrexate and increased anti-tumor action against pulmonary tumor cells [237].

4.4.3.3.3 Cell membrane-coated nanoparticles

A different approach for creating nanoparticles for tumor diagnosis and therapy is to blend natural biological substances with either organic or inorganic nanostructures. For example, there has been increased focus on encapsulating natural cell membranes with nanoparticles. By encasing the nanostructures in these cell membranes, this technique tends to provide more efficacy and protection to traditional nanoplatforms while also directly imparting biological features [238]. This naturally manifested membrane can be formed by a wide range of cells, comprising tumor cells, leukocytes, platelets, mesenchymal stromal cell membranes, and red blood cells. As per the research findings, the cell membrane derived from leukocyte was effectively coated upon porous silicon nanoparticles. This combination exhibits delayed phagocytic elimination, prolonged drug flow, and enhanced tumor area accumulation [239]. The durability and tumor-targeting capabilities of drug vehicles may be enhanced by mesoporous silica nanoparticles, which have been employed in previous investigations to cure tumors [240].

Moreover, the development of dual-membrane-coated nanoparticles can enhance their functionality [241]. Additionally, Wong and team suggested a multifaceted nanoparticle route of administration by modulating the dimensions and properties of nanomaterials at multiple stages in order to facilitate deep absorption into tumors. Their study utilized protease-induced breakdown of the 100 nm gelatin nanoparticles cores to liberate 10 nm quantum dot nanoparticles, resulting in a size shift of the nanoparticles inside the cancerous microbial environment [242].

4.4.4 Detection of biomarkers

Biomarkers are biological molecules present in blood, and other biological fluids, which indicate the normal or abnormal processes going on in living systems, or of a condition or illness, like tumor/malignancy [243]. Usually, biomarkers help in distinguishing between the normal and diseased person. Numerous mechanisms, such as post-translational alterations, transcriptional modifications, and constitutional or somatic variants, may be responsible for the abnormalities. Biomarkers come in a wide range of forms and can be classified as proteins (such as an enzyme or receptor), nucleic acids/genetic material (like an mRNA), and immunoglobulins, as depicted in figure 4.10. These cancer biomarkers are investigated to obtain detailed information about the cancer in a living system and this process is known as biomarker testing. Each and every tumor patient has a different sequence of biomarkers. Some specific biomarkers influence the efficacy of particular tumor treatments.

Clinical procedures benefit greatly from preliminary cancer detection and diagnosis, which may also raise the patient's survival rate. Despite this, low drug adherence, misdiagnosed treatment, poor sensitivity and accuracy of markers, etc make conventional cancer screening methods like mammography, Pap tests, prostate-specific antigen tests, fecal occult blood (FOB) tests, etc, insufficient for precise preliminary identification. However, because of their poor sensitivity and specificity, the biomarker assessments now utilized in clinics may be modified. As a new method, studies based on nanoparticles are offering excellent specificity as well as sensitivity in the identification of cancer biomarkers. The identification and measurement of specific tumor biomarkers is crucial to clinical diagnostics and

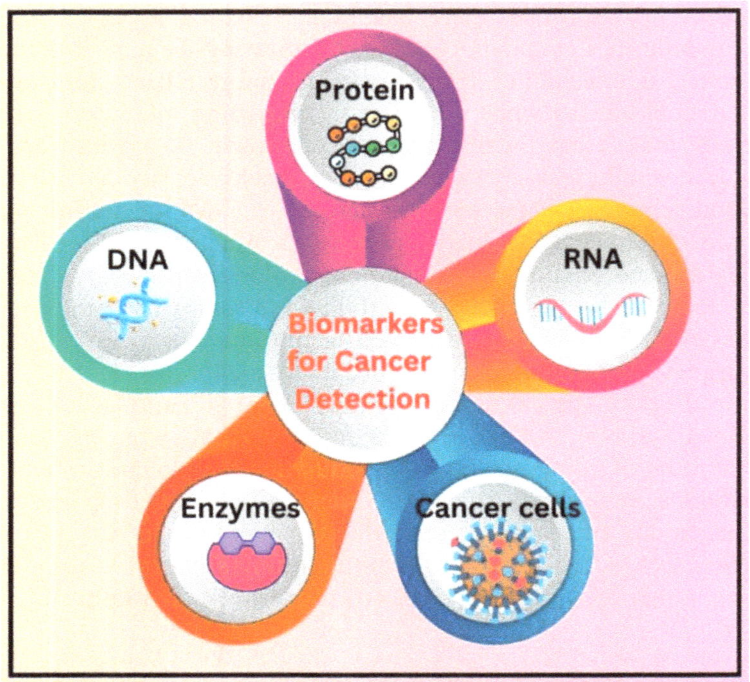

Figure 4.10. Types of biomarkers for cancer detection.

preliminary tumor detection. Whether nanoparticles can be utilized to recognize specific tumor biomarkers using intensified signals has been investigated. For example, miRNA-21 has been found to be a biological marker for breast tumor, and for better identification or diagnostics nano-genosensors were developed to intensify its signals [244]. Similarly, nano-immunosensors were used to hyper-sensitively find tumor antigen in breast cancer patients' plasma samples [245].

4.5 Nanotechnology in cancer therapy

Battles against cancer are like wars against nations. Thus, it is necessary to utilize a variety of weaponry, effective ammunition, and combat tactics [246]. The two main objectives of cancer therapy are first to eradicate the cancerous cells and resume normal life and second to ease the severity of the pain or disease in cases where a cure is impossible due to severe illness. Cancer therapy employs a range of methods, including radiation, chemotherapy, surgery, and other forms of treatment, to completely destroy or drastically diminish the cancerous cells in order to halt the cancer's progression. Based on the nature of illness, its location, and its stage of advancement, different treatment modalities will be chosen and implemented [247].

Cancer therapies are split into three categories: primary, adjuvant, and palliative therapy. The objective of primary therapy is to entirely eradicate the disease or destroy all cancerous cells in the patient's body. This can be achieved most commonly by surgical treatment. It also includes chemotherapy, radiation therapy, etc individually. Adjuvant therapy aims to eliminate all cancer cells that might survive despite primary therapy with the goal of minimizing the possibility of recurrence. This therapy involves chemotherapy, radiation therapy, and hormone therapy alone or as a combination treatment modality. Palliative therapy assists in minimizing the negative consequences of primary or adjuvant therapy as well as cancer-related indications and symptoms. Palliative therapy is performed along with other cancer-curing therapies.

Many malignancies have been treated with a variety of treatment methods that have evolved from traditional techniques like biopsy, antineoplastic therapy, and radiotherapy to considerably more specialized and focused therapeutics like immune therapy, gene therapy, hormonal treatment, and targeted therapy, as depicted in figure 4.11. The current and future treatment strategies with a higher probability of curing various cancers in association with nanotechnology are discussed below.

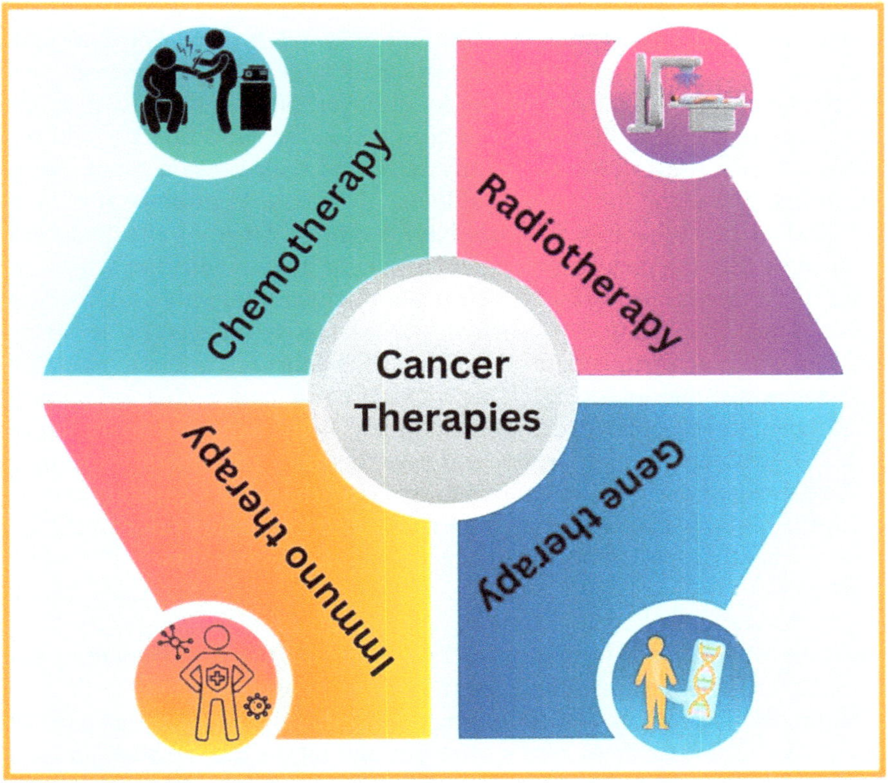

Figure 4.11. Types of cancer therapy.

4.5.1 Chemotherapy

Chemotherapy is an effective chemical treatment for cancer that targets cancerous cells at particular stages of their cell cycle. Chemotherapy was first used for treating cancer around the turn of the 20th century. The acceptability of pharmaceuticals as a treatment for complex malignancies was influenced by two diseases: advanced Hodgkin's disease and acute pediatric leukemia, which were both treated with combination chemotherapy in the 1960s and 1970s [248].

Bleomycin, vinblastine, and cisplatin [249] became breakthrough medications utilized in chemotherapy in the final stages of the 1970s; nevertheless, they had significant side effects, such as vomiting up to 12 times a day, etc. In the case of normal cells the body's natural biological processes remove damaged or surplus cells from the body, allowing new cells to proliferate. Tumor cells, on the other hand, are not subject to cell death, which gives them the ability to multiply more freely with eternal nature. Thus, in malignant masses, the ratio of cell growth to cell death is high, in contrast to normal bodies wherein cell division is proportionate and regulated by apoptosis [250]. Chemotherapy works to stop the tumor from spreading further either by ceasing cell proliferation or by inducing cell death. Thus chemotherapy is the process of killing cancerous cells using chemicals and thereby preventing the growth, division, and proliferation of cancer cells.

Chemotherapeutic drugs can be administered using a variety of methods, although they are often taken intravenously or by tablet. Within the last few years, substantial attempts have been made to discover powerful curative medicines. However, existing chemotherapy for cancer is less safe and effective since along with affected cells it also attacks healthy cells, and may cause a range of adverse consequences, including tiredness, baldness, dizziness, vomiting, and increased toxicity [251]. Chemotherapeutic drugs have a limited range of effectiveness [252]. This indicates that the concentration ranges where these medications substantially impact a tumor are in proximity to the ranges at which intolerable toxic side effects manifest. Thus, balancing the positive and negative effects of a variety of medications given at various doses throughout the course of a therapy period leads to more successful therapies [253]. This is called combination chemotherapy. High doses of chemotherapeutic drugs and complete body exposure to radiation are required to treat certain leukemias and lymphomas. This therapy destroys the connective tissue known as bone marrow, reducing the body's capacity to heal and replenish the blood. As a result, bone marrow collection occurs prior to the surgical portion of the therapy, allowing for recovery after the course of treatment is administered.

Despite technological breakthroughs in many areas of diagnosis, the detection and imaging of human cancer are still remaining inadequate. Presently, curative alternatives for advanced malignancies are limited to chemotherapy with combination treatments. The majority of traditional chemotherapy medications have a small therapeutic index due to haphazard spread throughout the human body and so cause cytotoxicity along with significant side effects while achieving sufficient anti-cancer effectiveness. The purpose of chemotherapeutic medication is to accomplish the beneficial outcomes of therapy objectives while adhering to all of the limits. Thus to tackle the challenges in cancer therapy, different nanoparticle systems for cancer screening and therapies have been widely developed. Nanoplatforms have enormous promise in cancer detection and therapies. Nanotechnology can improve the selectivity of anti-cancer drugs, boost tumor killing efficacy, and minimize toxicity and side effects [254].

Nanoplatforms possess a high surface area-to-volume ratio, unique dimensions, and specific designs, allowing nanoparticles to adsorb and hold a wide range of chemotherapy drugs, including anti-cancer medicines, proteins, and genetic materials [255]. A number of compositions utilizing nanoplatforms for distributing chemotherapy medicines are now in clinical testing, with numerous others being researched in studies. Liposomes, polymeric nanoparticles, metallic nanoparticles, micelles, dendrimers, quantum dots, etc are various types of nanoplatforms that are utilized to create multiple kinds of drug delivery vehicles that are effective against specific types of tumor cells.

Han *et al* [256] studied anti-tumor activity of paclitaxel-loaded liposomes for the treatment of breast cancer. They examined the anti-cancer effects of this novel paclitaxel-loaded liposome on breast tumors *in vitro* and *in vivo*. Their findings demonstrated that these liposomal nanoplatforms have an excellent chance of enhancing breast cancer therapy, consequently increasing the prognosis for patients as well as standard of life. Saneja *et al* [257] developed gemcitabine and betulinic acid co-encapsulated PLGA-PEG polymer nanoparticles to improve the effectiveness of chemotherapy. The results from this research suggested that PLGA-PEG nanoparticles may be employed to co-deliver various chemotherapy agents with varying characteristics, hence increasing anti-tumor efficiency. Zhang *et al* [258] demonstrated that doxorubicin is conjugated to methoxy-poly (ethylene glycol)-b-poly(amidoamine) (MPEG-b-PAMAM) via the acid-labile hydrazone, which is easily cleaved in the acidic environment of tumor locations. They focused on the manufacture of amphiphilic prodrugs, which are self-assembled nanoparticles in deionized water that efficiently encapsulate the hydrophobic anti-cancer medication 10-hydroxycamptothecin (HCPT). Their findings showed that HCPT-loaded nanoparticles inhibit cancer cell proliferation more effectively than HCPT-free nanoparticles.

4.5.2 Radiotherapy

A newer method of treating early-stage and metastatic cancer is called radiotherapy, which uses ionizing radiation in order to destroy cancerous cells locally [259]. Radiotherapy may harm DNA by physically ionizing it instantly and by utilizing radicals that are free through water ionization. To maximize its efficacy for managing tumors, radiation treatment must be made more effective. Nanoparticles have been increasingly employed in the field of radiotherapy because of their potential for effective radiosensitization and delivery of radiosensitizing drugs to the affected tumor areas, as well as their provision of an image-guided response to treatment [260]. A substance known as a radiosensitizer increases the sensitivity of cancerous cells to radiation treatment, thus enhancing the therapeutic index. While many medications and chemical substances have been studied as radiosensitizers thus far, nanotechnology-based radiosensitizers have been attracting much interest [261].

Numerous investigations have employed metallic nanoplatforms, like iron oxides, hafnium oxide (HfO_2), gadolinium [262], quantum dots, gold [263], titanium [264], and non-metallic nanoplatforms, which include fullerenes and silica as radiosensitizers for destroying the cancerous cells. Compton scattering is the primary mode of interaction that occurs between materials and x-ray radiation in ordinary clinical settings, where x-ray-generated radiation is typically employed for radiotherapy.

Radiosensitizers may enhance the effects of radiation therapy if they augment the Compton phenomenon. Gold nanoparticles are useful when low-frequency x-rays [265] are employed because of their high atomic number, which increases the photoelectric effect. Even though gold nanoparticles have other benefits, such as showing inert behavior, being environmentally friendly, and having favorable shape and size properties [266], nanoparticles of superparamagnetic iron oxide and gadolinium have the potential to serve as versatile theranostic agents. Additionally, they can be employed in conjunction with radiation or photothermal treatment in CT or MRI scans [267]. Moreover, it has been found that HfO_2 plays an important role in enhancing the Compton and photoelectric phenomenon owing to its higher atomic number and electron density, which makes radiation-based therapies more efficient. It is also speculated to have minimal dissolution, it does not participate in redox reactions, and it exhibits inert behavior in biological systems [268].

Additionally, the possible significance of silica nanoparticles in radiosensitization has been investigated. ROS generation is not greatly increased by exposing silica NPs to x-rays; however, the formation of ROS is substantially greater in amino-silane functionalized silicon nanoparticles [269]. Researchers have shown that irradiation by nano-C_{60}-gamma radiation results in increased destruction of diseased cancer cells and triggers apoptosis [270].

Quantum dots are another of the most studied radiosensitizers, which can be employed independently or in combination with photosensitizers [271]. The radiosensitizing activity of photosensitizer-conjugated quantum dots is boosted because of both the Compton phenomenon and the fluorescence resonance energy transfer (FRET) effect [272].

4.5.3 Gene therapy

In the 1980s, gene therapy was developed as a novel method of treating monogenic illnesses. It entails altering the genetic makeup of the cell by introducing new genes via integrative or non-integrative vector delivery to permanently fix the diseased gene and thus offers a conclusive treatment. Gene therapy, a cutting-edge medical treatment approach, when accompanied by radio and chemotherapy, becomes more effective in nucleic acid distribution to regulate the gene activity involved in cancer cell proliferation [273]. Nevertheless, the benefits of gene therapy are limited because of the specific endothelial system's rapid nucleic acid breakdown and the target cells' limited accessibility of DNA or RNA [274]. Furthermore, non-targeted administration, cytotoxicity, and quick immune system elimination are some of the challenges that conventional gene therapy may encounter.

Nanoparticles have been specifically engineered to transport therapeutic genes to cancerous cells with little damage to healthy cells, lower immunogenicity, and enhanced circulation time, to achieve successful gene therapies [275]. For instance, MRI-detectable gene therapy for hepatocellular carcinoma has been achieved by the use of polymer-based nanoparticles inserting particular targeting pullulans [276], and tumor-specific transport of small interfering RNA to glioblastoma cancers through the use of RGD-decorated lipid nanoparticles [277].

On the other hand, brain cancers are among the most dangerous illnesses now affecting people very frequently. Additionally, the blood–brain barrier makes treating brain tumors difficult in addition to the problem of drugs resistance. The blood–brain barrier is made up of multiple molecular structures and transport mechanisms that together produce efflux machinery or block the brain's ability to absorb various medications [278].

The blood–brain barrier's presence makes treating brain tumors difficult in addition to drug resistance. Yang *et al* synthesized lipid–polymer-based hybrid nanoparticles to achieve efficient and precise transportation of CRISPR–Cas9 plasmids that target the O6-methylguanine-DNA methyltransferase (MGMT) gene, which is immune to the temozolomide drug. According to their study this system could become an alternative to facilitate gene delivery across the blood–brain barrier for treating glioblastoma [279].

4.5.4 Immunotherapy

Currently, efforts are being made by scientific and clinical organizations to develop non-traditional tumor medicines that can completely kill tumor cells while minimizing harm or loss of good tissues. In recent decades, cancer immunotherapy has emerged as a prominent therapeutic modality that boosts the host's anti-cancer reaction by augmenting the quantity of healthy cells, boosting the congenital immune system, and reducing the host's immunosuppressive mechanisms [280]. Thus, a significant benefit over conventional tumor therapy is that cancer immunotherapy addresses metastasis and reappearance, in addition to eradicating malignancies.

As nanotechnology has advanced, there have been many studies utilizing nanomaterials for cancer immunotherapy because of their exceptional physiochemical qualities, which include large surface area, targeted delivery, and tunable surface chemistry.

For example, nanoparticles such as micelles, dendrimers, liposomes, poly (lactic-co-glycolic acid), and gold nanoparticles can be used as immunotherapeutic agents by transporting tumor-associated antigens (TAAs) into the cytoplasm of dendrimetic cells. This triggers the body's defense to destroy malignant cells [281].

Immunotherapy in conjunction with chemotherapy appears to be a suitable therapeutic strategy for cancer patients. For example, an investigation coupled GM-CSF in spermine adorned AcDEX nanoparticles and Nutlin-3a, an anti-cancer drug. This boosted the proliferation of apoptotic CD8+ T cells and triggered an immunological reaction that ultimately led to the cancerous cells apoptosis [282]. An additional investigation detailed the concurrent loading of pharmacological agents and antibodies into mesoporous silicon nanocarriers, inducing immunological activation and antibody-dependent chemotherapeutic activity in cancerous cells [283].

4.6 Clinical studies in nanoplatform-based cancer imaging

Since the early 1990s, nanoparticle-based techniques for delivering drugs have been successfully employed in clinical trials. Since then, the use of nanomedicine has grown in tandem with expanding technological demands to improve medicinal delivery. Novel types of nanomaterials have arisen that are capable of accomplishing extra delivery tasks and might facilitate novel methods of therapy. Numerous nanoparticles have gone through a number of clinical investigations and are being authorized for diverse applications in today's healthcare system. Over the past couple of decades nanomaterials have proven to be extraordinarily successful in fighting cancer as a great vehicle for securely delivering medications to cancer cells in order to accomplish targeted cancer treatment. A number of clinical investigations and some preliminary research works on nanoparticle-conjugated medications have yielded encouraging findings.

It was observed by Ryosuke and his coworkers that nanoparticles made of ZnO are poisonous to tiny cell lung carcinomas. It was observed during trials that these nanoparticles may decrease tumor cell proliferation in mice, without any noticeable adverse effects, thus making ZnO nanoparticles a promising medicine for curative use against small cell lung carcinomas [284].

Because of their distinct physical features, liposomes and polymer nanoparticles are commonly employed as medication delivery vehicles. In the research study performed by Lei Wei and colleagues, doxorubicin and infrared dye were encased by PD-L1 antibody-linked liposome–polymer nanoparticles (named PD-L1 antibody nanoparticles). By using mini-animal scanning strategies, they revealed in their experiments that nanoparticles based on PD-L1 antibody were successfully focused on malignant cells. Another study discovered that nanoparticles (PD-L1 antibody) identified A549 cells and were responsible for killing tumor cells and efficiently suppressing tumor development. These nanoparticles were discovered to be superior drug delivery vehicles as a result of this research [285].

Studies suggest that the tumor's environment varies from the standard tissue surroundings. Thus nanoparticles that are responsive to tumor microenvironmental indications are currently being extensively investigated in the therapy of malignancies. Glutathione (GSH)-sensitive polyurethane nanoparticles loaded with cisplatin (cisplatin-GPUs) were created by Roshni Iyer *et al.* As the cisplatin-GPUs approach the microenvironment of the tumor with a high GSH level, the cisplatin may be released. Cisplatin-GPUs effectively decrease tumor development when compared to free cisplatin in the xenograft A549 lung tumor mouse model [286].

A chitosan-based nanoparticulate system was engineered by Guo and colleagues [287], who studied the targeted drug delivery of methotrexate drug to the tumor site. In their designed nanoparticulate system, drug is hydrophobically linked with chitosan nanoparticles. Methotrexate was significantly collected at tumor regions and reduced tumor development was observed in BALB/c mice following IV (intravenous) administration of such nanoparticles. These findings point to the use of nanoparticles for targeted medicine delivery to reduce tumor cells for medicinal purposes.

Another reported example of biodegradable nanomaterials is black phosphorus quantum dots (BPQDs), which have high photothermal conversion capability and can effectively target tumor cells by simplifying the release of loaded granulocyte-macrophage colony-stimulating factor (GM-CSF) and lipopolysaccharide (LPS). As a cancer vaccine, Ye *et al* created BPQD nanovesicles encapsulated with tumor cell membranes, recognized as BPQD-CCNVs. BPQD-CCNVs were used in collaboration with programmed cell death (PD)-1 antibody, which is used to inhibit tumor invasion and its recurrence after surgery during immunotherapy [288].

Another reported nanoparticulate system that has reached clinical trial level is gold–silica core–shell nanoparticles. Recently, Riedel *et al* [289] successfully performed green synthesis of gold–silica core–shell nanoparticles having a particle size approximately in the range of 13.0 nm with a shell thickness of 2 nm using the pulsed-laser-ablation-in-liquid method. These have attracted much interest for implementation in biological applications due to their excellent ability to absorb NIR light and their transformation into a considerable amount of heat as well as remarkable cell visibility. The generated heat was utilized to induce highly confined hyperthermia for successful cancer photothermal therapy. These core–shell nanocarriers have been employed in a medical study to surgically remove benign tumors by applying a dual-modality imaging approach using MRI and ultrasonography. This anti-cancer loaded core–shell nanoparticle was investigated on 16 patients suffering from prostate cancer in a clinical trial. Under examination it was observed that patients were recovering and overall a 94% success rate achieved.

One more nanoparticulate system that has reached clinical trial level is a doxorubicin-loaded nanocarrier that later became the first nanomedicine approved by the US FDA for the treatment of ovarian carcinoma, Mediterranean (Kaposi) carcinoma, stage IV breast cancer, and myelomatosis [290]. It is a very effective anti-cancer medication that has grabbed the attention of researchers because of its outstanding effectiveness in spite of dose-limiting toxicity. Clinical research is being conducted on liposomal-derived therapeutic drugs, including doxil (liposomal doxorubicin) nano-based medicine. A variety of malignancies, including ovarian, stomach, and breast cancers, have been clinically studied using these preparations. In the first clinical trial of doxil, the pilot research was performed by incorporating nanoparticles of size 300–500 nm into hepatic cancer patients. In comparison to free doxorubicin, the FDA-approved formulations decreased hematological and cardiac damage [291]. Following that, a variety of liposome compositions and doses were further examined, and it was shown that hematologic toxicity occurs with increasing dosage levels. The attachment of targeted ligand to the drug-loaded nanomaterials has been utilized to minimize the poisoning caused by unidentified delivery. The pharmaceutical substance may be accurately delivered to the targeted malignant cells through these ligands, limiting unwanted harm to healthy tissues [292]. The European Medicine Agency (EMA) approved another PEGlylated liposomal formulation known as zolsketil in 2022 for treating breast and ovarian carcinomas, respectively [293]. Another PEGylated liposomal doxorubicin composition, namely JNS002, is being tested in a stage III clinical investigation on patients detected with fallopian canal cancer, abdominal tumor, and ovarian carcinoma [294]. Table 4.3 contains a few examples of FDA- or EMA-approved nanoplatform-based drugs used in cancer treatment (as of 2023).

A number of different nanoplatforms, including nanorods, micelles, polymeric nanoparticles, dendrimers, and gold nanocages, have also been studied both *in vitro* and *in vivo* and will shortly be put through clinical trials. According to previous investigations, it will take a number of years for more clinical trials to acquire faith and confidence in nanoplatforms for treating cancer.

4.7 Future direction and challenges

Clearly, nanotechnology is a game-changer in the field of cancer theranostics, and it could follow minimally invasive technologies such as automated and laparoscopic surgical procedures as another technical advancement in tumor cells surgery. The production costs, extensibility, complexity, individual safety, and possible toxicity of this innovative technology are some of its drawbacks. Additionally, various nano-theranostic materials are yet to be in the preliminary stages of experimental and clinical trials. To date, a large number of intensive research and clinical studies in the fields of targeted tumor nanotheranostics have produced encouraging and effective nanomaterials. Their effectiveness, however, is evaluated on the basis of the clinical results for cancer sufferers. Consequently, the next generation of diagnostics, combined treatments, and regional theranostics are dependent on the effective creation of nanoplatforms for improved healthcare.

4.8 Conclusion

Nanotechnology is a new scientific discovery with considerable implications across various industries, including engineering, medicine, and healthcare. Researchers have succeeded in disentangling the properties and behavior of nanomaterials offering novel solutions to persistent challenges in the healthcare business. Despite a handful of nanoparticles failing to reach clinical trial level, other novel and intriguing nanoparticles are already in development and displaying significant promis. Along with this, conventional techniques for secure and successful tumor theranostics were long-delayed, costly, showed weak scanning resolution, had large dose requirements, and showed rapid elimination. As a result, nanoplatform-based targeted cancer imaging and treatment have received much interest in recent years. This reduces the large dose requirement and time-consuming processes by targeted therapy along with thorough, accurate scanning and potential medication.

Table 4.3. FDA- or EMA-approved nanoplatform-based drugs used in cancer treatment (as of 2023).

S. no.	Types of nanoplatform	Clinical product/ trade name	Name of drug	Type of cancer	Findings	Clinical status	Approval year	References
1	Liposomes	Doxil/Caelyx	Doxorubicin	Kaposi's sarcoma, myeloid leukemia	Prolonged drug circulation time, drug loading, tumor targeting but long-term use may predispose female patients to oral squamous cell carcinoma	Approved by FDA	1995	[295]
2	Liposomes	Depocyt	Cytarabine/ Ara-C	Neoplastic meningitis	Extended the release time of drugs, reduced delivery and toxicity, but causes arachnoiditis and neurotoxicity	Approved by FDA	1999	[296]
3	Liposomes	Myocet	Doxorubicin	Combination therapy with cyclophosphamide in metastatic breast cancer	Less cardiotoxicity and equal anti-cancer activity but relative instability	Approved by FDA	2000	[297]
4	PLGA nanoparticles	Eligard	Leuprolide acetate	Prostate cancer	Controlled release and longer circulation time but some side effects: hot flushes followed by malaise/fatigue testicular atrophy, dizziness, gynecomastia and nausea	Approved by FDA	2002	[298]

(*Continued*)

Table 4.3. (*Continued*)

S. no.	Types of nanoplatform	Clinical product/ trade name	Name of drug	Type of cancer	Findings	Clinical status	Approval year	References
5	Albumin	Abraxane	Paclitaxel	Metastatic breast cancer		·	2005	[299]
6	mPEG-PLA micelle	Genexol PM	Paclitaxel	Metastatic breast cancer	Non-inferior efficacy and well tolerated	Approved by Republic of Korea	2007	[300]
7	Liposomes	Mepact	Mifamurtide	High-grade, resectable, non-metastatic osteosarcoma		Approved by EMA	2009	[301]
8	Liposome	Marqibo	Vincristine sulfate	Acute lymphoblastic leukemia	No polyethylene coating and slow release into circulation but drug toxicity and adverse side effects	Approved by FDA	2012	[302]
9	PEGylated liposomes	Onivyde	Irinotecan	Metastatic pancreatic cancer (secondary)	Enhanced delivery and reduced systemic toxicity but shows symptoms of diarrhea, nausea, vomiting, neutropenia	Approved by FDA	2015	[303]
10	Liposomes	Vyxeos	Daunorubicin	Acute myeloid leukemia	Significantly longer survival rate, but cause febrile neutropenia, fatigue, pneumonia, hypoxia, hypertension, bacteremia, sepsis	Approved by FDA and EMA	2017 2018	[304]

11	Magnetic Nano particles	Nano-therm	Iron oxide	Recurrent glioblastoma, prostate cancer	High EPR effect, heat production under stimulation with EMF and theranostic properties, with moderate adverse toxicity	Approved by FDA	2018	[305]
12	Micelle	Apealea	Paclitaxel	Ovarian, peritoneal and fallopian tube cancer	Improves progression-free survival in combination with carboplatin but causes side effects: neutropenia, diarrhea, nausea, vomiting, peripheral neuropathy	Approved by EMA	2018	[306]
13	Hafnium oxide nanoparticles	Hensify (NBTXR3)	Hafnium oxide nanoparticles stimulated with external radiation	Locally advanced soft tissue sarcoma (STS)	Radiotherapy enhancer but causes injection site pain, hypotension, radiation skin injury	Approved by CEMark	2019	[307]
14	Albumin	Pazenir	Paclitaxel	Metastatic breast cancer, metastatic adenocarcinoma of the pancreas, non-small cell lung cancer	High solubility, blood circulation time, tumor uptake (EPR), and less toxicity, but some side effects on non-cancer cells such as blood and nerve cells	Approved by EMA	2019	[308]

(*Continued*)

Table 4.3. (*Continued*)

S. no.	Types of nanoplatform	Clinical product/ trade name	Name of drug	Type of cancer	Findings	Clinical status	Approval year	References
15	Zolsketil	Zolsketil	Doxorubicin	Metastatic breast cancer, advanced ovarian cancer, multiple myeloma, AIDS-related Kaposi's sarcoma		Approved by EMA	2022	[309]
16	Liposomes	Thermodox	Doxorubicin	Hepatocellular carcinoma		Phase III		[310]

This chapter discusses the general introduction of cancer along with its classification. Furthermore, it also illustrates different routes of drug delivery, such as oral, transdermal, pulmonary, parenteral, nasal, sublingual, and rectal. Later it focuses on various types of nanoplatform and their specific tunable properties. Due to these unique properties, such as high surface-to-charge ratio, small particle size, scope of surface modification, distinct bond formation capability, etc, these nanoparticles are found to be suitable for medication delivery devices. These benefits allow for the widespread use of nanoplatform-based treatment modalities such as chemo, radio, immuono, and gene treatments. Additionally, this technology provides a system to achieve enhanced multitargeted therapy, which combats multidrug resistance, reduces tumor growth, and addresses malfunctioning apoptosis, proliferation of multidrug carrier, and hypoxic tumor surroundings.

The primary source of information for clinical diagnostic applications comes from medical imaging. The available molecular imaging modalities provide different information about the patient with different spatial and temporal resolution and sensitivity. For this reason, it is currently accepted that a single imaging modality cannot provide sufficient and exact information concerning the human body. Further, there is now increasing interest in merging diagnostic and therapeutic functions. This review briefly outlines the basic principles of the different imaging modalities, discussing how these imaging techniques have been used for response monitoring in preclinical and clinical studies using nanoplatforms known as nanotheranostics.

This chapter investigates the clinical development of cancer imaging that employs nanoplatforms, with particular emphasis on their capabilities, such as timely identification, precise diagnosis, and individualized therapy. However, a large number of distinct nanothernostic agents have undergone satisfactory clinical trials for the treatment of cancer. Many nanosystems are currently in the developmental stage for future translation to clinical investigations for improved cancer diagnosis and therapy.

References

[1] Ferlay J, Colombet M, Soerjomataram I, Parkin D M, Pineros M, Znaor A and Bray F 2021 Cancer statistics for the year 2020: an overview *Int. J. Cancer* **149** 778–89

[2] Foreword C M 2014 *World Cancer Report 2014* ed B W Stewart and C P Wild (Lyon: The International Agency for Research on Cancer)

[3] Martin T A, Ye L, Sanders A J *et al* 2000–2013 Cancer invasion and metastasis: molecular and cellular perspective *Madame Curie Bioscience Database* (Austin, TX: Landes Bioscience)

[4] Testa U, Pelosi E and Castelli G 2018 Colorectal cancer: genetic abnormalities, tumor progression, tumor heterogeneity, clonal evolution and tumor-initiating cells *Med. Sci. (Basel.)* **6** 31

[5] Mortezaee K, Salehi E, Mirtavoos-Mahyari H, Motevaseli E, Najaf M, Farhood B, Rosengren R J and Sahebkar A 2019 Mechanisms of apoptosis modulation by curcumin: implications for cancer therapy *J. Cell. Physiol.* **234** 12537–50

[6] Halazonetis T D, Gorgoulis V G and Bartek J 2008 An oncogene-induced DNA damage model for cancer development *Science* **319** 1352–5
[7] Vogelstein B, Papadopoulos N, Velculescu V E, Zhou S, Diaz L A and Kinzler K W 2013 Cancer genome landscapes *Science* **339** 1546–58
[8] Yan W, Wistuba I I, Emmert-Buck M R and Erickson H S 2011 Squamous cell carcinoma —similarities and differences among anatomical sites *Am. J. Cancer Res.* **1** 275–300
[9] Skoda J and Veselska R 2018 Cancer stem cells in sarcomas: getting to the stemness core *Biochim. Biophys. Acta Gen. Subj.* **1862** 2134–9
[10] Bispo J A B, Pinheiro P S and Kobetz E K 2020 Epidemiology and etiology of leukemia and lymphoma *Cold Spring Harb. Perspect. Med.* **10** a034819
[11] Galon J, Pages F, Marincola F M, Angel H K, Thurin M *et al* 2012 Cancer classifcation using the immunoscore: a worldwide task force *J. Transl. Med.* **10** 205
[12] Amin M B, Greene F L, Edge S B, Compton C C, Gershenwald J E, Brookland R K, Meyer L, Gress D M, Byrd D R and Winchester D P 2017 The eighth edition AJCC Cancer Staging Manual: continuing to build a bridge from a population-based to a more 'personalized' approach to cancer staging *CA Cancer J. Clin.* **67** 93–9
[13] Debela D T, Muzazu S G, Heraro K D, Ndalama M T, Mesele B W, Haile D C, Kitui S K and Manyazewal T 2021 New approaches and procedures for cancer treatment: current perspectives *SAGE Open Med.* **9** 1–10
[14] Nussbaumer S, Bonnabry P, Veuthey J L and Fleury-Souverain S 2011 Analysis of anticancer drugs: a review *Talanta* **85** 2265–89
[15] Arshad S, Sharif M and Naseer A 2016 A mini review on cancer and anticancer drugs *Indo Am. J. Pharm. Sci.* **3** 1383–8
[16] Kaur R, Singh J, Singh G and Kaur H 2011 Anticancer plants: a review *J. Nat. Prod. Plant Resour.* **1** 131–6
[17] Zhou X, Liu X and Huang L 2021 Macrophage-mediated tumor cell phagocytosis: opportunity for nanomedicine intervention *Adv. Funct. Mater.* **31** 2006220
[18] Zehnder A, Graham J, Reavill D R and McLaughlin A 2016 Neoplastic diseases in avian species *Current Therapy in Avian Medicine and Surgery* ed B L Speer (Philadelphia, PA: W B Saunders) pp 107–41 ch 3
[19] Thurston D E 2007 *Chemistry and Pharmacology of Anticancer Drugs* (Boca Raton, FL: CRC Press)
[20] Moretton A and Loizou J I 2020 Interplay between cellular metabolism and the dna damage response in cancer *Cancers* **12** 2051
[21] Kondo N, Takahashi A, Ono K and Ohnishi T 2010 DNA damage induced by alkylating agents and repair pathways *J. Nucl. Acids* 543531
[22] Wu H L, Gong Y, Ji P *et al* 2022 Targeting nucleotide metabolism: a promising approach to enhance cancer immunotherapy *J. Hematol. Oncol.* **15** 45
[23] Nitiss J L 2009 Targeting DNA topoisomerase II in cancer chemotherapy *Nat. Rev. Cancer* **9** 338–50
[24] Dhyani P, Quispe C, Sharma E *et al* 2022 Anticancer potential of alkaloids: a key emphasis to colchicine, vinblastine, vincristine, vindesine, vinorelbine and vincamine *Cancer Cell Int.* **22** 206
[25] Gao Y, Shang Q, Li W, Guo W, Stojadinovic A, Mannion C, Man Y G and Chen T 2020 Antibiotics for cancer treatment: a double-edged sword *J. Cancer* **11** 5135–49

[26] Alqahtani M S, Kazi M, Alsenaidy M A and Ahmad A Z 2021 Advances in oral drug delivery *Front Pharmacol.* **12** 618411
[27] Bhalani D V, Nutan B, Kumar A and Singh Chandel A K 2022 Bioavailability enhancement techniques for poorly aqueous soluble drugs and therapeutics *Biomedicines* **10** 2055
[28] Liu J, Leng P and Liu Y 2021 Oral drug delivery with nanoparticles into the gastrointestinal mucosa *Fundam. Clin. Pharmacol.* **35** 86–96
[29] Debele T A and Park Y 2022 Application of nanoparticles: diagnosis, therapeutics, and delivery of insulin/anti-diabetic drugs to enhance the therapeutic efficacy of diabetes mellitus *Life (Basel)* **12** 2078
[30] Malamatari M, Charisi A, Malamataris S, Kachrimanis K and Nikolakakis I 2020 Spray drying for the preparation of nanoparticle-based drug formulations as dry powders for inhalation *Processes* **8** 788
[31] Kumar A, Pandey A N and Jain S K 2016 Nasal-nanotechnology: revolution for efficient therapeutics delivery *Drug Deliv.* **23** 681–93
[32] Mohammed M A, Syeda J T M, Wasan K M and Wasan E K 2017 An overview of chitosan nanoparticles and its application in non-parenteral drug delivery *Pharmaceutics* **9** 53
[33] Kathe K and Kathpalia H 2017 Film forming systems for topical and transdermal drug delivery *Asian J. Pharm. Sci.* **12** 487–97
[34] Xu Y *et al* 2023 Applications and recent advances in transdermal drug delivery systems for the treatment of rheumatoid arthritis *Acta Pharm. Sin.* B **13** 4417–41
[35] Guillot A J, Navarrete M M, Garrigues T M and Melero A 2023 Skin drug delivery using lipid vesicles: a starting guideline for their development *J. Control. Release* **355** 624–54
[36] Etzioni R, Urban N, Ramsey S, McIntosh M, Schwartz S, Reid B, Radich J, Anderson G and Hartwell L 2003 *Nat. Rev. Cancer* **3** 243–52
[37] Sotiriou C and Piccart M J 2007 Taking gene-expression profiling to the clinic: when will molecular signatures become relevant to patient care? *Nat. Rev. Cancer* **7** 545–53
[38] Nie S, Xing Y, Kim G J and Simons J W 2007 Nanotechnology applications in cancer *Annu. Rev. Biomed. Eng.* **9** 257–88
[39] Cheng L, Wang X, Gong F, Liu T and Liu Z 2020 2D nanomaterials for cancer theranostic applications *Adv. Mater.* **32** e1902333
[40] Shepherd J, Fisher M, Welford A, McDonald D M, Kanthou C and Tozer G M 2017 The protective role of sphingosine-1-phosphate against the action of the vascular disrupting agent combretastatin A-4 3-ophosphate *Oncotarget.* **8** 95648–61
[41] Beyer T, Bidaut L, Dickson J *et al* 2020 What scans we will read: imaging instrumentation trends in clinical oncology *Cancer Imaging* **20** 38
[42] van Leeuwen F W B, Schottelius M, Mottaghy F M *et al* 2022 Perspectives on translational molecular imaging and therapy: an overview of key questions to be addressed *EJNMMI Res.* **12** 31
[43] Calatayud D G, Lledos M, Casarsa F and Pascu S I 2023 Functional diversity in radiolabeled nanoceramics and related biomaterials for the multimodal imaging of tumors *ACS Bio. Med. Chem. Au.* **3** 389–417
[44] Hasan M M, Alam M W, Wahid K A, Miah S and Lukong K E 2016 A low-cost digital microscope with real-time fluorescent imaging capability *PLoS One* **11** e0167863
[45] Dhawan A P, D'Alessandro B and Fu X 2010 Optical imaging modalities for biomedical applications *IEEE Rev. Biomed. Eng.* **3** 69–92

[46] Law G L and Wong W T 2014 An introduction to molecular imaging ed N Long and W T Wong *The Chemistry of Molecular Imaging* (Hoboken, NJ: Wiley) p 408
[47] Paola M D *et al* 2014 Echographic imaging of tumoral cells through novel nanosystems for image diagnosis *World J. Radiol.* **6** 459e70
[48] Wang A, Qi W, Gao T and Tang X 2022 Molecular contrast optical coherence tomography and its applications in medicine *Int. J. Mol. Sci.* **23** 3038
[49] Serganova I and Blasberg R G 2019 Molecular imaging with reporter genes: has its promise been delivered? *J. Nucl. Med.* **60** 1665–81
[50] Stuker F, Ripoll J and Rudin M 2011 Fluorescence molecular tomography: principles and potential for pharmaceutical research *Pharmaceutics* **3** 229–74
[51] Koch M and Ntziachristos V 2016 Advancing surgical vision with fluorescence imaging *Annu. Rev. Med.* **67** 153–64
[52] Atreya R, Waldner M J and Neurath M F 2010 Molecular imaging: interaction between basic and clinical science *Gastroenterol. Clin. N. Am.* **39** 911–22
[53] Godet I, Shin Y J, Ju J A *et al* 2019 Fate-mapping post-hypoxic tumor cells reveals a ROS-resistant phenotype that promotes metastasis *Nat. Commun.* **10** 4862
[54] Kremers G J, Gilbert S G, Cranfill P J *et al* 2011 Fluorescent proteins at a glance *J. Cell Sci.* **124** 157–60
[55] Sakuda T, Kubo T, Johan M P *et al* 2019 Novel near-infrared fluorescence-guided surgery with vesicular stomatitis virus for complete surgical resection of osteosarcomas in mice *J. Orthop. Res.* **37** 1192–201
[56] Widder E A and Falls B 2014 Review of bioluminescence for engineers and scientists in biophotonics *IEEE J. Sel. Top. Quantum Electron.* **20** 232–41
[57] Adams S T and Miller S C 2014 Beyond D-luciferin: expanding the scope of bioluminescence imaging *in vivo Curr. Opin. Chem. Biol.* **21** 112–20
[58] Liu S, Su Y, Lin M Z and Ronald J A 2021 Brightening up biology: advances in luciferase systems for *in vivo* imaging *ACS Chem. Biol.* **16** 2707–18
[59] England C G, Ehlerding E B and Cai W 2016 NanoLuc: a small luciferase is brightening up the field of bioluminescence *Bioconjug. Chem.* **27** 1175–87
[60] Germain-Genevois C, Garandeau O and Couillaud F 2016 Detection of brain tumors and systemic metastases using NanoLuc and Fluc for dual reporter imaging *Mol. Imaging Biol.* **18** 62–9
[61] Gibbons A E, Luker K E and Luker G D 2018 Dual reporter bioluminescence imaging with NanoLuc and firefly luciferase *Methods Mol. Biol.* **1790** 41–50
[62] Mezzanotte L, Fazzina R, Michelini E *et al* 2010 *In vivo* bioluminescence imaging of murine xenograft cancer models with a red-shifted thermostable luciferase *Mol. Imaging Biol.* **12** 406–14
[63] Yeh H W, Karmach O, Ji A *et al* 2017 Red-shifted luciferase–luciferin pairs for enhanced bioluminescence imaging *Nat. Methods* **14** 971–4
[64] Du M, Wang T, Yang Y, Zeng F, Li Y and Chen Z 2022 Application of genetically encoded molecular imaging probes in tumor imaging *Contrast Media Mol. Imaging* **2022** 5473244
[65] Badr C E and Tannous B A 2011 Bioluminescence imaging: progress and applications *Trends Biotechnol.* **29** 624–33
[66] Luker K E, Lewin S A, Mihalko L A *et al* 2012 Scavenging of CXCL12 by CXCR7 promotes tumor growth and metastasis of CXCR4-positive breast cancer cells *Oncogene* **31** 4750–8

[67] Baklaushev V P, Kilpeläinen A, Petkov S, Abakumov M A, Grinenko N F *et al* 2017 Luciferase expression allows bioluminescence imaging but imposes limitations on the orthotopic mouse (4T1) model of breast cancer *Sci. Rep.* **7** 7715
[68] Shi Y, Riese D J and Shen J 2020 The role of the CXCL12/CXCR4/CXCR7 chemokine axis in cancer *Front. Pharmacol.* **11** 574667
[69] Su J L, Wang B, Wilson K E, Bayer C L, Chen Y S, Kim S *et al* 2010 Advances in clinical and biomedical applications of photoacoustic imaging *Expert Opin. Med. Diagn.* **4** 497–510
[70] Guggenheim J A *et al* 2017 Ultrasensitive plano-concave optical microresonators for ultrasound sensing *Nat. Photonics* **11** 714–9
[71] Xia J, Yao J and Wang L V 2014 Photoacoustic tomography: principles and advances *Electromagn. Waves (Camb.)* **147** 1–22
[72] Fernandes D A and Kolios M C 2018 Intrinsically absorbing photoacoustic and ultrasound contrast agents for cancer therapy and imaging *Nanotechnology* **29** 505103
[73] Upputuri P K and Pramanik M 2020 Recent advances in photoacoustic contrast agents for *in vivo* imaging *WIREs Nanomed. Nanobiotechnol.* **12** e1618
[74] Mallidi S, Luke G P and Emelianov S 2011 Photoacoustic imaging in cancer detection, diagnosis, and treatment guidance *Trends Biotechnol.* **29** 213–21
[75] Zhao Z, Swartchick C B and Chan J 2022 Targeted contrast agents and activatable probes for photoacoustic imaging of cancer *Chem. Soc. Rev.* **51** 829–68
[76] Liu Y, Bhattarai P, Dai Z and Chen X 2019 Photothermal therapy and photoacoustic imaging via nanotheranostics in fighting cancer *Chem. Soc. Rev.* **48** 2053–108
[77] Ogunlade O, Stowe C, Jathoul A, Kalber T, Lythgoe M, Beard P and Pule M 2020 *In vivo* photoacoustic imaging of a nonfluorescent E2 crimson genetic reporter in mammalian tissues *J. Biomed. Opt.* **25** 1–12
[78] Piatkevich K D, Suk H J, Kodandaramaiah S B, Yoshida F, DeGennaro E M, Drobizhev M, Hughes T E, Desimone R, Boyden E S and Verkhusha V V 2017 Near-Infrared fluorescent proteins engineered from bacterial phytochromes in neuroimaging *Biophys. J.* **113** 2299–309
[79] Yang Y M, Chen J, Shang X L, Feng Z J, Chen C, Lu J Y *et al* 2019 Visualizing the fate of intra-articular injected mesenchymal stem cells *in vivo* in the second near-infrared window for the effective treatment of supraspinatus tendon tears *Adv. Sci.* **6** 1901018
[80] Guo B, Feng Z, Hu D H, Xu S D, Middha E, Pan Y T *et al* 2019 Precise deciphering of brain vasculatures and microscopic tumors with dual NIR-II fluorescence and photo-acoustic imaging *Adv. Mater.* **31** e1902504
[81] Merbach A S, Helm L and Toth E 2013 *The Chemistry of Contrast Agents in Medical Magnetic Resonance Imaging* (Chichester: Wiley) ch 2 pp 25–81
[82] Cleary J O S H and Guimaraes A R 2014 Magnetic resonance imaging ed M Linda, Mc Manus and R N Mitchell *Pathobiology of Human Disease* (New York: Academic) pp 3987–4004
[83] Wallyn J, Anton N, Akram S and Vandamme T F 2019 Biomedical imaging: principles, technologies, clinical aspects, contraste agents, limitations and future trends in nano-medicines *Pharm. Res.* **36** 78
[84] Julia-Sape M, Coronel I, Majos C *et al* 2012 Prospective diagnostic performance evaluation of single-voxel 1H MRS for typing and grading of brain tumours *NMR Biomed.* **25** 661–73
[85] Hu H, Katyayan K K, Czeskis B A, Perkins E J and Kulanthaivel P 2017 Comparison between radioanalysis and (19)F nuclear magnetic resonance spectroscopy in the

determination of mass balance, metabolism and distribution of pefloxacin *Drug Metab. Dispos. Biol. Fate Chem.* **45** 399–408

[86] Cady E B 2012 *In Vivo Cerebral 31 P Magnetic Resonance Spectroscopy* (Berlin: Springer)

[87] Babsky A M, Hekmatyar S K, Zhang H, Solomon J L and Bansal N 2005 Application of ^{23}Na MRI to monitor chemotherapeutic response in RIF-1 tumors *Neoplasia* **7** 658–66

[88] Hu S, Balakrishnan A, Bok R A *et al* 2011 ^{13}C-pyruvate imaging reveals alterations in glycolysis that precede c-Myc-induced tumor formation and regression *Cell Metab.* **14** 131–42

[89] Ngen E and Artemov D 2017 Advances in monitoring cell-based therapies with magnetic resonance imaging: future perspectives *Int. J. Mol. Sci.* **18** 198

[90] Ladd M E, Bachert P, Meyerspeer M, Moser E, Nagel A M, Norris D G, Schmitter S, Speck O, Straub S and Zaiss M 2018 Pros and cons of ultra-high-field MRI/MRS for human application *Prog. Nucl. Magn. Reson. Spectrosc.* **109** 1–50

[91] Rowe S P and Pomper M G 2022 Molecular imaging in oncology: current impact and future directions *CA Cancer J. Clin.* **72** 333–52

[92] Dula A N, Smith S A and Gore J C 2013 Application of chemical exchange saturation transfer (CEST) MRI for endogenous contrast at 7 Tesla *J. Neuroimaging* **23** 526–32

[93] Wu B, Warnock G, Zaiss M *et al* 2016 An overview of CEST MRI for non-MR physicists *EJNMMI Phys.* **3** 19

[94] Zhang L, Liu R, Peng H, Li P, Xu Z and Whittaker A K 2016 The evolution of gadolinium based contrast agents: from single-modality to multi-modality *Nanoscale* **8** 10491–510

[95] Sahraei Z, Mirabzadeh M, Fouladi D F, Eslami N and Eshraghi A 2014 Magnetic resonance imaging contrast agents: a review of literature *J. Pharm. Care* **2** 177–82

[96] Vinogradov E, Sherry A D and Lenkinski R E 2013 CEST: from basic principles to applications, challenges and opportunities *J. Magn. Reson.* **229** 155–72

[97] Longo D L, Busato A, Lanzardo S *et al* 2013 Imaging the pH evolution of an acute kidney injury model by means of iopamidol, a MRI-CEST pH-responsive contrast agent *Magn. Reson. Med.* **70** 859–64

[98] Namestnikova D *et al* 2017 Methodological aspects of MRI of transplanted superparamagnetic iron oxide-labeled mesenchymal stem cells in live rat brain *PLoS One* **12** e0186717

[99] Birkhuuser F D, Studer U E, Froehlich J M *et al* 2013 Combined ultrasmall superparamagnetic particles of iron oxide enhanced and diffusion-weighted magnetic resonance imaging facilitates detection of metastases in normal-sized pelvic lymph nodes of patients with bladder and prostate cancer *Eur. Urol.* **64** 953–60

[100] Triantafyllou M, Studer U E, Birkhauser F D *et al* 2013 Ultrasmall superparamagnetic particles of iron oxide allow for the detection of metastases in normal sized pelvic lymph nodes of patients with bladder and/or prostate cancer *Eur. J. Cancer* **49** 616–24

[101] Fortuin A S, Bruggemann R, van der Linden J *et al* 2018 Ultrasmall superparamagnetic iron oxides for metastatic lymph node detection: back on the block *Wiley Interdiscip. Rev. Nanomed. Nanobiotechnol.* **10** e1471

[102] Esposito A, Buscarino V, Raciti D, Casiraghi E, Manini M, Biondetti P and Forzenigo L 2019 Characterization of liver nodules in patients with chronic liver disease by MRI: performance of the liver imaging reporting and data system (LI-RADS v.2018) scale and its comparison with the Likert scale *Radiol. Med.* **125** 15–23

[103] Czarniecki M, Pesapane F, Wood B J, Choyke P L and Turkbey B 2018 Ultra-small superparamagnetic iron oxide contrast agents for lymph node staging of high-risk prostate cancer *Transl. Androl. Urol.* **7** S453–61
[104] Akhtar A M, Schneider J E, Chapman S J, S J *et al* 2010 *In vivo* quantification of VCAM-1 expression in renal ischemia reperfusion injury using non-invasive magnetic resonance molecular imaging *PLoS One* **5** e12800
[105] Sargsyan S A, Serkova N J, Renner B *et al* 2012 Detection of glomerular complement C3 fragments by magnetic resonance imaging in murine lupus nephritis *Kidney Int.* **81** 152–9
[106] Tolmachev V and Vorobyeva A 2022 Radionuclides in diagnostics and therapy of malignant tumors: new development *Cancers* **14** 297
[107] Ebhart G, Lamberts L E, Wimana Z, Garcia C, Emonts P, Ameye L, Stroobants S, Huizing M, Aftimos P, Tol J *et al* 2016 Molecular imaging as a tool to investigate heterogeneity of advanced HER2-positive breast cancer and to predict patient outcome under trastuzumab emtansine (T-DM1): the ZEPHIR trial *Ann. Oncol.* **27** 619–24
[108] Mankoff D A, Edmonds C E, Farwell M D and Pryma D A 2016 Development of companion diagnostics *Semin. Nucl. Med.* **46** 47–56
[109] van Dongen G A M S, Beaino W, Windhorst A D, Zwezerijnen G J C, Oprea-Lager D E, Hendrikse N H, van Kuijk C, Boellaard R, Huisman M C and Vugts D J 2021 The role of ^{89}Zr-immuno-PET in navigating and derisking the development of biopharmaceuticals *J. Nucl. Med.* **62** 438–45
[110] van der Heide C D and Dalm S U 2022 Radionuclide imaging and therapy directed towards the tumor microenvironment: a multi-cancer approach for personalized medicine *Eur. J. Nucl. Med. Mol. Imaging* **49** 4616–41
[111] Ferrier M G and Radchenko V 2019 An appendix of radionuclides used in targeted alpha therapy *J. Med. Imaging Radiat. Sci.* **50** S58–65
[112] Chien Y C, Chen J C H, Lin W C *et al* 2014 Using [^{18}F] FBAU for imaging brain tumor progression in an F98/tk-luc glioma-bearing rat model *Oncol. Rep.* **32** 691–9
[113] Zhang L, Suksanpaisan L, Jiang H *et al* 2019 Dual-isotope SPECT imaging with NIS reporter gene and duramycin to visualize tumor susceptibility to oncolytic virus infection *Mol. Ther. Oncol.* **15** 178–85
[114] Hussain S, Mubeen I, Ullah N, Shah S S U D, Khan B A, Zahoor M, Ullah R, Khan F A and Sultan M A 2022 Modern diagnostic imaging technique applications and risk factors in the medical field: a review *BioMed Res. Int.* 5164970**2022**
[115] Israel O *et al* 2019 Two decades of SPECT/CT—the coming of age of a technology: an updated review of literature evidence *Eur. J. Nucl. Med. Mol. Imaging* **46** 1990–2012
[116] Huellner M W and Strobel K 2014 Clinical applications of SPECT/CT in imaging the extremities *Eur. J. Nucl. Med. Mol. Imaging* **41** 50–8
[117] Abrantes A M, Pires A S, Monteiro L, Teixo R, Neves A R, Tavares N T, Marques I A and Botelho M F 2020 Tumour functional imaging by PET *Biochim. Biophys. Acta (BBA)—Mol. Basis Dis.* **1866** 165717
[118] Giammarile F, Castellucci P, Dierckx R, Lobato E E, Farsad M, Hustinx R, Jalilian A, Pellet O, Rossi S and Paez D 2019 Non-FDG PET/CT in diagnostic oncology: a pictorial review *Eur. J. Hybrid Imaging* **3** 20
[119] Sachpekidis C, Goldschmidt H, Kopka K *et al* 2018 Assessment of glucose metabolism and cellular proliferation in multiple myeloma: a first report on combined ^{18}F-FDG and ^{18}F-FLT PET/CT imaging *EJNMMI Res.* **8** 28

[120] Badawi R D, Shi H, Hu P *et al* 2019 First human imaging studies with the EXPLORER total-body PET scanner *J. Nucl. Med.* **60** 299–303
[121] Sarikaya I 2021 Breast cancer and PET imaging *Nucl. Med. Rev.* **24** 16–26
[122] Degrauwe N, Hocquele A, Digklia A, Schaefer N, Denys A and Duran R 2019 Theranostics in interventional oncology: versatile carriers for diagnosis and targeted image-guided minimally invasive procedures *Front. Pharmacol.* **10** 450
[123] Langbein T, Weber W A and Eiber M 2019 M. Future of theranostics: an outlook on precision oncology in nuclear medicine *J. Nucl. Med.* **60** 13S–9S
[124] Hosseini S M, Mohammadnejad J, Salamat S, Beiram Zadeh Z, Tanhaei M and Ramakrishna S 2023 Theranostic polymeric nanoparticles as a new approach in cancer therapy and diagnosis: a review *Mater. Today Chem.* **29** 101400
[125] Kaur J, Gulati M, Jha N K, Disouza J, Patravale V, Dua K and Singh S K 2022 Recent advances in developing polymeric micelles for treating cancer: breakthroughs and bottlenecks in their clinical translation *Drug Discov. Today* **27** 1495–512
[126] Lamichhane N, Udayakumar T S, D'Souza W D, Simone C B, Raghavan S R, Polf J and Mahmood J 2018 Liposomes: clinical applications and potential for image-guided drug delivery *Molecules* **23** 288
[127] Bober Z, Bartusik-Aebisher D and Aebisher D 2022 Application of dendrimers in anticancer diagnostics and therapy *Molecules* **27** 3237
[128] Beygi M, Oroojalian F, Hosseini S S, Mokhtarzadeh A, Kesharwani P and Sahebkar A 2023 Recent progress in functionalized and targeted polymersomes and chimeric polymeric nanotheranostic platforms for cancer therapy *Prog. Mater Sci.* **140** 101209
[129] Sanchez-Lopez E, Guerra M, Dias-Ferreira J, Lopez-Machado A, Ettcheto M, Cano A, Espina M, Camins A, Garcia M L and Souto E B 2019 Current applications of nanoemulsions in cancer therapeutics *Nanomaterials (Basel)* **9** 821
[130] Kulkarni N S, Guererro Y, Gupta N, Muth A and Gupta V 2019 Exploring potential of quantum dots as dual modality for cancer therapy and diagnosis *J. Drug Deliv. Sci. Technol.* **49** 352–64
[131] Mohkam M, Sadraeian M, Lauto A *et al* 2023 Exploring the potential and safety of quantum dots in allergy diagnostics *Microsyst. Nanoeng.* **9** 145
[132] Farzin A, Etesami S A, Quint J, Memic A and Tamayol A 2020 Magnetic nanoparticles in cancer therapy and diagnosis *Adv. Healthc. Mater* **9** e1901058
[133] Chen F, Hableel G, Zhao E R and Jokerst J V 2018 Multifunctional nanomedicine with silica: role of silica in nanoparticles for theranostic, imaging, and drug monitoring *J. Colloid Interface Sci.* **521** 261–79
[134] Kulkarni S, Kumar S and Acharya S 2022 Gold nanoparticles in cancer therapeutics and diagnostics *Cureus* **14** e30096
[135] Loh K P, Ho D, Chiu G N C, Leong D T, Pastorin G and Chow E K H 2018 Clinical applications of carbon nanomaterials in diagnostics and therapy *Adv. Mater.* 1–21
[136] Mousavi S M, Hashemi S A, Mazraedoost S, Yousefi K, Gholami A, Behbudi G, Ramakrishna S, Omidifar N, Alizadeh A and Chiang W H 2021 Multifunctional gold nanorod for therapeutic applications and pharmaceutical delivery considering cellular metabolic responses, oxidative stress and cellular longevity *Nanomaterials* **11** 1868
[137] Xu P, Wang R, Yang W *et al* 2021 A DM1-doped porous gold nanoshell system for NIR accelerated redox-responsive release and triple modal imaging guided photothermal synergistic chemotherapy *J. Nanobiotechnol.* **19** 77

[138] Gajbhiye K R, Salve R, Narwade M *et al* 2023 Lipid polymer hybrid nanoparticles: a custom-tailored next-generation approach for cancer therapeutics *Mol. Cancer* **22** 160
[139] Yanar F, Carugo D and Zhang X 2023 Hybrid nanoplatforms comprising organic nanocompartments encapsulating inorganic nanoparticles for enhanced drug delivery and bioimaging applications *Molecules* **28** 5694
[140] Hapuarachchige S and Artemov D 2020 Theranostic pretargeting drug delivery and imaging platforms in cancer precision medicine *Front. Oncol.* **10** 1131
[141] Yordanova A, Eppard E, Kurpig S, Bundschuh R A, Schonberger S, Gonzalez-Carmona M *et al* 2017 Theranostics in nuclear medicine practice *Onco. Targets Ther.* **10** 4821–8
[142] Duan H and Iagaru A 2023 Theranostic imaging and radiopharmaceutical therapy ed L Bodei, J S Lewis and B M Zeglis *Radiopharmaceutical Therapy* (Cham: Springer) pp 455–81
[143] Solnes L B, Werner R A, Jones K M, Sadaghiani M S, Bailey C R, Lapa C, Pomper M G and Rowe P 2020 Theranostics: leveraging molecular imaging and therapy to impact patient management and secure the future of nuclear medicine *J. Nucl. Med. Mar.* **61** 311–8
[144] Strosberg J, El-Haddad G, Wolin E *et al* 2017 Phase 3 trial of ^{177}Lu-dotatate for midgut neuroendocrine tumors *N. Engl. J. Med.* **376** 125–35
[145] Singh A and Amiji M M 2022 Application of nanotechnology in medical diagnosis and imaging *Curr. Opin. Biotechnol.* **74** 241–6
[146] Siafaka P I, Okur N U, Karavas E and Bikiaris D N 2016 Surface modified multifunctional and stimuli responsive nanoparticles for drug targeting: current status and uses *Int. J. Mol. Sci.* **17** 1440
[147] Chen X, Wang T, Le W, Huang X, Gao M and Chen Q 2020 Smart sorting of tumor phenotype with versatile fluorescent Ag nanoclusters by sensing specific reactive oxygen species *Theranostics* **10** 3430–50
[148] Chouhan R and Bajpai A K 2009 Real time *in vitro* studies of doxorubicin release from PHEMA nanoparticles *J. Nanobiotechnol.* **7** 1–12
[149] Desai N 2012 Challenges in development of nanoparticle-based therapeutics *Am. Assoc. Pharm. Sci. J.* **14** 282–95
[150] Abu-Salah K M, Zourob M M, Mouffouk F, Alrokayan S A, Alaamery M A and Ansari A A 2015 DNA-based nanobiosensors as an emerging platform for detection of disease *Sensors* **15** 14539–68
[151] Qin D, Xia Y and Whitesides G M 2010 Soft lithography for micro- and nanoscale patterning *Nat. Protoc.* **5** 491–502
[152] Bhatnagar A, Tripathi M, Na S and Prajapati A 2022 *Nanotechnology for Batteries In Nanotechnology for Electronic Applications* (Singapore: Springer Nature) pp 29–48
[153] McDonald S A, Konstantatos G, Zhang S, Cyr P W, Klem E J, Levina L and Sargent E H 2005 Solution-processed PbS quantum dot infrared photodetectors and photovoltaics *Nat. Mater.* **4** 138–42
[154] Sebastian P J and Gamboa S A 2005 Nanotechnology applied to thin film solar cells *Sol. Energy Mater. Sol. Cells* **88** 129–30
[155] Chen H C and Cheng C J 2022 Holographic optical tweezers: techniques and biomedical applications *Appl. Sci.* **12** 10244
[156] Begines B, Ortiz T, Perez-Aranda M, Martínez G, Merinero M, Arguelles-Arias F and Alcudia A 2020 Polymeric nanoparticles for drug delivery: recent developments and future prospects *Nanomaterials (Basel)* **10** 1403
[157] Liu C H and Grodzinski P 2021 Nanotechnology for cancer imaging: advances, challenges, and clinical opportunities *Radiol. Imaging Cancer* **3** 200052

[158] Nelson N R, Port J D and Pandey M K 2020 Use of superparamagnetic iron oxide nanoparticles (SPIONs) via multiple imaging modalities and modifications to reduce cytotoxicity: an educational review *J. Nanotheranost.* **1** 105–35

[159] Tandale P *et al* 2021 Fluorescent quantum dots: an insight on synthesis and potential biological application as drug carrier in cancer *Biochem. Biophys. Rep.* **26** 100962

[160] Yusuf A, Almotairy A R Z, Henidi H, Alshehri O Y and Aldughaim M S 2023 Nanoparticles as drug delivery systems: a review of the implication of nanoparticles' physicochemical properties on responses in biological systems *Polymers* **15** 1596

[161] Waite C L and Roth C M 2012 Nanoscale drug delivery systems for enhanced drug penetration into solid tumors: current progress and opportunities *Crit. Rev. Biomed. Eng.* **40** 21–41

[162] Anjum S, Ishaque S, Fatima H, Farooq W, Hano C, Abbasi B H and Anjum I 2021 Emerging applications of nanotechnology in healthcare systems: grand challenges and perspectives *Pharmaceuticals (Basel)* **14** 707

[163] Ashfaq A, Khursheed N, Fatima S, Anjum Z and Younis K 2022 Application of nanotechnology in food packaging: pros and cons *J. Agric. Food Res.* **7** 100270

[164] Kalita D and Baruah S 2019 The impact of nanotechnology on food ed R Fereira do Nascimento, O P Ferreira, A J De Paula and V O Sousa Neto *Advanced Nanomaterials, Nanomaterials Applications for Environmental Matrices* (Amsterdam: Elsevier) ch 11 pp 369–79

[165] Malik S, Singh J, Goyat R, Saharan Y, Chaudhry V, Umar A, Ibrahim A A, Akbar S, Ameen S and Baskoutas S 2023 Nanomaterials-based biosensor and their applications: a review *Heliyon* **9** 19929

[166] Saleem H, Zaidi S J, Ismail A F and Goh P S 2022 Advances of nanomaterials for air pollution remediation and their impacts on the environment *Chemosphere* **287** 132083

[167] Jangid N K, Yadav A, Jadoun S, Srivastava A and Srivastava M 2020 Outdoor pollution management by nanotechnology *Impact of Textile Dyes on Public Health and the Environment* (Hershey, PA: IGI Global) pp 258–77

[168] Joudeh N and Linke D 2022 Nanoparticle classification, physicochemical properties, characterization, and applications: a comprehensive review for biologists *J. Nanobiotechnol.* **20** 262

[169] Behzadi S, Serpooshan V, Tao W, Hamaly M A, Alkawareek M Y, Dreaden E C, Brown D, Alkilany A M, Farokhzad O C and Mahmoudi M 2017 Cellular uptake of nanoparticles: journey inside the cell *Chem. Soc. Rev.* **46** 4218–44

[170] Mazumdar S, Chitkara D and Mittal A 2021 Exploration and insights into the cellular internalization and intracellular fate of amphiphilic polymeric nanocarriers *Acta Pharm. Sin.* B **11** 903–24

[171] Shi L, Zhang J, Zhao M, Tang S, Cheng X, Zhang W, Li W, Liu X, Peng H and Wang Q 2021 Effects of polyethylene glycol on the surface of nanoparticles for targeted drug delivery *Nanoscale* **13** 10748

[172] Khan I, Saeed K and Khan I 2019 Nanoparticles: properties, applications and toxicities *Arab. J. Chem.* **12** 908–31

[173] Hoshyar N, Gray S, Han H and Bao G 2016 The effect of nanoparticle size on *in vivo* pharmacokinetics and cellular interaction *Nanomedicine (Lond)* **11** 673–92

[174] Oh N and Park J H 2014 Endocytosis and exocytosis of nanoparticles in mammalian cells *Int. J. Nanomed.* **9** 51–63

[175] Forest V, Leclerc L, Hochepied J F, Trouve A, Sarry G and Pourchez J 2017 Impact of cerium oxide nanoparticles shape on their *in vitro* cellular toxicity *Toxicol. in Vitro* **38** 136–41

[176] Li Y, Kroger M and Liu W K 2015 Shape effect in cellular uptake of PEGylated nanoparticles: comparison between sphere, rod, cube and disk *Nanoscale* **7** 16631–46
[177] Augustine R, Hasan A, Primavera R, Wilson R J, Thakor A S and Kevadiya B D 2020 Cellular uptake and retention of nanoparticles: insights on particle properties and interaction with cellular components *Mater. Today Commun.* **25** 101692
[178] Guerrini L, Alvarez-Puebla R A and Pazos-Perez N 2018 Surface modifications of nanoparticles for stability in biological fluids *Materials (Basel)* **11** 1154
[179] Khan Y, Sadia H, Ali Shah S Z, Khan M N, Shah A A, Ullah N, Ullah M F, Bibi H, Bafakeeh O T, Khedher N B *et al* 2022 Classification, synthetic, and characterization approaches to nanoparticles, and their applications in various fields of nanotechnology: a review *Catalysts* **12** 1386
[180] Yagublu V, Karimova A, Hajibabazadeh J, Reissfelder C, Muradov M, Bellucci S and Allahverdiyev A 2022 Overview of physicochemical properties of nanoparticles as drug carriers for targeted cancer therapy *J. Funct. Biomater.* **13** 196
[181] Baranwal J, Barse B, Di Petrillo A, Gatto G, Pilia L and Kumar A 2023 Nanoparticles in cancer diagnosis and treatment *Materials (Basel)* **16** 5354
[182] Chenthamara D, Subramaniam S, Ramakrishnan S G *et al* 2019 Therapeutic efficacy of nanoparticles and routes of administration *Biomater. Res.* **23** 20
[183] Zielinska A *et al* 2020 Polymeric nanoparticles: production, characterization, toxicology and ecotoxicology *Molecules* **25** 3731
[184] Chouhan R and Bajpai A K 2009 An *in vitro* release study of 5-fluoro-uracil (5-FU) from swellable poly-(2-hydroxyethyl methacrylate) (PHEMA) nanoparticles. *J. Mater. Sci.: Mater. Med.* **20** 1103–14
[185] Xiao X, Teng F, Shi C, Chen J, Wu S, Wang B, Meng X, EssietImeh A and Li W 2022 Polymeric nanoparticles-promising carriers for cancer therapy *Front. Bio. Eng. Biotechnol.* **10** 1024143
[186] Ghezzi M, Pescina S, Padula C, Santi P, Del Favero E, Cantu L and Nicoli S 2021 Polymeric micelles in drug delivery: an insight of the techniques for their characterization and assessment in biorelevant conditions *J. Control. Release* **332** 312–36
[187] Hanafy A F, Abdalla A M, Guda T K, Gabr K E, Royall P G and Alqurshi A 2019 Ocular anti-inflammatory activity of prednisolone acetate loaded chitosan-deoxycholate self-assembled nanoparticles *Int. J. Nanomed.* **14** 3679–89
[188] Bozzuto G and Molinari A 2015 Liposomes as nanomedical devices *Int. J. Nanomed.* **10** 975
[189] Nakhaei P, Margiana R, Bokov D O, Abdelbasset W K, Jadidi Kouhbanani M A, Varma R S, Marofi F, Jarahian M and Beheshtkhoo N 2021 Liposomes: structure, biomedical applications, and stability parameters with emphasis on cholesterol *Front. Bioeng. Biotechnol.* **9** 705886
[190] Mukherjee S, Mukherjee S, Abourehab M A S, Sahebkar A and Kesharwani P 2022 Exploring dendrimer-based drug delivery systems and their potential applications in cancer immunotherapy *Eur. Polym. J.* **177** 111471
[191] Gholap A D, Bhowmik D D, Deshmukh A Y and Hatvate N T 2023 Quintessential impact of dendrimer bioconjugates in targeted drug delivery ed S K Verma and A Das *Comprehensive Analytical Chemistry* (Amsterdam: Elsevier) vol 103 pp 257–302
[192] Bacha K, Chemotti C, Mbakidi J P, Deleu M and Bouquillon S 2023 Dendrimers: synthesis, encapsulation applications and specific interaction with the stratum corneum—a review *Macromol* **3** 343–70

[193] Chis A A *et al* 2020 Applications and limitations of dendrimers in biomedicine *Molecules* **25** 3982
[194] Christian D A, Cai S, Bowen D M, Kim Y, Pajerowski J D and Discher D E 2009 Polymersome carriers: from self-assembly to siRNA and protein therapeutics *Eur. J. Pharm. Biopharm.* **71** 463–74
[195] Zhang X Y and Zhang P Y 2017 Polymersomes in nanomedicine—a review *Curr. Med. Chem.* **13** 124–9
[196] Fonseca M, Jarak I, Victor F, Domingues C, Veiga F and Figueiras A 2024 Polymersomes as the next attractive generation of drug delivery systems: definition, synthesis and applications *Materials* **17** 319
[197] Bhatti R, Shakeel H, Malik K, Qasim M, Khan M A, Ahmed N and Jabeen S 2022 Inorganic nanoparticles: toxic effects, mechanisms of cytotoxicity and phytochemical interactions *Adv. Pharm. Bull.* **12** 757–62
[198] Zhou H, Ge J, Miao Q, Zhu R, Wen L, Zeng J and Gao M 2020 Biodegradable inorganic nanoparticles for cancer theranostics: insights into the degradation behavior *Bioconjug. Chem.* **31** 315–31
[199] Sanmartin-Matalobos J, Bermejo-Barrera P, Aboal-Somoza M, Fondo M, Garcia-Deibe A M, Corredoira-Vazquez J and Alves-Iglesias Y 2022 Semiconductor quantum dots as target analytes: properties, surface chemistry and detection *Nanomaterials* **12** 2501
[200] Gil H M, Price T W, Chelani K, Bouillard J S G, Calaminus S D J and Stasiuk G J 2021 NIR-quantum dots in biomedical imaging and their future *iScience* **24** 102189
[201] Voura E B, Jaiswal J K, Mattoussi H and Simon S M 2004 Tracking metastatic tumor cell extravasation with quantum dot nanocrystals and fluorescence emission-scanning microscopy *Nat. Med.* **10** 993
[202] Mandriota G, Di Corato R, Benedetti M, De Castro F, Fanizzi F P and Rinaldi R 2019 Design and application of cisplatin-loaded magnetic nanoparticle clusters for smart chemotherapy *ACS Appl. Mater. Interfaces* **11** 1864–75
[203] Legge C J, Colley H E, Lawson M A and Rawlings A E 2019 Targeted magnetic nanoparticle hyperthermia for the treatment of oral cancer *J. Oral Pathol. Med.* **48** 803–9
[204] Roy K and Roy I 2022 Therapeutic applications of magnetic nanoparticles: recent advances *Mater. Adv.* **3** 7425–44
[205] Lei W, Sun C, Jiang T, Gao Y, Yang Y, Zhao Q *et al* 2019 Polydopamine-coated mesoporous silica nanoparticles for multi-responsive drug delivery and combined chemo-photothermal therapy *Mater. Sci. Eng. C: Mater. Biol. Appl.* **105** 110103
[206] Xu C, Lei C and Yu C 2019 Mesoporous silica nanoparticles for protein protection and delivery *Front. Chem.* **7** 290
[207] Fontana F, Shahbazi M A, Liu D, Zhang H, Makila E, Salonen J, Hirvonen J T and Santos H A 2017 Multistaged nanovaccines based on porous silicon@acetalated dextran@cancer. Cell membrane for cancer immunotherapy *Adv. Mater.* **29** 1603239
[208] Zhang C, Xie H, Zhang Z, Wen B, Cao H, Bai Y, Che Q, Guo J and Su Z 2022 Applications and biocompatibility of mesoporous silica nanocarriers in the field of medicine *Front. Pharmacol* **13** 829796
[209] Yang W, Liang H, Ma S, Wang D and Huang J 2019 Gold nanoparticle based photothermal therapy: development and application for effective cancer treatment *Sustain. Mater. Technol.* **22** e00109

[210] Wang J, Potocny A M, Rosenthal J and Day E S 2020 Gold nanoshell-linear tetrapyrrole conjugates for near infrared-activated dual photodynamic and photothermal therapies *ACS Omega* **5** 926–40

[211] Kong F Y, Zhang J W, Li R F, Wang Z X, Wang W J and Wang W 2017 Unique roles of gold nanoparticles in drug delivery, targeting and imaging applications *Molecules* **22** 1445

[212] Riley R S and Day E S 2019 Gold nanoparticle-mediated photothermal therapy: applications and opportunities for multimodal cancer treatment *Wiley Interdiscip. Rev. Nanomed. Nanobiotechnol.* **9** e1449

[213] Clarance P *et al* 2020 Green synthesis and characterization of gold nanoparticles using endophytic fungi *Fusarium solani* and its *in-vitro* anticancer and biomedical applications *Saudi J. Biol. Sci.* **27** 706–12

[214] Tomoaia G, Horovitz O, Mocanu A, Nita A, Avram A *et al* 2015 Effects of doxorubicin mediated by gold nanoparticles and resveratrol in two human cervical tumor cell lines *Colloids Surf.* B **135** 726–34

[215] Mahmood M, Karmakar A, Fejleh A, Mocan T, Iancu C *et al* 2009 Synergistic enhancement of cancer therapy using a combination of carbon nanotubes and anti-tumor drug *Nanomedicine* **4** 883–93

[216] Huo D, He J, Li H, Yu H, Shi T *et al* 2014 Fabrication of Au@Ag core–shell NPs as enhanced CT contrast agents with broad antibacterial properties *Colloids Surf.* B **117** 29–35

[217] Gupta T, Pawar B, Vasdev N, Pawar V and Tekade R K 2023 Carbonaceous nanomaterials for phototherapy of cancer *Technol. Cancer Res. Treat.* **22** 15330338231186388

[218] Madani S Y, Naderi N, Dissanayake O, Tan A and Seifalian A M 2011 A new era of cancer treatment: carbon nanotubes as drug delivery tools *Int. J. Nanomed.* **6** 2963–79

[219] Luo C, Tian Z, Yang B, Zhang L and Yan S 2013 Manganese dioxide/iron oxide/acid oxidized multi-walled carbon nanotube magnetic nanocomposite for enhanced hexavalent chromium removal *Chem. Eng. J.* **234** 256–65

[220] Fernandes N B, Shenoy R U K, Kajampady M K, DCruz C E M, Shirodkar R K, Kumar L and Verma R 2020 Fullerenes for the treatment of cancer: an emerging tool *Environ. Sci. Pollut. Res. Int.* **29** 58607–27

[221] Huang H J, Kraevaya O A, Voronov I I, Troshin P A and Hsu S H 2020 Fullerene derivatives as lung cancer cell inhibitors: investigation of potential descriptors using QSAR approaches *Int. J. Nanomed.* **15** 2485–99

[222] Bilal M, Cheng H, Gonzalez R B G, Parra-Saldivar R and Iqbal H M N 2021 Bio-applications and biotechnological applications of nanodiamonds *J. Mater. Res. Technol.* **15** 6175–89

[223] Mochalin V, Shenderova O, Ho D *et al* 2012 The properties and applications of nanodiamonds *Nat. Nanotechnol.* **7** 11–23

[224] Magne T M, de Oliveira Vieira T, Alencar L M R *et al* 2022 Graphene and its derivatives: understanding the main chemical and medicinal chemistry roles for biomedical applications *J. Nanostruct. Chem.* **12** 693–727

[225] Rhazouani A, Gamrani H, El Achaby M, Aziz K, Gebrati L, Uddin M S and Aziz F 2021 Synthesis and toxicity of graphene oxide nanoparticles: a literature review of *in vitro* and *in vivo* studies *BioMed. Res. Int.* **2021** 5518999

[226] Yang K, Wan J, Zhang S, Zhang Y, Lee S T and Liu Z 2011 *In vivo* pharmacokinetics, long-term biodistribution, and toxicology of PEGylated graphene in mice *ACS Nano* **5** 516–22

[227] Mottaghitalab F, Farokhi M, Fatahi Y, Atyabi F and Dinarvand R 2019 New insights into designing hybrid nanoparticles for lung cancer: diagnosis and treatment *J. Control. Release* **295** 250–67
[228] Gao F, Zhang J, Fu C, Xie X, Peng F, You J *et al* 2017 iRGD-modified lipid–polymer hybrid nanoparticles loaded with isoliquiritigenin to enhance anti-breast cancer effect and tumor-targeting ability *Int. J. Nanomed.* **12** 4147–62
[229] Zhao X, Li F, Li Y, Wang H, Ren H, Chen J *et al* 2015 Co-delivery of HIF1α siRNA and gemcitabine via biocompatible lipid–polymer hybrid nanoparticles for effective treatment of pancreatic cancer *Biomaterials* **46** 13–25
[230] Wang Q, Alshaker H, Bohler T, Srivats S, Chao Y, Cooper C *et al* 2017 Core–shell lipid–polymer hybrid nanoparticles with combined docetaxel and molecular targeted therapy for the treatment of metastatic prostate cancer *Sci. Rep.* **7** 5901
[231] Zhang R X, Ahmed T, Li L Y, Li J, Abbasi A Z and Wu X Y 2017 Design of nanocarriers for nanoscale drug delivery to enhance cancer treatment using hybrid polymer and lipid building blocks *Nanoscale* **9** 1334–55
[232] Su X, Wang Z, Li L, Zheng M, Zheng C, Gong P *et al* 2013 Lipid–polymer nanoparticles encapsulating doxorubicin and 2′-deoxy-5-azacytidine enhance the sensitivity of cancer cells to chemical therapeutics *Mol. Pharm.* **10** 1901–9
[233] Hu Y, Hoerle R, Ehrich M and Zhang C 2015 Engineering the lipid layer of lipid–PLGA hybrid nanoparticles for enhanced *in vitro* cellular uptake and improved stability. *Acta Biomater.* **28** 149–59
[234] Colapicchioni V, Palchetti S, Pozz D, Marini E S, Riccioli A, Ziparo E *et al* 2015 Killing cancer cells using nanotechnology: novel poly(I:C) loaded liposome-silica hybrid nanoparticles *J. Mater. Chem.* B **3** 7408–16
[235] Meng H, Wang M, Liu H, Liu X, Situ A, Wu B *et al* 2015 Use of a lipid-coated mesoporous silica nanoparticle platform for synergistic gemcitabine and paclitaxel delivery to human pancreatic cancer in mice *ACS Nano* **9** 3540–57
[236] Kong F, Zhang X, Zhang H B, Qu X M, Chen D, Servos M *et al* 2015 Inhibition of multidrug resistance of cancer cells by co-delivery of DNA nanostructures and drugs using porous silicon nanoparticles@giant liposomes *Adv. Funct. Mater.* **25** 3330–40
[237] Park H, Yang J, Lee J, Haam S, Choi I H and Yoo K H 2009 Multifunctional nanoparticles for combined doxorubicin and photothermal treatments *ACS Nano* **3** 2919–26
[238] Fang R H, Kroll A V, Gao W and Zhang L 2018 Cell membrane coating nanotechnology *Adv. Mater.* **30** e1706759
[239] Parodi A, Quattrocchi N, van de Ven A L, Chiappini C, Evangelopoulos M, Martinez J O *et al* 2013 Synthetic nanoparticles functionalized with biomimetic leukocyte membranes possess cell-like functions *Nat. Nanotechnol.* **8** 61–8
[240] Liu C M, Chen G B, Chen H H, Zhang J B, Li H Z, Sheng M X *et al* 2019 Cancer cell membrane-cloaked mesoporous silica nanoparticles with a pH-sensitive gatekeeper for cancer treatment *Colloids Surf. B Biointerfaces* **175** 477–86
[241] Jiang Q, Liu Y, Guo R, Yao X, Sung S, Pang Z *et al* 2019 Erythrocyte-cancer hybrid membrane-camouflaged melanin nanoparticles for enhancing photothermal therapy efficacy in tumors *Biomaterials* **192** 292–308
[242] Wong C, Stylianopoulos T, Cui J, Martin J, Chauhan V P, Jiang W *et al* 2011 Multistage nanoparticle delivery system for deep penetration into tumor tissue *Proc. Natl. Acad. Sci. USA* **108** 2426–31

[243] Ahmad A, Imran M and Ahsan H 2023 Biomarkers as biomedical bioindicators: approaches and techniques for the detection, analysis, and validation of novel biomarkers of diseases *Pharmaceutics* **15** 1630

[244] Salahandish R, Ghaffarinejad A, Omidinia E, Zargartalebi H, Majidzadeh A K, Naghib S M and Sanati-Nezhad A 2018 Label-free ultrasensitive detection of breast cancer miRNA-21 biomarker employing electrochemical nano-genosensor based on sandwiched AgNPs in PANI and N-doped graphene *Biosens. Bioelectron.* **120** 129–36

[245] Hasanzadeh M, Solhi E, Jafari M, Mokhtarzadeh A, Soleymani J, Jouyban A and Mahboob S 2018 Ultrasensitive immunoassay of tumor protein CA 15.3 in MCF-7 breast cancer cell lysates and unprocessed human plasma using gold nanoparticles doped on the structure of mesoporous silica *Int. J. Biol. Macromol.* **120** 2493–508

[246] Surh Y J 2021 The 50-year war on cancer revisited: should we continue to fight the enemy within? *J. Cancer Prev* **26** 219–23

[247] Abbas Z and Rehman S 2018 An overview of cancer treatment modalities *Neoplasm* (Rijeka: InTech)

[248] DeVita V T and Chu E 2008 A history of cancer chemotherapy *Cancer Res.* **68** s8643–8653

[249] Falzone L, Salomone S and Libra M 2018 Evolution of cancer pharmacological treatments at the turn of the third millennium *Front. Pharmacol., Sec. Exp. Pharmacol. Drug Discov.* **9** 1300

[250] Wang R A, Li Q L, Li Z S, Zheng P J, Zhang H Z, Huang X F, Chi S M, Yang A G and Cui R 2013 Apoptosis drives cancer cells proliferate and metastasize *J. Cell. Mol. Med.* **17** 205–11

[251] Schirrmacher V 2019 From chemotherapy to biological therapy: a review of novel concepts to reduce the side effects of systemic cancer treatment (review) *Int. J. Oncol.* **54** 407–19

[252] Mondal J, Panigrahi A K and Khuda-Bukhsh A R 2014 Conventional chemotherapy: problems and scope for combined therapies with certain herbal products and dietary supplements *Austin J. Mol. Cell Biol.* **1** 10

[253] Saini R K, Chouhan R, Bagri L P and Bajpai A K 2012 Strategies of targeting tumors and cancers *J. Cancer Res. Update.* **1** 129–52

[254] Elumalai K, Srinivasan S and Shanmugam A 2024 Review of the efficacy of nanoparticle-based drug delivery systems for cancer treatment *Biomed. Technol.* **5** 109–22

[255] Sebastian R 2017 Nanomedicine—the future of cancer treatment: a review *J. Cancer Prev. Curr. Res.* **8** 204–8

[256] Han B *et al* 2020 Preparation, characterization, and pharmacokinetic study of a novel long-acting targeted paclitaxel liposome with antitumor activity *Int. J. Nanomed.* **15** 553–71

[257] Saneja A, Kumar R, Mintoo M J, Dubey R D, Sangwan P L, Mondhe D M, Panda A K and Gupta P N 2019 Gemcitabine and betulinic acid co-encapsulated PLGA-PEG polymer nanoparticles for improved efficacy of cancer chemotherapy *Mater. Sci. Eng. C: Mater. Biol. Appl.* **98** 764–71

[258] Zhang Y, Xiao C, Li M, Chen J, Ding J, He C, Zhuang X and Chen X 2013 Co-delivery of 10-hydroxycamptothecin with doxorubicin conjugated prodrugs for enhanced anticancer efficacy *Macromol. Biosci.* **13** 584–94

[259] Baskar R, Lee K A, Yeo R and Yeoh K W 2012 Cancer and radiation therapy: current advances and future directions *Int. J. Med. Sci.* **9** 193–9

[260] Boateng F and Ngwa W 2019 Delivery of nanoparticle-based radiosensitizers for radiotherapy applications *Int. J. Mol. Sci.* **21** 273

[261] Karabuga M, Erdogan S, Filikci K, Hazıroglu R, Tuncel M and Cengiz M 2023 Evaluation of efficacy of tumor-specific nanoliposomalradiosensitizer in radiotherapy *J. Drug Deliv. Sci. Technol.* **86** 104586
[262] Nosrati H, Salehiabar M, Charmi J, Yaray K, Ghaffarlou M, Balcioglu E and Ertas Y N 2023 Enhanced *in vivo* radiotherapy of breast cancer using gadolinium oxide and gold hybrid nanoparticles *ACS Appl Bio Mater* **6** 784–92
[263] Penninckx S, Heuskin A C, Michiels C and Lucas S 2020 Gold nanoparticles as a potent radiosensitizer: a transdisciplinary approach from physics to patient *Cancers (Basel)* **12** 2021
[264] Morita K *et al* 2021 Titanium oxide nano-radiosensitizers for hydrogen peroxide delivery into cancer cells *Colloids Surf.,* B **198** 111451
[265] Konefał A, Lniak W, Rostocka J, Orlef A, Sokol M, Kasperczyk J, Jarząbek P, Wronska A and Rusiecka K 2020 Influence of a shape of gold nanoparticles on the dose enhancement in the wide range of gold mass concentration for high-energy X-ray beams from a medical linac *Rep. Pract. Oncol. Radiother.* **25** 579–85
[266] Hammami I, Alabdallah N M, Al Jomaa A and Kamoun M 2021 Gold nanoparticles: synthesis properties and applications *J. King Saud. Univ.—Sci.* **33** 101560
[267] Daems N, Michiels C, Lucas S, Baatout S and Aerts A 2021 Gold nanoparticles meet medical radionuclides *Nucl. Med. Biol.* **100–1** 61–90
[268] Huang Y, Hu H, Li R Q, Yu B and Xu F J 2016 Versatile types of MRI-visible cationic nanoparticles involving pullulan polysaccharides for multifunctional gene carriers *ACS Appl. Mater. Interfaces* **17** 3919–27
[269] Erel-Akbaba G, Carvalho L A, Tian T, Zinter M, Akbaba H, Obeid P J, Chiocca E A, Weissleder R, Kantarci A G and Tannous B A 2019 Radiation-induced targeted nanoparticle-based gene delivery for brain tumor therapy *ACS Nano* **13** 4028–40
[270] Arif M, Nawaz A F, Ullah Khan S, Mueen H, Rashid F, Hemeg H A and Rauf A 2023 Nanotechnology-based radiation therapy to cure cancer and the challenges in its clinical applications *Heliyon* **9** e17252
[271] Uprety B and Abrahamse H 2022 Semiconductor quantum dots for photodynamic therapy: recent advances *Front. Chem.* **10** 946574
[272] Yao B, Liu X, Zhang W and Lu H 2023 X-ray excited luminescent nanoparticles for deep photodynamic therapy *RSC Adv.* **13** 30133–50
[273] Azevedo A, Farinha D, Geraldes C and Faneca H 2021 Combining gene therapy with other therapeutic strategies and imaging agents for cancer theranostics *Int. J. Pharm.* **606** 120905
[274] Uddin F, Rudin C M and Sen T 2020 CRISPR gene therapy: applications, limitations, and implications for the future *Front Oncol.* **10** 1387
[275] Mirza Z and Karim S 2021 Nanoparticles-based drug delivery and gene therapy for breast cancer: recent advancements and future challenges *Semin. Cancer Biol.* **69** 226–37
[276] Varzandeh M, Sabouri L, Mansouri V, Gharibshahian M, Beheshtizadeh N, Hamblin M R and Rezaei N 2023 Application of nano-radiosensitizers in combination cancer therapy *Bioeng. Transl. Med.* **8** e10498
[277] Zhao N, Yang Z, Li B, Meng J, Shi Z, Li P and Fu S 2016 RGD-conjugated mesoporous silicaencapsulated gold nanorods enhance the sensitization of triplenegative breast cancer to megavoltage radiation therapy *Int. J. Nanomed.* **11** 5595–610
[278] Bhowmik A, Khan R and Ghosh M K 2015 Blood brain barrier: a challenge for effectual therapy of brain tumors *BioMed Res. Int.* **2015** 320941

[279] Yang Q, Zhou Y, Chen J, Huang N, Wang Z and Cheng Y 2021 Gene therapy for drug-resistant glioblastoma via lipid–polymer hybrid nanoparticles combined with focused ultrasound *Int. J. Nanomed.* **16** 185–99

[280] Zhang F, Correia A, Makila E, Li W, Salonen J, Hirvonen J J, Zhang H and Santos H A 2017 Receptor-mediated surface charge inversion platform based on porous silicon nanoparticles for efficient cancer cell recognition and combination therapy *ACS Appl. Mater. Interfaces* **9** 10034–46

[281] Guo Y, Wang D, Song Q, Wu T, Zhuang X, Bao Y, Kong M, Qi Y, Tan S and Zhang Z 2015 Erythrocyte membrane-enveloped polymeric nanoparticles as nanovaccine for induction of antitumor immunity against melanoma *ACS Nano* **9** 6918–33

[282] Bauleth-Ramos T *et al* 2017 Nutlin-3a and cytokine co-loaded spermine-modified acetalated dextran nanoparticles for cancer chemo-immunotherapy *Adv. Funct. Mater.* **27** 1703303

[283] Li Y, Xiao Y, Lin H P, Reichel D, Bae Y, Lee E Y, Jiang Y, Huang X, Yang C and Wang Z 2019 *In vivo* β-catenin attenuation by the integrin α5-targeting nano-delivery strategy suppresses triple negative breast cancer stemness and metastasis *Biomaterials* **188** 160–72

[284] Tanino R, Amano Y, Tong X, Sun R, Tsubata Y, Harada M, Fujita Y and Isobe T 2020 Anticancer activity of ZnO nanoparticles against human small-cell lung cancer in an orthotopic mouse model *Mol. Cancer Ther.* **19** 502–12

[285] Wei L, Yu F and Meng Y 2021 Preparation of programmed cell death-ligand 1 antibody nanoparticles based on nude mouse model and its therapeutic effect on lung cancer *J. Nanosci. Nanotechnol.* **212** 895–902

[286] Iyer R, Nguyen T, Padanilam D, Xu C, Saha D, Nguyen K T and Hong Y 2020 Glutathione-responsive biodegradable polyurethane nanoparticles for lung cancer treatment *J. Control. Release* **321** 363–71

[287] Guo X, Zhuang Q, Ji T, Zhang Y, Li C, Wang Y, Li H, Jia H, Liu Y and Du L 2018 Multi-functionalized chitosan nanoparticles for enhanced chemotherapy in lung cancer *Carbohydr. Polym.* **195** 311–20

[288] Ye X, Liang X, Chen Q, Miao Q, Chen X, Zhang X and Mei L 2019 Surgical tumor-derived personalized photothermal vaccine formulation for cancer immunotherapy *ACS Nano* **13** 2956–68

[289] Riedel R, Mahr N, Yao C, Wu A, Yang F and Hampp N 2020 Synthesis of gold–silica core–shell nanoparticles by pulsed laser ablation in liquid and their physico-chemical properties towards photothermal cancer therapy *Nanoscale* **12** 3007–18

[290] Zhu L and Lin M 2021 The synthesis of nano-doxorubicin and its anticancer effect *Anticancer Agents Med. Chem.* **21** 2466–77

[291] Aloss K and Hamar P 2023 Recent preclinical and clinical progress in liposomal doxorubicin *Pharmaceutics* **15** 893

[292] Aldughaim M S, Muthana M, Alsaffar F and Barker M D 2020 Specific targeting of pegylated liposomal doxorubicin (Doxil®) to tumour cells using a novel TIMP3 peptide *Molecules* **26** 100

[293] Talens-Visconti R, Diez-Sales O, de Julian-Ortiz J V and Nacher A 2022 Nanoliposomes in cancer therapy: marketed products and current clinical trials *Int. J. Mol. Sci.* **23** 4249

[294] Motohashi T *et al* 2021 Randomized phase III trial comparing pegylated liposomal doxorubicin (PLD) at 50 mg/m^2 versus 40 mg/m^2 in patients with platinum-refractory and -resistant ovarian carcinoma: the JGOG 3018 trial *J. Gynecol. Oncol.* **32** e9

[295] Jensen G M and Hodgson D F 2020 Opportunities and challenges in commercial pharmaceutical liposome applications *Adv. Drug Deliv. Rev.* **154–155** 2–12

[296] Ventola C L 2017 Progress in nanomedicine: approved and investigational nanodrugs *PT* **42** 742–55

[297] Nirmala M J, Kizhuveetil U, Johnson A, Balaji G, Nagarajan R and Muthuvijayan V 2023 Cancer nanomedicine: a review of nano-therapeutics and challenges ahead *RSC Adv.* **13** 8606–29

[298] Tran S, DeGiovanni P J, Piel B and Rai P 2017 Cancer nanomedicine: a review of recent success in drug delivery *Clin. Transl. Med.* **6** 44

[299] Desai N 2016 *Nanoparticle Albumin-Bound Paclitaxel (Abraxane®): Albumin in Medicine: Pathological and Clinical Applications* (Berlin: Springer) pp 101–19

[300] Bobo D, Robinson K J, Islam J *et al* 2016 Nanoparticle-based medicines: a review of FDA-approved materials and clinical trials to date *Pharm. Res.* **33** 2373–87

[301] Lombardo D, Kiselev M A and Caccamo M T 2019 Smart nanoparticles for drug delivery application: development of versatile nanocarrier platforms in biotechnology and nanomedicine *J. Nanomater.* **2019** 1–26

[302] Caster J M, Patel A N, Zhang T and Wang A 2017 Investigational nanomedicines in 2016: a review of nanotherapeutics currently undergoing clinical trials *Wiley Interdiscip. Rev. Nanomed. Nanobiotechnol.* **9** e1416

[303] Noble J M, Chen L, Jog R, Kozak D and Zheng J 2019 Characterization of encapsulated liposomal irinotecan *Microsc. Microanal.* **25** 1274–5

[304] Krauss A C *et al* 2019 FDA approval summary: (daunorubicin and cytarabine) liposome for injection for the treatment of adults with high-risk acute myeloid leukemia *Clin. Cancer Res.* **25** 2685–90

[305] Regenold M, Bannigan P, Evans P J C, Waspe A, Temple M J and Allen C 2022 Turning down the heat: the case for mild hyperthermia and thermosensitive liposomes *Nanomedicine* **40** 102484

[306] Borga O, Lilienberg E, Bjermo H, Hansson F, Heldring N and Dediu R 2019 Pharmacokinetics of total and unbound paclitaxel after administration of paclitaxel micellar or nab-paclitaxel: an open, randomized, cross-over, explorative study in breast cancer patients *Adv. Ther.* **36** 2825–37

[307] Pavelic K, Kraljevic Pavelic S, Bulog A, Agaj A, Rojnic B, Čolic M and Trivanovic D 2023 Nanoparticles in medicine: current status in cancer treatment *Int. J. Mol. Sci.* **24** 12827

[308] Rodriguez F *et al* 2022 Nano-based approved pharmaceuticals for cancer treatment: present and future challenges *Biomolecules* **12** 784

[309] Fulton M D and Najahi-Missaoui W 2023 Liposomes in cancer therapy: how did we start and where are we now *Int. J. Mol. Sci.* **24** 6615

[310] Lyon P C, Griffiths L F, Lee J, Chung D, Carlisle R, Wu F, Middleton M R, Gleeson F V and Coussios C C 2017 Clinical trial protocol for TARDOX: a phase I study to investigate the feasibility of targeted release of lyso-thermosensitive liposomal doxorubicin (ThermoDox(R)) using focused ultrasound in patients with liver tumours *J. Ther. Ultrasound* **5** 28

www.ingramcontent.com/pod-product-compliance
Ingram Content Group UK Ltd.
Pitfield, Milton Keynes, MK11 3LW, UK
UKHW051857100926
8556IPUK00005B/663

9 780750 358620